WITHDRAWN

rsing Process
and
ing Diagnosis

Nursing Process and Nursing Diagnosis

SECOND EDITION

PATRICIA W. IYER, R.N., M.S.N., C.N.A.

President, Patricia Iyer Associates
Med League Support Services
Stockton, New Jersey

BARBARA J. TAPTICH, R.N., M.A.

Program Director, Heart Institute
Saint Francis Medical Center
Trenton, New Jersey

DONNA BERNOCCHI-LOSEY, R.N., M.A.

Office Nurse
San Jose, California;
Formerly Faculty, School of Nursing
University of Nevada at Las Vegas
Las Vegas, Nevada

1991

W.B. SAUNDERS COMPANY

Harcourt Brace Jovanovich, Inc.
Philadelphia, London, Toronto, Montreal, Sydney, Tokyo

W. B. SAUNDERS COMPANY

Harcourt Brace Jovanovich, Inc.

The Curtis Center
Independence Square West
Philadelphia, PA 19106

Library of Congress Cataloging-in-Publication Data

Iyer, Partricia W.
    Nursing process and nursing diagnosis / Patricia W. Iyer, Barbara
J. Taptich, Donna Bernocchi-Losey.—2nd ed.
        p.   cm.
    Includes bibliographical references and index.
    ISBN 0-7216-3421-4
    1. Nursing. 2. Nursing diagnosis. I. Taptich, Barbara J.
II. Bernocchi-Losey, Donna.   III. Title.
    [DNLM: 1. Nursing Assessment. WY 100 I97n]
RT41.I94   1991
610.73—dc20
DNLM/DLC   90-0145
for Library of Congress   CIP

Sponsoring Editor: Thomas Eoyang

Manuscript Editor: Elisa Costanza Affanato

Designer: Lorraine B. Kilmer

Production Manager: Frank Polizzano

Illustration Coordinator: Joan Sinclair

NURSING PROCESS AND NURSING DIAGNOSIS   ISBN   0-7216-3421-4

Last digit is the print number: 9   8   7   6   5   4   3   2   1

To our family members
who supported our ability to complete this edition:

Raj, Raj Jr., and Nathan Iyer
Bob, Bobby, and Michael Taptich
Michael, David, Heather, and Robert Louis Losey

About the Authors . . .

Patricia W. Iyer, RN, MSA, CNA is president of two businesses: Patricia Iyer Associates, providing nursing consulting and educational services, and Med League Support Services, assisting attorneys with malpractice cases. She has a diploma from Muhlenberg Hospital School of Nursing, a Bachelor of Science in Nursing, and a Master of Science in Nursing from University of Pennsylvania, Philadelphia. She is certified in nursing administration. Correspondence may be directed to the author at P.O. Box 231, Stockton, NJ 08559-0231.

Barbara J. Taptich, RN, MA, is Program Director for the Heart Institute at Saint Francis Medical Center, Trenton, New Jersey. She has a diploma from Saint Joseph's Hospital School of Nursing, Reading, Pennsylvania, a Bachelor of Arts in Health Education and School Nursing from Glassboro State College, Glassboro, New Jersey, and a Master of Arts in Health Care Administration from Rider College, Lawrenceville, New Jersey. Correspondence may be directed to the author at 20 Martin Lane, Mercerville, NJ, 08619.

Donna Bernocchi-Losey, RN, MA, practices jointly with Michael C. Losey, an Internal Medicine Specialist in San Jose, California. She has a Bachelor of Science in Nursing from Seton Hall University, South Orange, New Jersey, and a Master of Arts in Nursing from New York University, New York, New York. Correspondence may be directed to the author's office at 2895 The Villages Parkway, San Jose, CA 95135.

PREFACE

The nursing process is the foundation on which nursing practice is based. *Nursing Process and Nursing Diagnosis* began as a self-learning module designed to introduce the concept of nursing diagnosis within the framework of the nursing process. We identified the need for a current, comprehensive presentation of the nursing process with an emphasis on the diagnostic phase. This text evolved from that need.

The book provides a comprehensive presentation of each of the five phases of the nursing process. The continuing emphasis on nursing diagnosis within the nursing community has been reinforced by professional standards, regulatory agencies, reimbursement systems, and the desire for a nomenclature specific to the profession. The text is particularly strong in its comprehensive discussion and utilization of the concept of nursing diagnosis.

Nursing Process and Nursing Diagnosis is designed for nursing students and nursing practitioners wishing to learn or review nursing process theory. The material is presented in a clear, understandable manner and provides guidelines for the development of nursing diagnoses, outcomes, and interventions. Exercises and case studies in a self-test format provide the learner with an opportunity to apply these concepts. The appendices include additional information that expands upon the theory contained in the text.

This second edition reflects the changes that have occurred within nursing and the health care environment since the first edition was published in 1986. All the chapters have been reviewed, revised, and rewritten. Many of the examples have been altered to reflect the decreasing length of stay and increasing acuity of hospitalized clients. The nursing diagnoses used throughout the text have been updated to include the most current listing of diagnoses available at the time of publication. Case management has been added to the discussion of nursing care delivery systems in Chapter 8. The chapter on evaluation has been rewritten to further clarify the steps in evaluation and to update the quality assurance content. A new chapter on legal and ethical issues has been included.

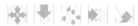
Additional exercises have been incorporated into the appendices to provide further opportunity to develop nursing diagnoses, outcomes, and interventions.

The authors wish to thank the following reviewers, whose valuable suggestions helped to refine the content of the second edition: Dickie H. Gerig, RN, MS, Grayson County College, Denison, Texas; Carolyn Holder, BSN, Summa Health Care Systems, Akron City Hospital, Akron, Ohio; Mary Ann Kathrein, RN, EdD, Kathrein & Associates, Villa Park, Illinois; Charlotte Lebsack, RN, BSN, Spokane Community College, Spokane, Washington; and Sara D. Sierra, RN, MS, Massachusetts Bay Community College, Wellesley Hills, Massachusetts.

We would also like to thank Thomas Eoyang, Senior Editor, and Michael Brown, Editor-in-Chief, W. B. Saunders Company, for their support and encouragement.

CONTENTS

Nursing Process
and
Nursing Diagnosis

1 THE NURSING PROCESS

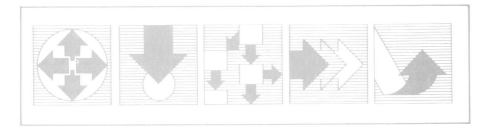

INTRODUCTION

Early nursing practice encompassed many roles. The nurse focused on comfort measures and maintaining a sanitary environment. In addition, the roles of pharmacist, dietitian, physical therapist, and social worker were part of nursing practice. The nurse as a health care provider met the total needs of the client. Since that time, there have been a number of factors that have altered the dimensions of nursing practice. These include social, scientific/technological, educational, economic, and political changes. During the evolutionary process, the common thread that has remained is the nurse's focus on the total needs of the client. However, the previously identified factors have also changed the complexion of health care in general. A variety of disciplines—physical therapy, social services, and dietetics—have evolved to assist in meeting client needs. The role of the nurse in the delivery of these ancillary services has shifted from provider to coordinator. This allows the nurse to concentrate on the body of knowledge unique to nursing in the resolution of client problems. The method by which this is accomplished is the *nursing process*. It may be helpful to explore some definitions of nursing prior to examining the nursing process in detail.

DEFINITIONS OF NURSING

The profession of nursing has been defined by nursing leaders, by professional organizations, and according to functions.

Nursing Leaders

The earliest definition of nursing was provided by Florence Nightingale in 1859. Nightingale's *Notes on Nursing—What It Is, What It Is Not*—defined nursing as having "charge of the personal health of somebody . . . and what nursing has to do . . . is to put the patient in the best condition for nature to act upon him." The nature of nursing is complex, and efforts to define it have continued. A frequently quoted definition, used internationally, was formulated by Henderson (1961). She viewed nursing as assisting "the individual, sick or well, in the performance of those activities contributing to health or its recovery (or to peaceful death) that he would perform unaided if he had the necessary strength, will or knowledge."

Fagin (1978) suggests that "nursing is defined as including the promotion and maintenance of health, prevention of illness, care of persons during acute phases of illness, and rehabilitation and restoration of health." Orlando (1961) viewed nursing as providing "the help the patient may require for his needs to be met, that is, for his physical and mental comfort to be assured as far as possible."

Rogers (1970) describes nursing as both an art and a science. She further identifies the existence of a unique knowledge base "growing out of scientific research and logical analysis and capable of being translated into nursing practice."

These definitions are just a sample of the many descriptions of nursing. It could be summarized that nursing is both a science and an art. Nursing has its own body of knowledge based on scientific theory and focuses on the health and well-being of the client. Nursing is concerned with the psychological, spiritual, social, and physical aspects of the person, rather than only the client's diagnosed medical condition. In other words, the focus is on the responses of the total person interacting with the environment. These responses may be influenced by past experiences, the physical environment, the social situation, and family dynamics. Nursing is an art that involves caring for the client during times of illness and assisting the client to achieve maximum health potential throughout the life cycle. Nursing strives to adapt to the needs of people in a variety of settings—home, work, clinics, and hospitals—through personal interaction with individuals, families, and communities.

Professional Organizations

The mission of defining nursing has been undertaken by others in addition to nurse leaders. In 1979, the American Nurses' Association, the professional organization for nursing in the United States, defined nursing and established the scope of nursing practice. The end result of the ANA's efforts was the publication of "Nursing: A Social Policy Statement (1980)". The definition of nursing presented in this document reflected the historical evolution of the profession and its theoretical base: "Nursing is the diagnosis and treatment of human responses to actual or potential health problems."

Human Responses

Human responses are the phenomena of concern to nurses. The nurse focuses on two types of responses: "(1) reactions of individuals and groups to actual health problems (health-restoring responses), such as the impact of ill-

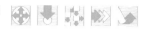

ness—effects upon the self and family, and self-care needs; and (2) concerns of individuals and groups about potential health problems (health supporting responses), such as monitoring and teaching in populations or communities at risk in which educative needs for information, skill development, health-oriented attitudes and related behavioral changes arise" (ANA, 1980). More simply, this means that the scope of nursing practice includes the tasks of assessing, diagnosing, planning, treating, and evaluating the responses observed in both sick and well persons. Nursing interventions can be directed to the management of the response to an actual problem, such as an illness or disease, or the prevention of a health problem in a client at risk. In short, the nurse deals with the client's response to the health problem. The nurse is concerned with the effect of the disease or health problem on the client's life. These human responses are dynamic in nature and change as the client and/or family progresses along the continuum between health and illness. The client usually has one or more human responses to an acute illness or long-term disease. The human responses are diverse and vary in nature because each client is a unique individual, and the response to the health problem or potential health problem will be a reflection of the individual's interaction with the environment. Consider the following situation.

Example. Mr. Vegas is a 52 year old cross-country truck driver. While driving his truck 1000 miles from home, he began to develop some tightness in his chest. At first, he passed it off as indigestion. When the discomfort failed to dissipate, he drove to the nearest hospital. Mr. Vegas was admitted to the intensive care unit with severe chest pain. He was restless and withdrawn. Later, he said that this was his first time in the hospital and he was afraid he might die. He asked the nurse to call his wife to ask her to come as quickly as possible. Fortunately, Mr. Vegas had an uncomplicated heart attack. After a few days, he was transferred to another floor. While the nurse was transferring him, Mr. Vegas expressed his concern over the fact that he was going to a new unit. Once on the unit, the physician informed him that it would be in his best interest to change his lifestyle and perhaps retire from truck driving. Mr. Vegas stated that this was impossible for he had no other way to support his wife and four children.

This example demonstrates some of the human responses Mr. Vegas had to the health problem of a heart attack. During his hospitalization, the medical diagnosis remained the same from the time of admission to discharge. However, the human responses were multiple in nature and varied based on his progress along the health care continuum. Upon admission, the responses exhibited were those of pain, fear of death, and loneliness. As his health status improved, he exhibited fear about his transfer and had difficulty in accepting the major change in lifestyle suggested by the physician. The nurse's role was to identify the responses of pain, fear, loneliness, and anxiety and to assist the client in managing them. These are the types of human responses that are within the realm of nursing practice.

Table 1–1 is an illustration of some of the human responses that are the focus for nursing intervention.

TABLE 1–1. HUMAN RESPONSES

1. Self-care limitations

2. Impaired functioning in areas such as rest, sleep, ventilation, circulation, activity, nutrition, elimination, skin, sexuality

3. Pain and discomfort

4. Emotional problems related to illness and treatment, life-threatening events, or daily experiences, such as anxiety, loss, loneliness, and grief

5. Distortion of symbolic functions, reflected in interpersonal and intellectual processes, such as hallucinations

6. Deficiencies in decision-making and ability to make personal choices

7. Self-image changes required by health status

8. Dysfunctional perceptual orientation to health

9. Strains related to life processes, such as birth, growth and development, and death

10. Problematic affiliative relationships

Reprinted with permission of the American Nurses' Association. From Nursing: A Social Policy Statement. Kansas City, MO: American Nurses' Association, 1980.

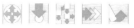

1-1 TEST YOURSELF

HUMAN RESPONSES

After reading the situation below, identify four human responses to actual or potential health problems.

Mrs. Hart was a 32 year old white female admitted to the acute care facility for removal of her right breast. Mrs. Hart informed the nurse that her husband had noticed the lump in her breast approximately six months ago. She had put off going to the doctor because she was afraid that it might be cancer. She explained that she had a two year old child at home and was hoping to become pregnant in the near future, but now that the lump had been discovered, her own future was in doubt. She had delayed childbirth because of her career as an accountant. During the conversation she became teary-eyed. After questioning her, the nurse determined that she was anxious about receiving anesthesia.

Mrs. Hart underwent a right modified mastectomy. On her first day after surgery, she experienced much pain, and because of the nature of the surgery her ability to move her right arm was impaired. This was disturbing to her since she was right-handed. She was not accustomed to being so dependent. On the fourth day after surgery, the physician informed Mrs. Hart that because the disease had spread to two lymph nodes she would require chemotherapy, radiation therapy, or both. After the physician left, Mrs. Hart broke down and started to cry. She told the nurse that she was afraid she would never be able to have another child or see her little girl grow up. She also refused to look at her incision when the dressing was changed and expressed that she was scarred for life and would never be attractive to her husband again.

HUMAN RESPONSES

1.

2.

3.

4.

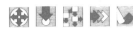

 1–1 TEST YOURSELF □ ANSWERS

1. Self-care limitations
2. Pain
3. Fear of anesthesia
4. Fear of death
5. Change in self-image
6. Change in relationship with husband
7. Impaired sexuality
8. Grief

Nursing Functions

Nursing has also been defined in terms of functions or roles. In nursing practice, the roles can be divided into three areas: independent, interdependent, and dependent functions.

Independent Functions

Independent functions are those activities that are considered to be within nursing's scope of diagnosis and treatment. These actions do not require a physician's order. Some examples include:

1. Assessment of the client/family through health history and physical examination to ascertain health status;

2. Diagnosis of responses requiring nursing interventions;

3. Identification of nursing actions that are likely to maintain or restore health;

4. Implementation of measures designed to motivate, guide, support, counsel, or teach the client/family;

5. Referral to other members of the health care team when indicated and allowed by individual state nurse practice acts;

6. Evaluation of the client's response to nursing and medical interventions;

7. Participation with consumers or other health care providers in the improvement of health care systems.

Interdependent Functions

Interdependent functions of the nurse are those that are carried out in conjunction with other health team members. For example, in the case of a pregnant woman with diabetes in a high-risk clinic, the nurse and dietician collaborate to develop a plan for meeting the nutritional needs of the expectant mother and developing fetus. The dietician contributes in meal planning and teaching, while the nurse reinforces the teaching and monitors the client's ability to incorporate the diet into daily food selection. Another example might be seen in the physician's office. The physician diagnoses the medical problem of hypertension and

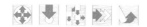

orders medications and dietary modifications in an elderly client. In response to the physician's findings, the office nurse evaluates the client's reaction to the diagnosis and initiates teaching about the disease, drugs, and diet. These are examples of interdependent functions of the nurse.

Dependent Functions

Dependent functions of the nurse are the activities performed based on the physician's orders. These include the administration of medications or specific treatments. For example, in a hospital pediatric unit, the nurse recognizes an elevated temperature in a child with gastroenteritis. In this setting, it is not within the scope of nursing practice to order antipyretics and intravenous fluids. However, when these treatment modalities are ordered by the physician, it is the nurse's responsibility to administer the medication and initiate intravenous therapy. These are the dependent functions of the nurse.

It is important to note that each state has legally defined the practice of nursing in its Nursing Practice Act. Once licensed, the nurse is responsible and accountable for practicing nursing within the state's legal definition. For example, the practice of nursing, as described by the New Jersey State Board of Nursing in its Nurse Practice Act (1975), is clearly defined in terms of its independent, interdependent, and dependent roles. It states:

Independent and Interdependent Functions	"The practice of nursing as a registered professional nurse is defined as diagnosing and treating human responses to actual or potential physical and emotional health problems through such services as case-finding, health teaching, health counseling, and provision of care supportive to or restorative of life and well being . . .
Dependent Functions	. . . and executing medical regimen as prescribed by a licensed or otherwise legally authorized physician or dentist."

CASE STUDY

Mr. Rubin Paul, age 64, had surgery five days ago for cancer. While caring for Mr. Paul, the nurse noted he was withdrawn and non-communicative. The client's wife verbalized her concern about this dramatic change in her husband's behavior. The nurse discussed this information with the surgeon, and they reached a mutual agreement that a psychiatric evaluation would benefit Mr. Paul. The client and his wife agreed, and the physician ordered a psychiatric consultation. The nurse notified the consultant and shared information pertinent to Mr. Paul's physical and psychological status. The psychiatrist evaluated the client, confirmed the diagnosis of postop depression, and ordered medications. The nurse incorporated the administration of this medication along with the use of therapeutic communication into the client's plan of care. In addition, the nurse monitored Mr. Paul's response to both of these modalities.

The following lists identify the independent, interdependent, and dependent functions that the nurse perfomed in this case study.

INDEPENDENT	INTERDEPENDENT	DEPENDENT
1. Assessment of psychological status (withdrawn and noncommunicative)	1. Discussion with surgeon regarding psychiatric evaluation	1. Administration of medication
2. Therapeutic communication	2. Communication with psychiatrist about physical and psychological status	
3. Evaluation for response to medication and therapeutic communication		

In conclusion, the practice of nursing has been defined by nursing leaders, by professional organizations, and according to function to include independent, interdependent, and dependent components. This definition will continue to evolve in response to nursing research and theory building as well as to the increasing complexity of health care. However, meeting the total needs of the client will continue to be the focus of nursing practice.

1–2 TEST YOURSELF

NURSING FUNCTIONS

The following situation will give you a chance to practice identifying the independent, interdependent, and dependent functions of the registered nurse. After reading the scenario, identify three independent, one interdependent, and three dependent functions of the nurse.

Mr. Ease was an 84 year old white male admitted to your unit at 6 AM. The night charge nurse reported that Mr. Ease had a history of urinary incontinence at home. His skin was intact, but she noted a reddened area approximately two inches in diameter at the base of his spine. He had limited range of motion in all his extremities and was unable to reposition himself in bed.

On first rounds, the nurse found Mrs. Ease, his 80 year old wife, outside the room crying. She stated that she was worried about what was going to happen to her husband since they had no children and she could no longer care for him.

Based on the physician's physical examination and information obtained from the nurse, some of the physician's orders included: intravenous therapy, vital signs every four hours, two acetaminophen (Tylenol) by mouth every four hours for a temperature elevation above 102°F, insertion of Foley urinary catheter, and consultation with physical therapy.

During the course of the day, Mr. Ease's temperature rose to 103°F (rectally). The nurse administered the Tylenol and decided to monitor the client's vital signs every hour for the next three hours. The nurse inserted the Foley catheter and established a turning schedule. Intravenous therapy and intake and output recording were initiated. The physical therapy department was notified, and a social service referral was made by the nurse. After consultation with a physical therapist, a regimen for range of motion exercises was established. This included bedside physical therapy twice a day on the day shift by the therapist and specific active and passive exercises on the evening shift by the nursing staff.

INDEPENDENT	INTERDEPENDENT	DEPENDENT
1.	1.	1.
2.		2.
3.		3.

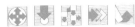

1–2 TEST YOURSELF □ ANSWERS

INDEPENDENT	INTERDEPENDENT	DEPENDENT
1. Increasing frequency of vital sign measurements	1. Performing active and passive range of motion exercises as suggested by physical therapy	1. Measuring and recording vital signs every four hours
2. Initiating intake and output recording		2. Administering medications
3. Assessing need for skin protection measures		3. Initiating intravenous therapy
4. Social service referral		4. Inserting Foley catheter

THE NURSING PROCESS

The science of nursing is based on a broad theoretical framework. The nursing process is the method by which this framework is applied to the practice of nursing. It is a deliberative problem-solving approach that requires cognitive, technical, and interpersonal skills and is directed to meeting the needs of the client/family system (Smith and Germain, 1975). The nursing process consists of five sequential and interrelated phases—assessment, diagnosis, planning, implementation, and evaluation. These phases integrate the intellectual functions of problem-solving in an effort to define nursing actions.

History

The nursing process has evolved into a five phase process consistent with the developing nature of the profession. It was first described as a distinct process by Hall (1955). Johnson (1959), Orlando (1961), and Wiedenbach (1963) each developed a different three phase process that contained rudimentary elements of the five phase process. In 1967, Yura and Walsh authored the first text that described a four phase process—assessment, planning, implementation, and evaluation. In the mid-1970s, Bloch (1974), Roy (1975), Mundinger and Jauron (1975), and Aspinall (1976) added the diagnostic phase, resulting in a five phase process.

Since that time, the nursing process has been legitimized as the framework of nursing practice. The American Nurses' Association used the nursing process as a guideline in developing the Standards of Nursing Practice. The nursing process has been incorporated into the conceptual framework of most nursing curriculums. It has also been included in the definition of nursing in the majority of nurse practice acts. More recently, the state board licensing examinations were revised to test the ability of the aspiring registered nurse to utilize the steps of the nursing process.

Definition

The nursing process can be defined in terms of three major dimensions: purpose, organization, and properties.

Purpose

The major purpose of the nursing process is to provide a framework within which the individualized needs of the client, family, and community can be met. Yura and Walsh (1988) state that "the nursing process is the designated series of actions intended to fulfill the purpose of nursing—to maintain the client's optimal wellness—and, if this state changes, to provide the amount and quality of nursing care his situation demands to direct him back to wellness. If wellness cannot be achieved, the nursing process should contribute to the client's quality of life, maximizing his resources to achieve the highest quality of living possible for as long a time as possible."

The nursing process involves an interactional relationship between the client and the nurse, with the client as the focus. The nurse validates observations with the client, and together they utilize the process. This assists the client to deal with actual or potential changes in health and results in individualized care.

Organization

As previously noted, the nursing process is organized into five identifiable phases—assessment, diagnosis, planning, implementation, and evaluation. Each can be further described as follows.

Assessment.　Assessment is the first phase of the nursing process. Its activities are focused on gathering information regarding the client, the client/family system, or the community for the purpose of identifying the client's needs, problems, concerns, or human responses. Data are collected in a systematic fashion, utilizing the interview or nursing history, physical examination, laboratory results, and other sources.

Diagnosis.　During this phase, the data collected during assessment are critically analyzed and interpreted. Conclusions are drawn regarding the client's needs, problems, concerns, and human responses. Nursing diagnoses are identified and provide a central focus for the remainder of the phases. Based on the nursing diagnoses, the plan of care is designed, implemented, and evaluated.

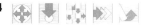

The nursing diagnoses supply an efficient method of communicating the client's problems.

Planning. In the planning phase, strategies are developed to prevent, minimize, or correct the problems identified in the nursing diagnosis. The planning phase consists of several steps:

1. Establishing priorities for the problems diagnosed
2. Setting outcomes with the client to correct, minimize, or prevent the problems
3. Writing nursing interventions that will lead to the achievement of the proposed outcomes
4. Recording nursing diagnoses, outcomes, and nursing interventions in an organized fashion on the care plan.

Implementation. Implementation is the initiation and completion of the actions necessary to achieve the outcomes defined in the planning stage. It involves communication of the plan to all those participating in the client's care. The interventions can be carried out by members of the health team, the client, or the client's family. The plan of care is used as a guide. The nurse continues to collect data regarding the client's condition and interaction with the environment. Implementation also includes recording the patient's care on the proper documents. This documentation verifies that the plan of care has been carried out and can be used as a tool to evaluate the plan's effectiveness.

Evaluation. The last phase of the nursing process is evaluation. It is an ongoing process that determines the extent to which the goals of care have been achieved. The nurse assesses the progress of the client, institutes corrective measures if required, and revises the nursing care plan.

This discussion has separated the nursing process into five distinct phases. In actual practice, it is impossible to separate the phases because they are interrelated and interdependent.

Properties

The nursing process has six properties. It is purposeful, systematic, dynamic, interactive, flexible, and theoretically based. The nursing process can be described as purposeful because it is goal directed. The nurse utilizes the phases of the process to provide quality client-centered care. The process is systematic because it involves the use of an organized approach to achieve its purpose. This deliberate method promotes the quality of nursing and avoids the problems associated with intuition or traditional care delivery.

The nursing process is dynamic because it involves continuous change. It is an ongoing process focused on the changing responses of the client that are identified throughout the nurse-client relationship. The interactive nature of the nursing process is based on the reciprocal relationships that occur between the nurse and the client, family, and other health professionals. This component ensures the individualization of client care.

The flexibility of the process may be demonstrated in two contexts: (1) it can be adapted to nursing practice in any setting or area of specialization dealing with individuals, groups, or communities; (2) its phases may be used sequentially and concurrently. The nursing process is most frequently utilized in sequence; however, the nurse may utilize more than one step at a time. For example, while implementing the plan, the nurse may evaluate the plan's effectiveness.

Finally, the nursing process is theoretically based. The process is devised from a broad base of knowledge, including the sciences and humanities, and can be applied to any of the theoretical models of nursing.

IMPLICATIONS OF THE NURSING PROCESS

The use of the nursing process in practice has implications for the profession of nursing, the client, and the individual nurse.

Implications for the Profession

Professionally, the nursing process concretely demonstrates the scope of nursing practice. Through the five phases, nursing continues to define its role to the consumer and other health care professionals. This clearly points out that the realm of nursing is more than just implementing the plan of care as prescribed by the physician.

In addition, the nursing process has been incorporated into standards of practice. These standards were adopted and published by the American Nurses' Association (Table 1–2). Nurses are held accountable for practicing according to these standards regardless of the setting or their area of specialization. Ad-

TABLE 1–2. GENERIC STANDARDS OF PRACTICE

I. The collection of data about the health status of the client/patient is systematic and continuous. The data are accessible, communicated, and recorded.
II. The nursing diagnosis is derived from health status data.
III. The plan of nursing care includes goals derived from the nursing diagnosis.
IV. The plan of nursing care includes priorities and prescribed nursing approaches or measures to achieve goals derived from the nursing diagnosis.
V. Nursing actions provide for patient participation in health promotions, maintenance, and restoration.
VI. Nursing actions assist the patient to maximize his health capabilities.
VII. The patient's progress or lack of progress toward goal achievement is determined by the patient and the nurse.
VIII. The patient's progress or lack of progress toward goal achievement directs reassessment, recording of priorities, new goal setting, and revision of the plan of nursing care.

Reprinted with permission of the American Nurses' Association. From Standards of Nursing Practice. Kansas City, MO: American Nurses' Association, 1973.

ditional standards have been formulated by the ANA Divisions of Practice (Maternal-Child Health, Gerontology, Psychiatric Mental Health, Community Health, and so on).

Implications for the Client

The use of the nursing process benefits the client and family. It encourages them to participate actively in care by involving them in all five phases of the process. The client provides assessment data, validates the nursing diagnosis, confirms outcomes and interventions, assists with implementation, and provides feedback for evaluation. In addition, the written plan promotes continuity of care, which results in a safe, therapeutic environment. The absence of this continuity may cause problems similar to those described in the following situation.

Example. Verna MacCarthy was a nursing supervisor of a medical-surgical unit. On rounds, she encountered Mrs. Martin, the wife of one of the clients, who stated that she had some complaints concerning the care of her husband. She explained that her husband developed an infection of his incision following bowel surgery. The doctor told her the dressing had to be changed and the wound irrigated three times daily. She indicated that this procedure was being done but that each nurse did it differently. Some even asked her or her husband how to do the procedure. "How come the nurses don't all do it the same? Who is doing it right? Shouldn't it be written somewhere? How will my husband ever get better?"

This situation demonstrates that when nursing care is uncoordinated, the family loses confidence in the staff's ability to meet the client's needs. An anxiety-producing environment is created rather than a therapeutic one.

The use of a systematic method of providing nursing care also improves the quality of that care. The absence of this type of approach can lead to error, omissions, and duplications in care.

Example. Lucille Rosso, a 30 year old teacher, delivered her second child a week ago. Usually the public health nurse's first visit includes teaching about growth and development and contraception. However, the nurse's assessment of this client's learning needs revealed adequate understanding in both of these areas. Therefore teaching focused on providing information about infant nutrition—a topic of concern to the client.

The use of the nursing process in this situation ensured a thorough assessment of the client's learning needs and involved her in planning approaches to meet them. Failure to do so might have resulted in a frustrating experience for the client, which could also compromise the quality of care delivered.

Individualized care is also promoted by the use of the nursing process. For example, the priorities of care for a client with pneumonia frequently focus on temperature monitoring, hydration, and antibiotic therapy. When Bonnie

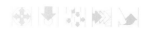

O'Malley was admitted for pneumonia, her three preschool children were left with a 15 year old baby sitter. The physician's plan of care included temperature control, intravenous therapy, and antibiotics. In the assessment phase, the nurse identified Bonnie's concern about her children. Because of her child care problem, Bonnie felt she had no choice but to leave the hospital against medical advice. The nurse initiated a social service consultation that resolved Bonnie's dilemma. This allowed Bonnie to remain in the hospital and to participate in those measures designed to restore her health. By addressing Bonnie's special needs, the nurse was able to provide quality individualized care.

Implications for the Nurse

The nursing process increases job satisfaction and enhances professional growth. The development of meaningful nurse-client relationships is facilitated by the nursing process. The rewards obtained from nursing practice are frequently derived from the nurse's ability to assist the client to meet identified needs. The genuine "thank you," regardless of the manner in which it is expressed by clients and their families, often outweighs any other type of recognition.

The nursing process encourages innovation and creativity in solving nursing care problems. This prevents the boredom that could result from a repetitive, task-oriented approach.

Example. Consider the case of Karen and Glenn Stanton, who were seen in the emergency department with multiple injuries after a car accident. The nurse determined that Mr. and Mrs. Stanton were extremely apprehensive about being separated from each other. The traditional approach of admitting them to separate rooms would add additional stress and interfere with their recuperation. Therefore, the nurse requested that the admitting department place the couple in the same room. Upon discharge, the couple expressed their appreciation.

This creative intervention hastened their recovery and provided the nurse with a sense of accomplishment.

Job satisfaction may also be increased through the use of the care plan developed from the nursing process. Well-written care plans save time and energy and prevent the frustration that is generated by trial and error nursing. Consider this situation.

Example. Mr. Lodge was a 300 lb man who had a right total hip replacement three days ago. Today the nurse caring for him must get him out of bed. The nurse giving change of shift report stated that yesterday was his first time out of bed. The nurse was concerned about how she was going to accomplish this task. She knew that Mr. Lodge was overweight, could not bear weight on the right leg, and was at risk for dislocating his hip. She was familiar with several recommended procedures for getting the client out of bed safely; however, the chart and care plan gave no indication of which method was successfully used on the previous day. Mr. Lodge was unable to describe the method used, and the nurses who assisted him were not available. The nurse finally selected a strategy, chose a chair, and estimated the amount of assistance she would need to move Mr. Lodge.

This situation illustrates how the nursing care plan can save time and decrease frustration. In this instance, if the care plan had specified directions on how to get Mr. Lodge out of bed, the nurse would not have experienced frustration and anger. She would have been able to get Mr. Lodge out of bed more efficiently. As demonstrated here, coordinating a client's nursing care through the use of a care plan greatly increases the chances of achieving the desired outcome.

The nursing process enhances professional growth. The application of the nursing process encourages the development of cognitive, technical, and interpersonal skills. The nurse accumulates additional knowledge through interaction with colleagues, clients, and other health care providers. The nursing process increases the potential for accurate identification of the client's response and implementation of appropriate actions. Quality assurance activities are used to examine the care provided, compare it to predetermined standards, and identify strengths and weaknesses. This assures quality care and suggests areas requiring additional education or development. Interaction with a variety of clients and other health care professionals encourages refinement of the nurse's verbal and nonverbal communication skills. The effectiveness of the nurse in daily practice is therefore enhanced.

SUMMARY

The dimensions of nursing practice have evolved in response to the scientific/technological, educational, economic, and political changes in society. The practice of nursing has been defined by nursing leaders, by professional organizations, and by regulatory agencies.

The nursing process is the method by which the theoretical frameworks of nursing are applied to actual practice. It can be defined in terms of three major dimensions: purpose, organization, and properties. The nursing process provides the framework to meet the individualized needs of the client, family, and community. It can be organized into five phases—assessment, diagnosis, planning, implementation, and evaluation. It has been characterized as purposeful, systematic, dynamic, interactive, flexible, and theoretically based.

The use of the nursing process has implications for the profession of nursing, the client, and the individual nurse. Professionally the nursing process defines the scope of nursing practice and identifies standards of nursing care. The client

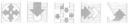

benefits by the use of the nursing process, since it ensures quality care while encouraging the client to participate in care. Finally, the benefits for the individual nurse are increased job satisfaction and enhancement of professional growth.

REFERENCES

American Nurses' Association: A Social Policy Statement. Kansas City, MO: American Nurses' Association, 1980.

American Nurses' Association: Standards of Nursing Practice. Kansas City, MO: American Nurses' Association, 1973.

Aspinall MJ: Nursing diagnosis—the weak link. Nursing Outlook 1976; 24:433–437.

Bloch D: Some crucial terms in nursing—what do they really mean? Nursing Outlook 1974; 22:689–694.

Fagin C: Primary care as an academic discipline. Nursing Outlook 1978; 26:750–753.

Hall LE: Quality of Nursing Care. Public Health News, June 1955.

Henderson V: Basic principles of nursing care. London: International Council of Nurses, 1961.

Johnson D: A philosophy for nursing diagnosis. Nursing Outlook 1959; 7:198–200.

Mundinger M and Jauron G: Developing a nursing diagnosis. Nursing Outlook 1975; 23:94–98.

Nightingale F: Notes on Nursing. What It Is, What It Is Not. New York: Dover Publications, 1969. (Originally published, 1859).

Orlando I: The Dynamic Nurse–Patient Relationship. New York: GP Putnam's Sons, 1961.

Rogers ME: Nursing Science: Introduction to the Theoretical Basis of Nursing. Philadelphia: FA Davis, 1970.

Roy C: The impact of nursing diagnosis. AORN Journal 1975; 21:1023–1030.

Smith DW, and Germain CP: Care of the Adult Patient. 4th ed. Philadelphia: JB Lippincott, 1975.

State of New Jersey Nursing Practice Act. Newark, NJ: New Jersey Board of Nursing, 1975.

Wiedenbach E: The helping art of nursing. American Journal of Nursing 1963; 63(11):544–557.

Yura H, and Walsh M: The Nursing Process: Assessing, Planning, Implementing, Evaluation, 1st ed. New York: Appleton-Century-Crofts, 1967.

Yura H, and Walsh M: The Nursing Process: Assessing, Planning, Implementing, Evaluation, 4th ed. New York: Appleton-Century-Crofts, 1988.

BIBLIOGRAPHY

Carlson JH, Craft C, and McGuire AD (eds): Nursing Diagnosis. Philadelphia: WB Saunders, 1982.

Griffith J, and Christensen P: Nursing Process: Application of Theories, Framework & Models, 2nd ed. St. Louis: CV Mosby, 1986.

Kanar RJ: Standards of nursing practice assessed through the application of the nursing process. Journal of Nursing Quality Assurance 1987; 1(2):72–78.

Kelly LY: Dimensions of Professional Nursing. 5th ed. New York: Macmillan, 1985.

LaMonica EL: The Humanistic Nursing Process. Boston: Jones & Bartlett, 1985.

McHugh MK: Has nursing outgrown the nursing process? Nursing 1987; 17(8):50–51.

2

ASSESSMENT

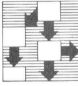

INTRODUCTION

PREREQUISITES
    Beliefs
    Knowledge
    Skills

DATA COLLECTION
    Types
    Sources
    Methods

DOCUMENTATION
    Purposes
    Guidelines

COMPUTERS AND NURSING ASSESSMENT
    Data Collection
    Documentation

SUMMARY

Assessment is the first step of the nursing process and can be described as the organized and systematic process of collecting data from a variety of sources to analyze the health status of a client. It consists of two components—data collection and documentation. The importance of this phase of the nursing process has been addressed specifically in the Standards of Nursing Practice of the American Nurses' Association. The first standard defines the need for the systematic collection of data that are accessible to health care providers (ANA, 1973). The fact that the assessment standard is the first of the eight standards is significant in reinforcing its importance as the key to the remaining steps of the nursing process.

The assessment phase provides a solid foundation that promotes the delivery of quality individualized care. Accurate, complete assessment is necessary to facilitate the diagnosis and treatment of human responses—the scope of nursing practice as defined by the ANA (1980). Assessment forms the basis for the identification of nursing diagnoses, development of outcomes, implementation of nursing interventions, and evaluation of nursing actions.

The initial assessment enables the nurse to accumulate comprehensive data about health responses. It also helps to identify the specific factors that contribute to the existence of these responses in an individual client. This encourages the nurse and client to develop outcomes. It also facilitates the implementation of nursing interventions designed to achieve the outcomes. Subsequent assessments validate the existence of previously identified concerns and document the client's progress toward the outcomes. These data also determine whether the nurse should change, expand, or discontinue nursing interventions. Since assessment is a continuous process, subsequent data also allow the nurse to identify additional problems that may have developed as a result of hospitalization, the disease process, or treatment modalities. This is accomplished through a process that compares current information to previously acquired baseline data.

PREREQUISITES

The assessment phase is influenced by the nurse's beliefs, knowledge, and skills. The nurse's beliefs and knowledge form the foundation for nurse-client interactions. Knowledge and skills are the tools that enable the nurse to acquire data, determine their significance, and develop interventions that promote quality individualized nursing care.

Beliefs

The nurses' beliefs include philosophies about nursing, health, the client as an individual and as a health care consumer, and the interactions between these factors. These become part of the theoretical framework upon which the nurse's practice is based. This framework is reflected not only in the assessment phase but also throughout the remaining components of the nursing process.

Example. Steven Bodine, age 25, is admitted to the hospital with a medical diagnosis of metastatic cancer of the lung. His primary site, testicular cancer, was diagnosed three years ago, and he has completed an extended series of both radiation and drug therapies. Steven and his wife have reached a mutual decision that his disease process and the need for continuing therapy have severely affected the quality of his life. Therefore, he has chosen to discontinue all therapy. This decision is supported by his physician.

The nurse believes that Steven has the right to make an informed decision and to control the manner in which he spends the remainder of his life. His nurse also believes that a nurse's role as a client advocate is to assist him in accomplishing these goals. The assessment phase identifies that Steven would like to be made comfortable and to die at home with the support of his family. The nurse's interventions would therefore focus on the implementation of a pain management regimen, patient/family teaching, and referral to a hospice program.

Knowledge

The process of assessment demands that the nurse possess an extensive body of knowledge from a variety of disciplines. This knowledge base includes both physical and behavioral sciences. The nurse is expected to master basic concepts of anatomy, physiology, chemistry, nutrition, microbiology, psychology, and sociology. The components of this scientific base allow the nurse to make the initial assessment of the client's physiological and psychological state. Such a body of knowledge also forms the basis for recognition of change during subsequent assessments. This facilitates the identification of contributing factors, both positive and negative, that determine the client's position on the health/illness continuum.

The nurse's knowledge base must also include the fundamentals of problem-solving analysis, and decision-making. The nurse must be able to analyze assessment data, recognize significant relationships among data, develop valid conclusions, and subsequently make sound nursing judgments that contribute to the client's progress.

Example. John Thomas is an obese 42 year old salesman who is admitted to the hospital for a cholecystectomy. On the third postop day, Mr. Thomas calls the nurse and indicates that he feels as though his "stitches are popping." The nurse notes that he is pale and diaphoretic, and further observation reveals four open sutures at the incisional area. A loop of bowel is protruding through the lower end of the opening. In addition, the client is hypotensive, with a blood pressure of 100/68.

Based on this assessment, the nurse instructs the client not to eat or drink, places a sterile saline-soaked dressing over his abdomen, and contacts Mr. Thomas's surgeon. The nurse's knowledge base is used to anticipate the need for further surgery. Her problem-solving skills resulted in prompt nursing actions that prevented more serious complications.

Skills

A variety of skills are necessary for the nurse to complete an effective assessment. These skills are related to the knowledge base and may be both technical and interpersonal in nature.

Technical skills associated with the assessment phase involve specific techniques and procedures that allow the nurse to collect the data. Some are associated with the use of equipment such as stethoscopes, sphygmomanometers, and thermometers for the measurement of vital signs. Other technical skills involve the performance of procedures such as palpation of pulses or auscultation of heart, lung, or bowel sounds. Both types of technical skills are required for accurate, complete assessment.

Interpersonal skills are important during all phases of the nursing process but are particularly critical to successful assessment. Since this is a communicative, interactive process, the nurse must have highly developed communication skills. These skills facilitate the development of positive relationships between the nurse and client or family. These positive relationships allow the nurse to

☐ Determine what the client/family sees as priorities

☐ Identify additional nursing concerns

☐ Create a therapeutic environment in which mutual outcomes may be accomplished.

The therapeutic environment begins to develop during assessment and requires the nurse to possess verbal and nonverbal communication abilities. Certainly, the nurse must be able to share information with the client by choosing language that accurately conveys the desired message at a level appropriate for the client. In addition, the nurse must have highly developed listening skills, which contribute to the therapeutic environment by allowing the client to feel comfortable expressing thoughts, feelings, and concerns. The nonverbal component of communication is of particular importance in the assessment process and the development of nurse-client relationships.

Creativity, common sense, and flexibility are additional interpersonal skills required when assessing the client or family. The nurse is frequently required to be creative in developing strategies to facilitate assessment. This is particularly important when clients are very young or frightened or have communication barriers.

Example.   Cindy is a three year old who was brought to the university clinic by her mother. She is complaining of abdominal pain and is obviously frightened. Cindy screams when the nurse attempts to examine her abdomen. The nurse asks Cindy to show where it hurts on her doll or on mommy. This creative approach allows the nurse to obtain information in a manner that is much less threatening to Cindy.

Common sense dictates that detailed nursing histories should be postponed on clients who are experiencing acute anxiety, pain, or dyspnea. This creates an environment of sensitivity and caring, which may also be evidenced by the nurse's flexibility in responding to client requests.

Example.   Nora York is a 61 year old woman admitted for elective knee joint replacement. The nurse greets her, makes her comfortable, and begins the nursing history. Mrs. York indicates that she would prefer that her daughter, a nurse, be with her during the interview and that she expects her within an hour.

In this situation, the nurse demonstrates flexibility in selecting the timing of the health history. This sensitivity puts Mrs. York at ease and strengthens the nurse's relationship with this client.

DATA COLLECTION

In the context of the nursing assessment, data might be defined as specific information obtained about a client. The nurse systematically accumulates the information required to diagnose the client's health responses and to identify contributing factors. This data base subsequently forms the foundation for the remaining phases of the nursing process—diagnosis, planning, implementation, and evaluation.

Types of Data

Four types of data are collected by the nurse during assessment—subjective, objective, historical, and current. A complete and accurate data base usually includes a combination of these types.

Subjective data might be described as the individual's view of a situation or a series of events. This information cannot be determined by the nurse independent of interaction or communication with the individual. Subjective data are frequently obtained during the nursing history and include the client's perceptions, feelings, and ideas about self and personal health status. Examples include the client's descriptions of pain, weakness, frustration, nausea, or embarrassment. Information supplied by sources other than the client—e.g., family, consultants, and other members of the health team—may also be subjective if based on the individual's opinion rather than substantiated by fact.

In contrast, objective data are both observable and measurable. This information is usually obtained through the senses—sight, smell, hearing, and touch—during the physical examination of the client. Examples of objective data include respiratory rate, blood pressure, edema, and weight.

During the assessment of a client, the nurse must consider both subjective and objective findings. Frequently, these findings substantiate each other, as in the case of John Thomas, the client whose incision opened three days after surgery. The subjective information provided by Mr. Thomas, "feels like my stitches are popping," was validated by the nurse's objective findings—pallor, diaphoresis, hypotension, and protrusion of the bowel through the incision.

In the case of Peggy Malletts, the nurse observes the client crying as she stands in front of the nursery two days after premature delivery of her first child. The nurse suggests that Peggy seems "upset," and the client validates that she is "afraid that her baby might die." Here, the objective data observed by the nurse (crying) were substantiated by subjective data obtained from the client (feelings of fear).

At times, subjective and objective data may be in conflict. Juan, a 16 year old client, denied that he was in pain after surgical repair of an inguinal hernia. Juan's denial would be considered subjective data, since it reflects his feelings of pain. However, the nurses documented several objective findings that are consistent with the usual response to pain (facial grimaces, elevated pulse rate, clutching incision area). In this case the subjective and objective data are in conflict; therefore the nurse must accumulate additional information to resolve the discrepancy.

Another consideration when describing data concerns the element of time. In this context, data may be either historical or current (Bellack and Bamford, 1984). Historical data involve information about events that have occurred prior to the present, which might include previous hospitalizations, normal elimination patterns, or chronic diseases. In contrast, current data refer to events that are occurring in the present—blood pressure, vomiting, postoperative pain. Again, a combination of both current and historical data may be used to verify problems or to identify discrepancies.

Example. A public health nurse visits John Kelly, age 62, at his home following his discharge from an extended care facility. During the initial interview, Mr. Kelly indicates that he has not moved his bowels for two days. When the nurse expresses concern, the client indicates that his normal pattern is every three days.

In this case, the current data (no BM for two days) are invalidated as a problem in view of the historical data (normal pattern every third day).

Example. Kelly O'Keefe, age five, is admitted for tonsillectomy. In the immediate postoperative period, her pulse rate ranges from 90 to 108. Four hours later, the nurse observes that Kelly is swallowing frequently and her pulse is 124.

In this situation, current data (pulse rate 124) substantiate the existence of a problem (bleeding) when compared with historical data (pulse rate 90 to 108).

For the data base to be complete, the nurse should collect all four types of data. Subjective and objective data provide specific information regarding the client's health status and help to identify problems. Additionally, current and historical data assist in this process by establishing time frames or usual behavioral patterns.

The following exercises are designed to assist you to recognize subjective, objective, historical, and current data.

2–1 TEST YOURSELF

TYPES OF DATA

The following is a list of data. Indicate by checking (✔) whether each item is subjective or objective.

DATA	SUBJECTIVE	OBJECTIVE
1. "I feel tired today."		
2. Blood pressure 180/96		
3. Speaks only when spoken to		
4. "She seems nervous."		
5. "My leg hurts."		
6. Dirt under nails		
7. Rash on flank		
8. "I need help."		
9. Absent bowel sounds		
10. Respiratory rate 24		

Now, identify each of the following as historical or current.

DATA	HISTORICAL	CURRENT
1. No prior surgery		
2. "I used to eat when I was nervous."		
3. Temperature 97.8°F		
4. "I'm allergic to sulfa."		
5. Weight 118 lb		
6. Smoked three packs of cigarettes a day until last month		
7. Warm, dry skin		
8. Worked part-time until one year ago		
9. Two episodes of nocturia six months ago		
10. Diminished breath sounds at base of right lung		

2–1 TEST YOURSELF □ ANSWERS

The following is a list of data. Indicate by checking (✔) whether each item is subjective or objective.

DATA	SUBJECTIVE	OBJECTIVE
1. "I feel tired today."	✔	
2. Blood pressure 180/96		✔
3. Speaks only when spoken to		✔
4. "She seems nervous."	✔	
5. "My leg hurts."	✔	
6. Dirt under nails		✔
7. Rash on flank		✔
8. "I need help."	✔	
9. Absent bowel sounds		✔
10. Respiratory rate 24		✔

Now, identify each of the following as historical or current.

DATA	HISTORICAL	CURRENT
1. No prior surgery	✔	
2. "I used to eat when I was nervous."	✔	
3. Temperature 97.8°F		✔
4. "I'm allergic to sulfa."		✔
5. Weight 118 lb		✔
6. Smoked three packs of cigarettes a day until last month	✔	
7. Warm, dry skin		✔
8. Worked part-time until one year ago	✔	
9. Two episodes of nocturia six months ago	✔	
10. Diminished breath sounds at base of right lung		✔

Sources of Data

During the assessment phase, data are collected from a variety of sources. These sources are classified as either primary or secondary. The client is the primary source and should be utilized to obtain pertinent subjective data. The client can most accurately (1) share personal perceptions and feelings about health and illness, (2) identify individual goals or problems, and (3) validate responses to diagnostic or treatment modalities.

Secondary sources are those other than the client. These are utilized in situations in which the client is unable to participate or when additional information is required to clarify or validate data supplied by the client. Secondary sources might include the client's family or significant other, individuals in the client's immediate environment, other members of the health team, and the medical record. Family, friends, and coworkers may also provide pertinent historical data regarding the client's normal patterns in the home, at work, and in recreational environments.

Example. Cathy Johnson, age 24, is admitted to the Intensive Care Unit following an automobile accident. Since Cathy is comatose, the nurse interviews her father. During this conversation, Mr. Johnson indicates that Cathy was hit in the eye when she was 13 and has a permanently dilated right pupil.

In this situation, the information obtained from the client's family provides historical data that clarify the nurse's physical findings. These are significant in view of the client's history.

Other members of the health team may also contribute significant data.

☐ Other nurses who have cared for the client during hospitalization may provide information concerning that client's responses.

☐ The physical therapist may be able to assist the nurse to compare the motor skills demonstrated by the client during therapy with those observed on the nursing unit.

☐ The physician may be able to describe the client's emotional response to a previous heart attack.

Each of these secondary sources may add to the nurse's knowledge base and therefore expand the data available for comparing and evaluating client responses.

The individuals in the client's immediate hospital environment may also provide additional information. Visitors may substantiate the nurse's view that the client is less communicative today than on a previous day. Other clients may be able to provide current data about events that occur when the nurse is not present. For example, the client in another bed may validate the nurse's impression that an elderly client climbed over the siderails and fell out of bed.

The medical record contains an abundance of demographic data—marital status, occupation, religion, insurance. This provides insight into the client's socioeconomic status. Additionally, the record contains current and historical data documented by personnel in other disciplines (physician, dietician, respiratory therapist, social worker, discharge planner). Diagnostic data are also available, including laboratory and radiological findings.

The nurse must carefully consider the client's rights to privacy and confidentiality when obtaining information from secondary sources. Additionally, these client rights may outweigh the needs of others to obtain sensitive data.

Example. Mr. Turi's employer brings him to the emergency department after he vomits blood while at work. The client tells the nurse that he has been drinking a fifth of Scotch a day for five years. While providing information to the nurse, Mr. Turi's employer states, "He drinks, doesn't he? That's why he's bleeding again!"

In this situation, the client's employer is attempting to obtain confidential information about the client's drinking patterns. The nurse should protect the client's privacy by tactfully focusing the conversation on other topics rather than confirm Mr. Turi's alcoholism without his approval.

2–2 TEST YOURSELF

SOURCES OF DATA

CASE STUDY

Mr. Ted Alexander, a 50 year old white divorced resident of Las Vegas, was on a business trip to Atlantic City when he developed pain in the right lower abdominal quadrant. He took Alka-Seltzer but obtained little relief, and the pain persisted for the next two days. He was busy with appointments during the day and evening and was able to ignore the pain. He ate very little and took two sleeping pills at night. On the afternoon of the third day, the pain became much more intense, and when it continued for several hours and he began to vomit repeatedly, he went to the emergency department.

Physical examination and laboratory data at this time revealed an alert, well-groomed male with generalized abdominal tenderness, rigidity of the abdominal wall, presence of a palpable mass in the right inguinal area, absent bowel sounds, and a white blood count (WBC) of 20,000/mm^3 (normal = 5000–9000). The diagnosis of ruptured appendix was made. He was admitted to the hospital for initial medical management with surgery anticipated at a later date.

Your examination of the patient reveals the following: B/P 140/80, P 116, R 26, T 101.2°F. The patient indicates that he is 6'2" tall and weighs 196 lb. He is alert and oriented and states "My gut is killing me." His skin is warm to the touch and slightly diaphoretic. The patient states that he had been a heavy drinker for 15 years and was admitted to the hospital with cirrhosis two years ago by his family doctor, Dr. Martland, but has never had surgery. He denies drinking for the past two years but smokes two packs of cigarettes daily.

Mr. Alexander is tense throughout your conversation but shares a number of concerns with you, including his separation from his two teenage children who live with him. He is also anxious about being cared for by an unfamiliar physician. The emergency department (ED) nurse indicates that he wears contact lenses and is concerned because he left his case and supplies as well as his glasses in his hotel. He gives you $75.00 in cash and traveler's checks to deposit in the hospital safe. He has a partial lower plate of dentures and caps on his four front teeth. Further inquiry reveals that the patient prefers a low fat diet, occasionally uses laxatives, and has had several occurrences of urinary urgency and nocturia in the last six months.

The physician states that his treatment plan includes gastric suction, antibiotics, and IV fluid therapy with electrolytes and vitamins until the patient is stabilized enough for exploratory surgery. Mr. Alexander agrees to this plan but is concerned about his job demands and wonders how he will deal with "getting back home when all of this is over."

Based on the case study, identify three examples of each subjective, objective, current, and historical data as well as three secondary sources of data.

SUBJECTIVE DATA

1.

2.

3.

OBJECTIVE DATA

1.

2.

3.

CURRENT DATA

1.

2.

3.

HISTORICAL DATA

1.

2.

3.

SECONDARY SOURCES

1.

2.

3.

2–2 TEST YOURSELF □ ANSWERS

SUBJECTIVE DATA
1. Abdominal pain.
2. Height and weight; concerns about separation from children and private MD
3. Low fat diet preference; smoking

OBJECTIVE DATA
1. Abdominal rigidity, inguinal mass, absent bowel sounds
2. B/P 140/80, P 116, R 26, T 101.2°F, skin warm and diaphoretic, WBC 20,000/mm^3
3. Partial dentures, caps

CURRENT DATA
1. Vital signs
2. Skin warm, diaphoretic
3. Smokes two packs of cigarettes daily

HISTORICAL DATA
1. Drinking heavily for 15 years
2. No previous surgery; occasional use of laxatives
3. Urgency and nocturia in last six months; pain for two days

SECONDARY SOURCES
1. Laboratory data
2. Emergency department nurse
3. Physician

Methods of Data Collection

There are three major methods that are utilized to gather information during a nursing assessment. These methods include interview, observation, and physical examination. These techniques provide the nurse with a logical, systematic approach to the collection of data required for subsequent nursing diagnosis and care planning.

Interview

The interview serves four purposes in the context of a nursing assessment: (1) it allows the nurse to acquire specific information required for diagnosis and planning; (2) it facilitates the nurse-client relationship by creating an opportunity for dialogue; (3) it allows the client to receive information and to participate in identification of problems and goal-setting; and (4) it assists the nurse to determine areas for specific investigation during the other components of the assessment process.

The nursing interview is a complex process that requires refined communication and interaction skills. It differs from the types of interviews performed by other members of the health team since it focuses on identification of client responses that may be treated through nursing intervention. It is a purposeful process designed to allow both nurse and client to give and receive information.

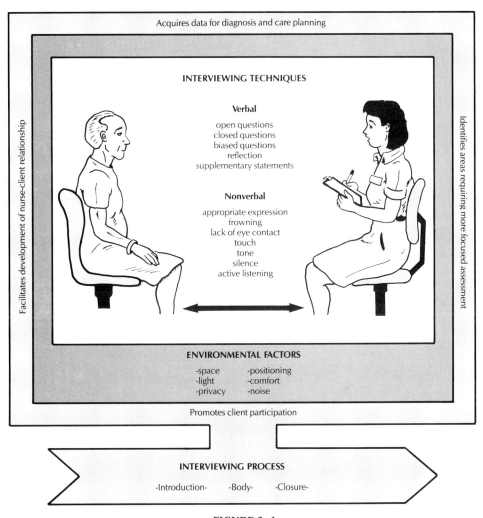

FIGURE 2–1.

Figure 2–1 illustrates the interview process including purposes, components, and factors affecting its success.

Segments of the Interview.   The interview consists of three segments— introduction, body, and closure.

INTRODUCTION.   In the introductory phase, nurse and client begin to develop a therapeutic relationship. The nurse's professional attitude is probably the most significant factor in creating an environment in which a positive relationship can be developed. The nurse's approach should convey respect for the client; therefore it is appropriate to share introductions. The client should be addressed by name—e.g., ''Mr. Jones'' rather than ''Bill'' or ''Pop.'' The nurse should explain the purpose of the interview, estimate the time required, and assess for factors that may inhibit involvement (e.g., pain, lack of privacy). All questions should be directed to the client. Family and other secondary sources should be utilized when the client is unable to respond. The client should be assured that the information gathered is confidential. These approaches create an atmosphere of trust and sensitivity in which the client may feel comfortable sharing information of a personal nature.

BODY.   During this second part of the interview, the nurse focuses the dialogue on specific areas designed to obtain the data required. This usually begins with the client's chief complaint and generally incorporates other areas such as past medical history, family history, and religious and cultural data. A more complete listing is seen in Table 2–1.

Interviews are done in a variety of settings, including the hospital, clinic, nursing home, physician's office, college infirmary, and client's home. The for-

TABLE 2–1. HEALTH HISTORY CONTENT

Client Profile

Brief statement about the client

Chief Complaint

Client's statement about reason for seeking medical assistance

History of Present Illness

Description of client's symptoms, including onset, location, duration, quality, intensity, aggravating, alleviating, and associated factors, course of illness, problem

Past Medical History

Summary of client's health, including major and minor adult illnesses, previous hospitalization and surgery, major injuries or accidents, drug or food allergies, usual response to illness

Family History

Identification of family members and health trends, including age, sex, and health status of living family members; age, sex, and cause of death of deceased family members; familial history of cancer, heart disease, hypertension, stroke, epilepsy, renal disorders, diabetes, arthritis, tuberculosis

Medication History

Listing of medications, including name, dosage, frequency of administration, duration of therapy, time of last dose (should include nonprescription drugs taken, including aspirin, laxatives, antihistamines, etc.)

Alcohol, Tobacco, and Drug History

Description of usual patterns of usage, including alcohol type, average consumption; tobacco type, amount per day, age started, stopped; drug type, frequency of use

Social History

Summary of employment, occupation, education, hobbies, living environment, recreation, religion

Patterns of Daily Living

Identification of client's usual patterns, including sleep/rest, hygiene, activity, elimination, diet/fluids, health practices

mat for collecting the health history is dependent on the type of setting and the purpose of the interview. Some nurses prefer to use a free-flow approach that begins with the client's chief complaint and extends to other areas based on individual client cues (Fig. 2–1). Others prefer a more structured approach that utilizes a specific format. Content areas are defined, and the nurse utilizes a form as a checklist to ensure that all content areas have been addressed (Fig. 2–2). The nurse should use the format that is found to be most comfortable and that results in a logical, systematic accumulation of pertinent information about the client.

CLOSURE.   The final phase of the interview is closure. During this phase, the nurse prepares the client for termination of the interview. ''Mrs. Black, we'll be finishing in a few minutes.'' The nurse should not introduce new material at this time; however, the client may want to discuss additional topics. If time allows, this may be accomplished, or the nurse may suggest a second interview at another time. The most significant points discussed during the interview should be summarized. This allows the client to verify or negate the nurse's perceptions of major problems, client concerns, and other pertinent data. This also lays the foundation for clarification and mutual goal-setting in the planning process. The nurse should attempt to end the interview in a manner that conveys warmth and appreciation. ''Mrs. Black, thanks for sharing this information about yourself—it will be very useful in helping us to plan your care.'' This may set the scene for future nurse-client interactions throughout their therapeutic relationships.

Factors Affecting the Interview.   There are a number of variables that affect the success of a nurse-client interview. These include environmental factors, interviewing techniques, and verbal and nonverbal communication.

ENVIRONMENTAL FACTORS.   An informative interview is dependent upon effective nurse-client interaction. The environment in which the interview takes place frequently affects the ability of the client and the nurse to participate in this process. The nurse can attempt to control the environment by manipulating several physical factors.

The interview area should be arranged to allow comfortable face-to-face interaction between the nurse and the client or family. The client should be positioned comfortably in bed or in a chair with the nurse seated opposite. Standing over the client should be avoided if possible, since this may convey superiority, disinterest, or haste.

Privacy should be assured, since the client is expected to answer many personal questions. This may be accomplished by pulling a curtain, finding a quiet spot, or closing a door. Privacy also increases the potential for accurate, complete information and assists in creating a trusting relationship. To facilitate the concentration of both nurse and client, the interview area should be free from noise, odors, and interruptions. The temperature of the area should be comfortable, and lighting should allow both participants to observe each other clearly.

MERCER MEDICAL CENTER
NURSING HISTORY AND PHYSICAL

Date _____ Time _____ A.M. P.M.

BP _____ TPR _____

Admitting Diagnosis _____

_____

PAST MEDICAL HISTORY (medical, surgical, trauma)

_____
_____
_____
_____
_____
_____
_____
_____
_____
_____
_____

Height _____ Weight _____
ALLERGIES AND REACTIONS _____

MEDICATIONS
Name & Dosage | Usual Time Taken | Time of Last Dose

REASONS FOR HOSPITALIZATION (onset, character, methods used to resolve problem)

_____
_____
_____
_____   Signature_____

	SUBJECTIVE		OBJECTIVE	
COMMUNICATION	☐ Hearing Loss ☐ Visual Changes ☐ Denied	Comments: _____ _____ _____ _____	☐ Glasses ☐ Contact Lens Pupil Size R___ L___ Reaction _____	☐ Language Barrier ☐ Hearing Aide ☐ Speech Difficulties
OXYGENATION	☐ Dyspnea ☐ Smoking History _____ ☐ Cough ☐ Sputum ☐ Denied	Comments: _____ _____ _____ _____ _____	Resp ☐ Regular ☐ Irregular Describe:_____ _____ R _____ L _____	
CIRCULATION	☐ Chest Pain ☐ Leg Pain ☐ Numbness of Extremities ☐ Denied	Comments: _____ _____ _____ _____	Heart Rhythm ☐ Regular ☐ Irregular Ankle Edema _____ Pulse Car. Rad. DP Fem.* R _____ L _____ Comments: _____ _____ *If applicable	
NUTRITION	Diet: _____ ☐ N ☐ V Character ☐ Recent change in weight, appetite ☐ Swallowing difficulty ☐ Denied	Comments: _____ _____ _____ _____ _____	☐ Dentures ☐ None Upper Lower	Full Partial With Patient ☐ ☐ ☐ ☐ ☐ ☐

RBG 13122 (11/84)

FIGURE 2–2. Sample structured nursing assessment form. (Courtesy of Mercer Medical Center, Trenton, NJ.)

	SUBJECTIVE		OBJECTIVE	
ELIMINATION	Usual bowel pattern	☐ Urinary Frequency	Comments: _____	Bowel Sounds _____
	☐ Constipation	☐ Urgency	_____	Abdominal distention present:
	Remedy	☐ Dysuria	_____	☐ Yes ☐ No
	_____	☐ Hematuria	_____	
	Date of last BM	☐ Incontinence	_____	Urine* (color, consistency, odor)
	_____	☐ Polyuria	_____	_____
	☐ Diarrhea	☐ Foley in place	_____	_____
	Character	☐ Denied	_____	*If foley in place

MGT. OF HEALTH AND ILLNESS	☐ Alcohol ☐ Denied	Briefly describe patient's ability to follow treatments (diet, meds, etc.) for chronic health problems (if present).
	(Amount, frequency)	_____
	_____	_____
	☐ BSE Last Pap Smear _____	_____
	LMP: _____	_____

SKIN INTEGRITY	☐ Dry	Comments: _____	☐ Dry	☐ Cold	☐ Pale
		_____	☐ Flushed	☐ Warm	
	☐ Itching	_____	☐ Moist	☐ Cyanotic	
		_____	*Rashes, ulcers, decubitus (describe size, location, drainage)		
	☐ Other	_____	_____		
		_____	_____		
	☐ Denied		_____		
	*Use Skin/body Stamp on Progress Notes		_____		

ACTIVITY/SAFETY	☐ Convulsions	Comments: _____	☐ LOC and Orientation _____
	☐ Dizziness	_____	_____
	☐ Limited motion	_____	Gait: ☐ Walker ☐ Cane ☐ Other
	of joints	_____	☐ Steady ☐ Unsteady _____
		_____	☐ Sensory and motor losses in face or extremities _____
	Limitations in	_____	_____
	ability to:	_____	_____
	☐ Ambulate	_____	☐ ROM limitations _____
	☐ Bathe self	_____	_____
	☐ Other	_____	_____
	☐ Denied		_____

COMFORT SLEEP/WAKE	☐ Pain	Comments: _____	☐ Facial Grimaces
	(Location,	_____	☐ Guarding
	frequency,	_____	☐ Other signs of pain _____
	remedies)	_____	_____
	☐ Nocturia	_____	
	☐ Sleep Difficulties	_____	☐ Siderail release form signed (60 + years)
	☐ Denied		

COPING	Occupation _____	Observed non-verbal behavior _____
	Members of household _____	_____
	_____	_____
	_____	Person and phone number that can be reached at any time
	Most supportive person _____	_____
	_____	_____

R.N. Signature _____

FIGURE 2–2 *Continued*

Interviewing Techniques. Interviews are most informative when the nurse utilizes both verbal and nonverbal techniques to obtain data. The combination of both approaches facilitates the acquisition of an accurate, complete data base.

VERBAL TECHNIQUES. The most commonly used verbal techniques include questioning, reflection, and supplementary statements. The nurse who uses all of these approaches during the interview is more likely to be successful in obtaining the most significant information from the client.

Questioning allows the nurse to obtain information from the client, clarify perceptions of client responses, and validate other subjective or objective data. Questions may be open, closed, or biased.

Open questions are those that by their nature elicit the client's perception of an event or description of concerns or feelings. Generally, these questions require more than a one or two word response.

Examples

"What happened today that made you come to the emergency department?"
"How did you feel when the doctor told you about your blood pressure?"
"Which medications do you take on a regular basis?"
"What do you usually do when the pain occurs?"

Questions beginning with "what," "how," or "which" tend to result in the most detailed client response. "Why" questions tend to put the client in a defensive position.

Examples

"Why did you do that?"
"Why didn't you see a doctor sooner?"

The following outlines the advantages and disadvantages of open questions.

ADVANTAGES	DISADVANTAGES
☐ Provide clients with the stimulus to express important concerns	☐ Tend to elicit lengthy or wordy responses in a limited time frame
☐ Help to facilitate communication by encouraging clients to respond	☐ Allow the client to stray from content of question or focus on irrelevant topics (particularly when client is not comfortable discussing topic)
☐ Tend to be less threatening and to elicit more honest replies	

Closed questions are those that require brief one or two word responses. They are used most frequently to obtain specific facts.

Examples

"Did you take your blood pressure medicine today?"
"How long did the pain last?"
"When was your last menstrual period?"
"How many times did you have diarrhea yesterday?"

Advantages	Disadvantages
☐ Avoid lengthy responses ☐ Allow the nurse to focus the interview ☐ Help to clarify responses to open-ended questions	☐ Discourage verbalization and limit the type and amount of data obtained (brief and superficial) ☐ Tend to make the client feel defensive

Example

Nurse: What do you usually do when the back pain occurs? (Open)
Client: Well, I usually lie down and take two pain pills.
Nurse: Did you do that today before you came to the hospital? (Closed)
Client: Yes

Biased questions are those that tend to elicit a specific response or reaction from a client. They may be either open or closed. The most commonly used are leading or loaded questions. Leading questions imply that a particular response is preferred. Clients tend to answer these questions with responses they feel are desirable.

Examples

"You don't take drugs, do you?"
"There's no history of mental illness in your family, is there?"
"You're feeling better today, aren't you?"

Loaded questions are used to elicit the client's reaction to a specific topic. The nurse is usually trying to evaluate the client's nonverbal response more than the content of the actual reply to the question.

Examples

"Do you think that your pain increases after your husband visits?"
"Does your drinking interfere with your work?"

When asking questions of this nature, the nurse is watching for squirming, lack of eye contact, or other signs of uneasiness. This nonverbal behavior may be more revealing than the client's verbal response. Biased questions tend to intimidate clients and frequently block the communication process. Clients often provide responses that they believe are expected; therefore, the information may be inaccurate. Biased questions should be used only when other techniques have been unsuccessful. Ideally, the use of a mixture of open and closed questioning will result in accurate, complete data, eliminating the need for biased questions.

The second verbal interviewing technique is the use of *reflection*. The nurse's perception of the client's response is repeated or rephrased. Repetition encourages the client to continue discussion of a particular area of content. The nurse repeats key words from the client's statement and assists the client to explore the topic more completely.

Example

Nurse: How did you feel when the doctor told you about your high blood pressure?
Client: I was really afraid.
Nurse: You were really afraid? (Repetition of key words.)
Client: Yes, I thought I might have a stroke and die or be an invalid.

Since rephrasing provides the client with the nurse's interpretation of the information discussed, this allows both nurse and client to expand, clarify, or correct the nurse's perception.

Example

Client: I found this lump in my breast last week when I was taking a shower. My mother had them too before she died from cancer.
Nurse: You're afraid that you might have cancer?
Client: Yes. I'm too young to die; my children need me.

In this case the nurse's perceptions were verified by the client.

Example

Client: I never had this dizziness or nausea until the doctor started me on that new blood pressure medicine.
Nurse: You think that the medicine is the cause of the problems you're having now?
Client: No, not really, but I think it may be part of the problem.

Here, the client clarified the nurse's interpretation of the initial statement.

After reflective statements, clients may seek advice or reassurance or ask the nurse to validate their feelings. The client might respond with "What do you think?" "It's OK, isn't it?" or "What would you do?" Such responses may also be the client's attempt to obtain additional information. The nurse should avoid providing advice, unrealistic reassurance, or opinions since this tends to shift the accountability for decision-making from the client to the nurse. The most effective method of dealing with this type of interaction is to use reflection to redirect the question.

Example

Client: The doctor told me that I can either have my hysterectomy the day after tomorrow or go home and come back in six weeks. What would you do, nurse?

Nurse: You're not sure whether you should have the surgery now or later? Let's look at the pros and cons of each.

This approach allowed the nurse to (1) rephrase the client's concerns, (2) clarify the decision that needed to be made by the client, and (3) create an environment that would encourage the client to look at her options objectively before making a decision.

The use of *supplementary statements* may encourage the client to continue verbalization throughout the interview. Short phrases such as "um-hm," "yes," "go on," "I see," and "what happened next?" send a clear message. These brief responses let the client know that the nurse is interested and they frequently stimulate further communication. They are particularly effective when accompanied by nonverbal cues such as touch, eye contact, and nodding the head.

 2–3 TEST YOURSELF

VERBAL TECHNIQUES

Read the following statements and identify them as open (O), closed (C), biased (B), reflective (R), or supplementary (S).

____ "When did you first notice the lump in your breast?"
____ "And then?"
____ "You don't really believe that old wives' tale, do you?"
____ "You're confused about how many times a day you should be taking this pill?"
____ "How do you know when your blood sugar is low?"
____ "When did you stop beating your wife?"
____ "Oh, when you went to India you got malaria?"
____ "What do you think you can do to assist in your recovery?"
____ "Do you have any questions about what will be happening to you tomorrow?"
____ "Go on."

2–3 TEST YOURSELF □ ANSWERS

Key—(O) open, (C) closed, (B) biased, (R) reflective, (S) supplementary

(C)   "When did you first notice the lump in your breast?"

(S)   "And then?"

(B)   "You don't really believe that old wives' tale, do you?"

(R)   "You're confused about how many times a day you should be taking this pill?"

(O)   "How do you know when your blood sugar is low?"

(B)   "When did you stop beating your wife?"

(R)   "Oh, when you went to India you got malaria?"

(O)   "What do you think you can do to assist in your recovery?"

(C)   "Do you have any questions about what will be happening to you tomorrow?"

(S)   "Go on."

NONVERBAL TECHNIQUES.   The nurse should be aware of a number of non-berbal methods that may facilitate or enhance communication during the interview. The nonverbal components of a nurse-client interaction frequently convey a message more effectively than the actual spoken words. In fact, if the verbal and nonverbal messages differ, the nonverbal message tends to be accepted more readily. The most common nonverbal components include facial expression, body position, touch, voice, silence, and active listening.

The client's *facial expressions* often reveal important information. The nurse should watch for appropriateness of expression, frowning, and lack of eye contact.

Appropriateness of expression suggests that facial expression should be congruent with the words being spoken and to the context of the conversation. The nurse should be particularly alert to situations in which the expression on the client's face does not match the verbal message. For example, when a client describes himself as depressed, the nurse would not expect to see a smile on his face. Similarly, when a woman talks about how happy she is in her marriage, her facial expression usually indicates sincerity. The nurse might question this sincerity if her statement is accompanied by a smirk.

The nurse should also be concerned if the facial expression is not appropriate to the context of the message. For example, sometimes a nurse will encounter a client who smiles when discussing a serious problem. The smile, which may be resulting from uneasiness, could mislead the nurse into believing that the client is not concerned about the problem.

Frowning may indicate disagreement, lack of understanding, pain, anger, or unhappiness. For example, when a nurse is explaining to Mrs. Kuroishi that she should take her pulse each day before taking her digoxin, the client frowns. The nurse might interpret this as an indication of unwillingness to carry out this step. In reality, Mrs. Kuroishi does not know how to take her pulse.

Lack of eye contact may mean that the client is uncomfortable, shy, nonassertive, bored, intimidated, or withdrawn. For example, in a venereal disease clinic, the nurse frequently questions clients about sexual contacts. In response to this question, Tyrell Williams turns his face away. The nurse might interpret this change in eye contact as embarrassment. In reality, Tyrell is trying to remember a number of names.

The nurse may want to clarify discrepancies between facial expressions and verbal messages or context. For example, the nurse might say, "I notice that you are smiling when you discuss your illness, but your words indicate your concern. I'm confused. Could you clarify this for me?"

Similarly, facial expression exhibited by the nurse may also convey mixed messages. For example, the nurse who smiles inappropriately when the client shares very personal or sensitive information may upset the client. In fact, the nurse may feel uncomfortable discussing the topic. Likewise, frowning after a client's comments may be seen as being judgmental, when in reality the nurse may have a headache. Lack of eye contact because of preoccupation with a confused client in the other bed may be interpreted as lack of interest.

Body position and stance are elements of interaction that convey a nonverbal message. The nurse should attempt to create an environment of warmth and trust. This is frequently accomplished by a calm, relaxed posture. This position communicates interest and caring and tends to help the client feel comfortable in disclosing personal information. A hurried approach, an inappropriately warm or cold attitude, or a rigid or overly casual posture communicate disinterest, boredom, or preoccupation. These nonverbal messages tend to confuse the client and inhibit the interview process.

The nurse should observe the nonverbal messages communicated by the client's posture or stance throughout the interview. The timing of specific behaviors may be particularly significant. A relaxed posture may indicate readiness to share information, just as a tense or rigid stance suggests unwillingness to share, pain, or anxiety. The relaxed client who tenses or shifts position when discussing family relationships or alcohol consumption may be communicating discomfort in discussing particularly sensitive information.

Gestures may also provide the nurse with information about the client.

Finger pointing		anger; control
Hand wringing	*may suggest*	anxiety
Nodding		agreement
Shoulder shrugging		uncertainty

The nurse should be particularly observant for discrepancies between the client's spoken words and the nonverbal messages communicated by posture or stance.

The use of *touch* may also significantly affect the interview process. The individual's use or response to touch may effectively communicate specific attitudes, feelings, or responses. Clients may vary in their degree of comfort with touching or being touched. The nurse's use of touch should be determined by the client's readiness to accept it. This is frequently evidenced by response to an introductory handshake or to the touching that accompanies taking a pulse or blood pressure. The client's tolerance of touch may be dependent upon cultural background, social maturity, and past experiences. Some clients consider even simple touch an intrusion, and withdrawal from touch may demonstrate fear, pain, or resentment. On the other hand, the client who grasps the nurse's arm, squeezes hands, or touches the face may be communicating warmth, appreciation, or the need for support or reassurance.

The nurse may convey caring, concern, and support by a simple touch on the client's arm, squeezing of a hand, or an arm around the shoulder. Similarly, rough, rushed, or insincere touch communicates the opposite message.

Although *voice* is usually considered to be a verbal technique, it will be discussed here because of the nonverbal messages that may be conveyed. There are a number of vocal characteristics that may be significant in determining the perceptions of both nurse and client. These include tone of voice, rate of speech, and volume. The nurse who speaks calmly, relatively slowly, and at a comfortable level communicates relaxation, patience, and concern with privacy. The client may be intimidated, embarrassed, or uncomfortable when interviewed by the overly excited nurse who is loud or speaks too rapidly.

The client who speaks slowly, in a monotone, or with a flat affect may be worried or depressed. Conversely, loud or rapid speech suggests anger, pain, impatience, or hearing deficits. These may be particularly significant if observed at specific points in the interview.

Example

> *Nurse:*   How do you feel about your surgery?
> *Client:*   I told you, it's nothing to worry about, it's only a cyst. (Spoken loudly, through clenched teeth.)

Clearly this client is communicating some type of distress. It may be anger or impatience in response to repeated questioning or anxiety about the possible outcome of surgery.

There are a number of other sounds that may convey meaning. They may indicate impatience, sarcasm, pain, anxiety, embarrassment, emphasis, agreement, or disagreement.

Nurses and clients are often uncomfortable when periods of *silence* occur during the interview. However, silence may be an important tool for the nurse. It provides an opportunity to (1) review what has transpired up to that point in the interview, (2) collect thoughts, and (3) begin to organize data. Frequently, inexperienced interviewers attempt to fill the gaps in conversation with multiple questions to avoid the discomfort associated with silence. This may communicate anxiety to the client and is often confusing. The client may feel pressured, rushed, or unable to respond.

Silence evidenced by the client may be significant in conveying discomfort, thoughtfulness, or embarrassment. The nurse should consciously avoid filling silent periods too quickly. This indicates an acceptance of the client's feelings and may strengthen the nurse-client relationship.

The verbal and nonverbal components of the interview process communicate vital messages to the participants. The most skilled interviewers use the technique of *active listening* to enhance interaction with clients. This method involves three stages—listening to the verbal component, identifying the existence of nonverbal cues, and carefully determining the significance of both. The nurse who learns to listen not only to what is spoken but also to what is left unsaid is able to interpret the client's feelings and responses effectively and to identify specific areas requiring further exploration. Consequently this (1) allows more accurate reflection of these perceptions to the client, (2) encourages clarification or validation by the client, and (3) promotes the acquisition of a more accurate and complete data base. Table 2–2 summarizes guidelines for interviewing.

Observation

The second method of data collection used during the assessment phase is observation. Systematic observation involves the use of the senses to acquire information about the client, significant other, the environment, and interactions among these three variables. Observation is a skill that requires discipline and

TABLE 2–2. GUIDELINES FOR INTERVIEWING

1. Select the environment carefully, assuring privacy and comfort. Avoid noises, odors, interruptions, inadequate lighting, and temperature extremes.
2. Defer the interview when indicated because of the client's condition or environmental barriers.
3. Create an environment of trust, caring, and concern with a calm unhurried approach.
4. Utilize the client as the primary source of data whenever possible, address by name, and avoid talking around the client to family or others.
5. Begin with introductions, a handshake, and an explanation of the purpose of the interview, including its relationship to nursing care.
6. Use terminology appropriate to the client's level of understanding. Speak clearly and distinctly.
7. Discuss the client's chief complaint early in the interview. Focus on this complaint and determine its effects on the client.
8. Encourage verbalization by using open-ended questions and supportive statements. Discuss general nonthreatening information before asking personal questions. Avoid interruptions, ''why'' questions, and biased questions.
9. Verify perceptions of the client's responses by using the reflective techniques of repetition and rephrasing.
10. Provide realistic reassurance if necessary. Avoid giving advice, opinions, or unrealistic reassurance.
11. Listen actively, maintain eye contact, and observe the nonverbal behavior of the client.
12. Conclude the interview with a brief summary of the client's problems, including anticipated nursing interventions.
13. Document as soon as possible away from the client's bedside, utilizing notations written briefly during the interview.

practice on the part of the nurse. It demands a broad knowledge base and conscious use of the senses—sight, smell, hearing, and feeling. Table 2–3 provides a list of the types of observations that can be obtained by the use of the senses.

The observations identified by the senses may be either positive or negative indices in the individual client. For example, crying may be viewed as a positive expression of grief in the parents of a terminally ill child, the odor of perfume may indicate progress in a woman after disfiguring breast surgery, or the presence of bowel sounds may signal the return of bowel function following abdominal surgery.

Each of the individual findings identified during observation requires further investigation, which may either substantiate or negate the nurse's initial impressions.

TABLE 2–3.   OBSERVATION: USE OF SENSES

Sight
Abrasions, absence of body part, absent or broken teeth, baldness, bandages, bitten nails, bleeding, blinking, blisters, boils, books, braces, bunions, burns, calluses, canes, casts, catheter, cleanliness of client or environment, clenched fists, clothing, convulsions, corns, crusting, crutches, crying, cyanosis, decubitus, dentures, diaphoresis, diarrhea, distention, drainage, drooling, ecchymosis, edema, eyeglasses, feces, fidgeting, fistula, flaking, flared nares, flies, flowers, frowning, gait, hangnail, hearing aids, hives, intravenous device, jaundice, jewelry, lighting, make-up, moles, monitor electrodes, mottling, newspaper, ostomy, paresis, petechiae, pimples, position—sitting, standing, or lying, posture, pregnancy, ptosis, purulent drainage, redness, room—type, size, and temperature, scabs, scars, scratches, scratching, shivering, significant other, skin color, slings, sneezing, squinting, stairs, sternal retraction, striae, support stockings, tatoo, telephone, television, tension, toilet articles, twitching, ulcerations, urine, vaccination, varicosities, vomiting, walker, warts, wheelchair, yawning

Hearing
Banging, barking, blood pressure, bruit, burping, clicking, coughing, crying, dripping, eructation, esophageal speech, expressions of pain, anger, sorrow, or depression, gargling, gasping, groaning, grunting, gurgling, harsh cough, heart rate and rhythm, hiccough, hissing, hoarseness, hyperactive or hypoactive bowel sounds, knocking, laughing, loudness, moaning, panting, radio, scratching, screaming, sighing, sirens, sneezing, squeaking, stammering, stuttering, sucking, telephone ringing, television, tone of voice, wheezing, whispering, whistling, yawning

Touch
Coarseness, coldness, dryness, edema, goose bumps, hardness, heat, lumps, masses, moisture, pain, pulsation, relaxation, roughness, skin texture, smoothness, softness, subcutaneous emphysema, swelling, tautness, temperature, tension, tremors, warmth, wetness

Smell
Alcohol, axillary odor, bleeding, breath or body odor, disinfectants, feces, flowers, foot odor, garlic, gas, hair spray, marijuana, medicine, onion, perfume, perspiration, pubic odor, purulent drainage, tobacco, urine, vomitus

Physical Examination

The third major method of collecting data during the assessment process is physical examination. The focus of the physician's physical examination is the diagnosis of disease. The nurse's examination concentrates on (1) further defining the client's response to the disease process, particularly those responses amenable to nursing actions, (2) establishing baseline data for comparison in evaluating the efficacy of nursing or medical interventions, and (3) substantiating subjective data obtained during interview or other nurse-client interactions.

Techniques.   The nurse uses four specific techniques during the examination—inspection, palpation, percussion, and auscultation.

Inspection refers to the visual examination of the client to determime normal, unusual, or abnormal conditions or responses. It is a type of observation that focuses on specific behaviors or physical features. Inspection is also more systematic and detailed than observation, since it defines characteristics such as size, shape, position, anatomical location, color, texture, appearance, movement, and symmetry.

Generally, inspection refers to the use of the unaided eye; however, the expanded role of the nurse in a variety of settings may incorporate the use of instruments. Those used most frequently are the otoscope and ophthalmoscope. These tools allow the nurse to complete a more comprehensive and accurate examination of the eye or ear when indicated.

Palpation is the use of touch to determine the characteristics of body structure under the skin. This technique allows the nurse to evaluate size, shape, texture, temperature, moisture, pulsation, vibration, consistency, and mobility. The nurse's hands are the tools of palpation, and specific parts are utilized to assess particular characteristics. The back of the hand is most useful in assessing temperature because the skin in this area is thinner and allows discrimination of temperature differences. The fingertips are used to determine texture and size, since nerve endings are concentrated there. The palmar surfaces of the metacarpal joints are the most sensitive to vibration and therefore are particularly useful in detecting phenomena such as thrills over the heart or peristalsis.

Light palpation is the method used to examine most body parts. The use of the nurse's dominant hand is preferred. The hand is held parallel to the body part being examined, with fingers extended. Gentle pressure is exerted downward while the nurse moves the hand in a circular motion. This technique is frequently used in breast examination to detect the presence and characteristics of abnormal masses. Deep palpation is particularly effective when examining the abdomen to locate organs or identify unusual masses. This technique requires both hands, one for pressure application and the other as a sensor. The nurse's dominant hand is placed over the area to be palpated and becomes the passive sensor. The other hand is positioned on top and is used to apply pressure. The client's facial expression and body movements during palpation provide the nurse with additional information to assist in evaluating variables such as the degree of pain or discomfort.

Percussion involves the nurse's striking of a body surface with a finger or fingers to produce sounds. This allows determination of size, density, organ boundaries, and location. Direct percussion occurs when the nurse strikes or taps the body surface directly with one or more fingers of one hand. This method is often used to define the cardiac border. Indirect percussion is used more frequently. The nurse places the index or middle finger of one hand firmly on the skin and strikes with the middle finger of the other hand.

The sounds resulting from percussion may be described as flat, dull, resonant, or tympanic. Flat sounds are low-pitched and abrupt and are produced when muscle or bone is percussed. Dull sounds are medium-pitched and thudding and may be heard over the liver and spleen. Resonance is a clear, hollow sound produced by percussion over a normal air-filled lung. Tympany is a loud, high-pitched sound heard over a gas-filled stomach or puffed-out cheek.

Auscultation involves listening to the sounds produced by the organs of the body. The nurse may use direct auscultation (with the unaided ear) to detect sounds such as wheezing. Generally, however, sounds are evaluated indirectly by using a stethoscope. This technique is used most frequently to determine the characteristics of lung, heart, and bowel sounds. The nurse identifies the frequency, intensity, quality, and duration of auscultated sounds.

Each of the four techniques—inspection, palpation, percussion, and auscultation—may be performed independently. However, the most effective method of physical examination is a comprehensive approach including a combination of techniques.

Examination Approaches. A systematic methodology is vital to accurate and complete physical examination. There are a variety of useful and practical approaches used by nurses to assess clients systematically. The head-to-toe, major body systems, functional health patterns, and human response patterns approaches are described below.

HEAD-TO-TOE. This approach begins with the client's head and systematically and symmetrically progresses down the body to the feet. The components of the physical examination are outlined in Figure 2–3. A more detailed guide is found in Appendix A.

MAJOR BODY SYSTEMS. In this approach, the nurse examines the body by systems rather than individual body parts. Information from the interview and observation assists the nurse to determine which systems require particular emphasis. The components of this system are identified in Figure 2–4, with a more detailed guide in Appendix B.

FUNCTIONAL HEALTH PATTERNS. This approach allows the nurse to collect data systematically by evaluating the functional health patterns of the client. The nurse attempts to identify patterns and to focus the physical examination on particular functional areas. The list in Table 2–4 identifies the patterns evaluated. A more detailed guide may be found in Appendix C.

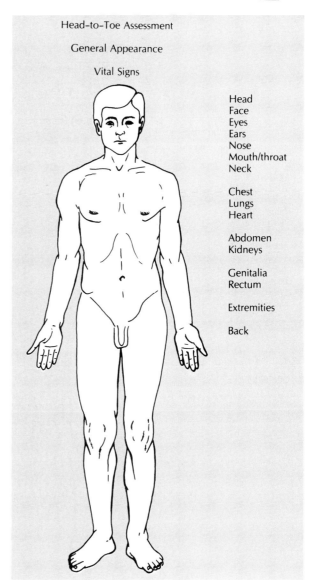

Head-to-Toe Assessment

General Appearance

Vital Signs

Head
Face
Eyes
Ears
Nose
Mouth/throat
Neck

Chest
Lungs
Heart

Abdomen
Kidneys

Genitalia
Rectum

Extremities

Back

FIGURE 2–3. Head-to-toe assessment.

HUMAN RESPONSE PATTERNS.   This methodology allows the nurse to examine the client based on the nine human response patterns that reflect the client's interaction with the environment. Table 2–5 lists assessment categories under each of the nine patterns. A more detailed guide may be found in Appendix D.

Comparison of these approaches reveals that the information obtained is identical. Therefore, the nurse should select the method that is found to be most

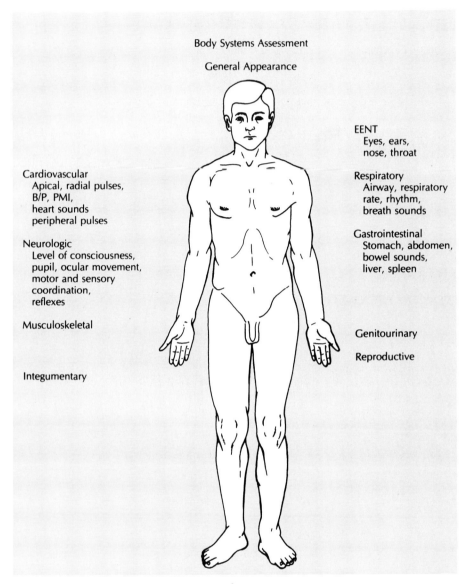

Body Systems Assessment

General Appearance

EENT
  Eyes, ears,
  nose, throat

Respiratory
  Airway, respiratory
  rate, rhythm,
  breath sounds

Gastrointestinal
  Stomach, abdomen,
  bowel sounds,
  liver, spleen

Cardiovascular
  Apical, radial pulses,
  B/P, PMI,
  heart sounds
  peripheral pulses

Neurologic
  Level of consciousness,
  pupil, ocular movement,
  motor and sensory
  coordination,
  reflexes

Musculoskeletal

Genitourinary

Reproductive

Integumentary

FIGURE 2–4. Body systems assessment.

effective or more appropriate to a particular practice setting. Regardless of the approach selected, skilled physical examination requires discipline and practice to perfect assessment techniques.

In summary, the first component of the assessment phase, data collection, involves the accumulation of subjective, objective, current, and historical information from primary and secondary sources. The nurse utilizes interviewing,

TABLE 2–4. FUNCTIONAL HEALTH PATTERNS ASSESSMENT GUIDE

Health perception/health management	General appearance
Nutritional/metabolic	Vital signs, height, weight
Elimination	Eyes
Activity/exercise	Mouth
Sleep/rest	Hearing
Cognitive/perceptual	Pulses
Self-perception	Respirations
Sexuality/sexual functioning	Skin
Coping/stress management	Functional ability
Value/belief systems	Mental status
Physical examination	

TABLE 2–5. HUMAN RESPONSE PATTERNS ASSESSMENT GUIDE

Exchanging

Cardiac	Cerebral
Peripheral	Skin Integrity
Oxygenation	Physical regulation
Nutrition	Elimination

Communicating

Read/write/understand English, other languages, impaired speech, other forms of communication

Relating

Relationships	Socialization

Valuing

Religious preference, important religious practices, spiritual concerns, cultural orientation, cultural practices

Choosing

Coping	Participation in health regimen
Judgment	

Moving

Activity	Rest
Recreation	Environmental maintenance
Health maintenance	Self-care
Meaningfulness	Sensory-perception

Perceiving

Self-concept	Meaningfulness
Sensory perception	

Knowing

Current health problems	Health history
Current medications	Risk factors
Readiness to learn	Mental status
Memory	

Feeling

Pain/discomfort associated/aggravating/alleviating factors
Emotional integrity/status

observation, and physical examination skills to acquire an organized, accurate, and systematic data base about the individual client.

DOCUMENTATION

The second component of the assessment phase is documentation of the data base. Although the following discussion of documentation is primarily directed toward the recording of data accumulated during the assessment, documentation is integral to all phases of the nursing process.

Purposes of Documentation

The recording of data in the client's medical record is an important part of the nursing process for a variety of reasons. First, it establishes a mechanism for communication among the members of the health team. This provides a variety of disciplines with pertinent, accurate, and current data about the client as an individual. A common frustration of clients in health systems is repeated questioning and examination by a variety of personnel—physicians, nurses, therapists, dieticians. Complete documentation assists in eliminating this repetition and prevents gaps in data. It also helps to create positive relationships between the client and health care providers.

Second, documentation of assessment data facilitates the delivery of quality client care. The information collected allows the nurse to develop preliminary nursing diagnoses, outcomes, and nursing interventions. Accurately documented baseline findings form the standard for comparison of subsequent data collection, allowing the nurse to validate, clarify, or update preliminary diagnoses and to facilitate the provision of consistent individualized care.

Third, documentation assures a mechanism for the evaluation of individual client care. Medical records are reviewed by a variety of internal systems and external regulatory agencies. These may include quality assurance and risk management committees, State Departments of Health (DOH), Professional Review Organizations (PRO), and the Joint Commission on Accreditation of Healthcare Organizations (JCAHO). These committees and organizations have developed standards for the delivery of nursing care. Careful documentation, beginning with the assessment data base, assists in demonstrating compliance with these accepted standards. Table 2–6 illustrates the JCAHO standards that relate to documentation.

Fourth, documentation creates a permanent legal record of the care provided to the client. Although the medical record is confidential, it is available as a legal document in a number of situations. Obviously, the chart may be utilized to evaluate liability in a malpractice litigation. However, it may also be used to document client competence, determine the extent of injury in accident or compensation claims, or substantiate the provision of specific treatment modalities

TABLE 2–6. JOINT COMMISSION STANDARDS THAT AFFECT DOCUMENTATION

STANDARD

NC.1   Patients receive nursing care based on a documented assessment of their needs.

REQUIRED CHARACTERISTICS

NC 1.1   Each patient's need for nursing care related to his/her admission is assessed by a registered nurse.*

   NC 1.1.1   The assessment is conducted either at the time of admission or within a time frame preceding or following admission that is specified in hospital policy.*

   NC 1.1.2   Aspects of data collection may be delegated by the registered nurse.

   NC 1.1.3   Needs are reassessed when warranted by the patient's condition.*

NC 1.2   Each patient's assessment includes consideration of biophysical, psychosocial, environmental, self-care, educational, and discharge planning factors.*

   NC 1.2.1   When appropriate, data from the patient's significant other(s) are included in the assessment.

NC 1.3   Each patient's nursing care is based on identified nursing diagnoses and/or patient care needs and patient care standards, and is consistent with the therapies of other disciplines.*

   NC 1.3.1   The patient and/or significant other(s) are involved in the patient's care, as appropriate.

   NC 1.3.2   Nursing staff members collaborate, as appropriate, with physicians and other clinical disciplines in making decisions regarding each patient's need for nursing care.

   NC 1.3.3   Throughout the patient's stay, the patient and, as appropriate, his/her significant other(s) receive education specific to the patient's health care needs.*

      NC 1.3.3.1   In preparation for discharge, continuing care needs are assessed and referrals for such care are documented in the patient's medical record.

   NC 1.3.4   The patient's medical record includes documentation of:*

      NC 1.3.4.1   the initial assessments and reassessments;

      NC 1.3.4.2   the nursing diagnoses and/or patient care needs;

      NC 1.3.4.3   the interventions identified to meet the patient's nursing care needs;

      NC 1.3.4.4   the nursing care provided;

      NC 1.3.4.5   the patient's response to, and the outcomes of, the care provided;

      NC 1.3.4.6   the abilities of the patient and/or, as appropriate, his/her significant other(s) to manage continuing care needs after discharge.

   NC 1.3.5   Nursing care data related to patient assessments, the nursing care planned, nursing interventions, and patient outcomes are permanently integrated into the clinical information system (for example, the medical record).*

      NC 1.3.5.1   Nursing care data can be identified and retrieved from the clinical information system.

STANDARD

NC 5   The nurse executive and other nursing leaders participate with leaders from the governing body, management, medical staff and other clinical areas in the hospital's decision-making structures and processes.*

REQUIRED CHARACTERISTICS

NC 5.5   The nurse executive, or a designee(s), participates in evaluating, selecting, and integrating health care technology and information management systems that support patient care needs and the efficient utilization of nursing resources.*

   NC 5.5.1   The use of efficient interactive information management systems for nursing, other clinical (for example, dietary, pharmacy, physical therapy) and other non-clinical information is facilitated wherever appropriate.

---

* The asterisked items are key factors in the accreditation decision process. Copyright 1990 by the Joint Commission on Accreditation of Healthcare Organizations, Oakbrook Terrace, IL. Reprinted with permission.

for reimbursement purposes. Therefore, detailed accurate documentation, beginning with assessment findings, may protect the client, the care providers (particularly nurses), and the institution or agency. Additional information on legal and ethical considerations can be found in Chapter 10.

Finally, documentation provides the foundation for nursing research. The information found in the medical record may be utilized as a source for identification of research topics specific to nursing practice. Validation of nursing diagnoses, comparison of client responses to nursing interventions, and development of nurse-client relationships are potential areas of exploration. The accumulation of a body of research associated with nursing practice helps to define nursing as a science and to refine the nursing process.

The documentation of the nursing assessment should clearly identify those findings that necessitate nursing interventions. These include a variety of factors affecting the client's health status or ability to function. The client's responses, perceptions, feelings, and coping mechanisms are particularly significant in the formulation of nursing diagnoses and the identification of specific nursing interventions.

Guidelines for Documentation

The format for recording the nursing assessment varies among practice settings. Regardless of the type and structure of the documentation tool, there are some general guidelines that should be considered.

1. The nurse's entries should be written objectively without bias, value judgments, or personal opinion. The subjective information provided by the client, family, and other members of the health team should be included. The nurse should use quotation marks to clearly identify these types of statements.

Example

Client's description of illness: "My diabetes is out of control, and I'm here to have tests and get it regulated."

2. Descriptions or interpretations of objective data should be supported by specific observations.

Example

Emotional status: Depressed, sits in darkened room with curtain pulled around bed, rarely initiates conversation, responds in monotone with short answers when questioned, limited eye contact, cries softly.

These findings support the nurse's interpretation of depression.

3. Generalizations should be avoided, including "basket terms" such as "good," "fair," "usual," "normal." These descriptions are open to broad interpretation based on the reader's point of reference.

Example

"Abdomen moderately distended" may be interpreted differently by each nurse reading the entry. More specific documentation might include the exact measurement of abdominal girth.

"Fair mobility" may suggest that the client was able to perform activities of daily living effectively. In reality, the nurse may mean that the client was able to turn independently in bed but required assistance with bathing, feeding, and ambulating.

"Normal bowel patterns" is more clearly defined by "moves bowels every other day without the use of laxatives."

4. Findings should be described as thoroughly as possible, including defining characteristics such as size and shape.

For example, the description of a client's decubitus ulcer should include measurements, depth, color, odor, and drainage. This is particularly important when documenting the initial assessment, since this information is the base line for evaluating the effectiveness of nursing interventions.

5. The nurse should document data clearly and concisely, avoiding superfluous information and long, rambling sentences.

Example

"The client indicates that she didn't feel good for five days, so she went to the doctor and told him about her symptoms. He gave her three medications, including antihistamine, antibiotic, and cough medicine. These didn't help so she went to the emergency room, and the doctor there admitted her."

This could be reworded as: "History of fever, cough, and nasal congestion × 5 days, unrelieved by antihistamine, antibiotic, antitussives prescribed by family physician."

6. The assessment should be written or printed legibly in nonerasable ink. Errors in documentation should be corrected in a manner that does not obscure the original entry. The most commonly used method involves drawing a single line through the incorrect item, writing "mistaken entry," and initialing the entry. The use of white-out, erasure, or crossing out to obliterate the entry is not acceptable.

7. Entries should be correct in grammar and spelling. The nurse should incorporate only those abbreviations approved for use in the particular practice setting. Slang, clichés, and labels should be avoided except in the context of a direct quotation.

Figure 2–5 demonstrates how the information obtained from Ted Alexander, the man described in 2–2 Test Yourself, would be documented.

I. GENERAL INFORMATION: Date: 3/30/91 Time: 11:00 am Informant: client

Primary Language: English   ID BAND: ☑ Yes ☐ No

Allergies: denied

Whom to Notify in Emergency: Jamie and Pam Alexander   children   702-788-8772
(Name)   (Relationship)   (Phone)

Mode of Admission: ☐ Ambulatory   ☐ Wheelchair   ☑ Stretcher   ☐ Oriented to Unit

☑ "Release of Personal Effects" form completed   Prosthesis: none

T: 101.2   P: 116   R: 26   B/P R: 140/80   L: _____   Ht.: 6'2 ft./in.(cm)   Wt.: 196 (lb.)(kg)

List of Personal Belongings Sent Home: _____

Kept by Patient: $75 cash and traveler's checks in safe

II. HEALTH HISTORY/HOSPITALIZATIONS:

Has had no surgery history of alcoholism for 15 years, hospitalized for cirrhosis 2 years ago

MEDICATIONS TAKEN AT HOME/DATE STARTED:

occasional laxative

Patient's understanding of reason for Hospitalization: "To fix the pain in my belly"

Personal Medication: ☑ none   ☐ sent to Pharmacy   ☐ sent home
☐ at bedside   ☐ "Receipt for Patient Medication" form signed

III. ACTIVITIES OF DAILY LIVING:
Smoking: ☑ Yes ☐ No Pack/Day: 2/day
ETOH: Daily Intake: stopped drinking 2 yrs ago
Diet Type: Low fat
Sleep/Risk patterns: No problems

Falls Risk: ☐ Yes ☑ No

DISCHARGE PLANNING:
☑ Anticipate return to self care
☑ Social Work referral
☐ Appliance/Equipment needs
☐ Home Health Care needs

Prevention of Falls protocol implemented: ☐ Yes ☑ No

IV. SOCIAL HISTORY (If pertinent: Home situation, occupation, education, cultural practices, etc.) Divorced father of 2 teenagers who live with them in Las Vegas. Does not know anyone in NJ. Anxious about being cared for by strange physician. Is a businessman who is concerned about job demands and how he will return to Nevada when discharged

Signature: W. Silverstein RN   , R.N.

*ITEMS TO BE COMPLETED FOR PATIENTS STAYING LESS THAN 48 HOURS

The Mount Vernon Hospital
NURSING ASSESSMENT & DATA BASE
Page 1

V-NUR-1689/R-1/87
PKGS. OF 100 SETS
CAT. #98-516V

FIGURE 2–5. Documentation of Client Ted Alexander. (Courtesy of The Mount Vernon Hospital, Alexandria, VA.)

V. PRESENT FINDINGS:

*Respiratory: Rhythm: _Regular_   ☐ cough

Breath sounds: ☑ clear   ☐ congested   ☐ wheeze

*Cardiovascular: Rhythm: _Regular_   ☐ chest pain   ☐ edema

Comments: _____

Mouth/Gums/Teeth: ☐ Intact   ☐ Odor   ☐ Bleeding   ☑ Dentures   Comments: _Has_
partial lower plate + caps on 4 front teeth

*Gastrointestinal: Usual Time & Frequency: _9 am every 1-2 days_ Time of Last B.M.: _930_ _3/29_
   ☐ Change in Bowel Habits   ☐ Constipation   ☐ Diarrhea   ☑ Bowel Sounds Absent   ☐ Bleeding
   ☐ Change in Appetite   ☐ Nausea   ☑ Vomiting   ☐ Weight Change
Comments: _Vomiting began today prior to admission. Has abd_
pain and a mass in right inguinal area
Genitourinary: Time of Last Voiding: _7:30 am_
   ☑ Change in Bladder Habits   ☐ Frequency   ☐ Retention   ☐ Incontinence
Comments: _Has had urgency and nocturia several times in last_
6 months

Reproductive: ☐ Change in Menstrual Cycle   LMP: _____
   ☐ Vaginal Discharge   ☐ Self Breast Exam   ☐ Breast Changes
Comments: _not applicable_
   ☐ Prostate Problems   ☐ Penile Discharge
Comments: _denied_

*Musculoskeletal: ☑ Independent   ☐ Needs Assistance   ☐ Change in Mobility   ☐ Fractures
   ☐ Paralysis   ☐ Prosthesis
Comments: _____

*Integumentary: ☐ Intact   ☐ Lacerations   ☐ Discolorations   ☐ Rash   ☐ Dry   ☑ Warm
   ☐ Cool   ☑ Diaphoretic
Comments: _____

Neurological: L.O.C.   ☐ Alert   ☐ Lethargic   ☐ Comatose
Oriented: ☑ Person   ☑ Place   ☑ Time   Pupils: _Equal & reactive to light_   ☐ Paresis
*Vision: ☐ No difficulty   ☐ Blurred   ☐ Diplopia   ☐ Blind   ☐ Glasses   ☑ Contact Lenses
   ☐ Artificial Eye
*Hearing: ☑ No difficulty   ☐ Limited   ☐ Deaf   ☐ Tinnitus   ☐ Hearing Aide
*Speech: ☑ No difficulty   ☐ Slurred   ☐ Aphasic
Comments: _____

Appearance/Behavior: Affect: ☑ Appropriate   ☐ Flat   ☐ Agitated
Comments: _____

* VI. IDENTIFIED PROBLEMS (Consider Discharge Concerns): _Provide pain relief_
Assist pt to make arrangements for care of
children + return to Nevada

Signature: _W. Silverstein RN_ _____ , R.N.
*ITEMS TO BE COMPLETED FOR PATIENTS STAYING LESS THAN 48 HOURS

The Mount Vernon Hospital
NURSING ASSESSMENT & DATA BASE
Page 2

V-NUR-1690/R-1/87
PAD OF 50
CAT. #98-507V

FIGURE 2–5   _Continued_

COMPUTERS AND NURSING ASSESSMENT

Computer applications that automate all phases of the nursing process have been designed and implemented. These applications include both components of the assessment phase—data collection and documentation.

Data Collection

Many automated systems provide for computerized history-taking. This may be accomplished directly or indirectly. In direct systems, the client uses a computer terminal to respond to a series of questions. These histories have been demonstrated to be valid when compared with those taken indirectly and are frequently more complete and accurate (Andreoli and Musser, 1985). In indirect systems, the nurse obtains the information from the client and enters it into a bedside terminal.

Computerized systems are particularly valuable in automating physical examination. Computer terminals located at the bedside prompt the nurse to complete examinations using the body systems, head-to-toe, functional health, or human response patterns. Figure 2–6 demonstrates a sample screen used in a body systems approach.

Computers frequently provide objective data when located in technologically advanced areas, such as critical care units. Automated readings of vital signs and abnormal heart rhythms are frequently utilized by critical care nurses to provide both initial and subsequent data. "The computer can detect arrhythmias, generate alarms for vital signs ranging out of safe bound[s], store records of unusual events, provide graphic representation of vital sign trends and correlate vital signs to reveal unsuspected relationships" (Tamarisk, 1982).

Documentation

Nurses may also use computers to document the data obtained in the interview or examination. The nurse enters the data either at the bedside or in a central location. When a significant health problem is identified, the computer assists the nurse to document it accurately and completely. For example, if the nurse enters data indicating a reddened area on the client's skin, the computer will prompt for information such as location, size, and drainage (Tamarisk, 1982). Figure 2–7 demonstates a sample of a documented nursing assessment.

The principal advantages of computerized data collection are thoroughness and ease of recording data. The step-by-step design of the assessment process ensures that no significant areas are overlooked. Use of the computer reduces the amount of clinical time required to enter information using the traditional pen and paper format, thus improving efficiency.

The primary disadvantages of computerized client records include the expense, the time required to develop or adapt program components, and the training required prior to use. Additionally, some object to the restrictions imposed by standardized screens, formats, and limited vocabulary (Gluck, 1980).

```
17WES-0301              NYUMC HOSP 4
MATRIX # .1107     HOSP# 04     03/29/85
DYNAMIC MATRIX


(N)         PHYSICAL ASSESSMENT         PG1     01
                    SKIN                         02
        *SKIN ASSESSMENT UNREMARKABLE            03
*SKIN ASSESS'T UNCHANGED FROM PREV. NOTE         04
                                                 05
    (SKIN COLOR)        (TEMP)(MOISTURE)         06
NORMAL      JAUNDICE     COOL   NORMAL           07
ASHEN       PALE         HOT    DRY              08
DUSKY       PURPLISH     WARM   OILY             09
CYANOTIC                        DIAPHORETIC      10
ERYTHEMATOUS                                     11
                                EDEMA            12
    (TEXTURE)     (TURGOR)      ANKLE            13
    LEATHERY      ELASTIC       ARM              14
    ROUGH        INELASTIC      HAND             15
    SMOOTH        LOOSE         PERIORBITAL      16
    THICK         TAUT          SACRAL           17
    THIN                        PEDAL            18
                                 *SKIN PG2       19
            *BACK      *NEXT     *ANATOMY         20
--------------------------------------------
   RETURN                       REVIEW
ERR         TYPE        RETRIEVE

17WES-1019              NYUMC HOSP 4
MATRIX # 1108      HOSP# 04     05/28/85
DYNAMIC MATRIX


(N)         PHYSICAL ASSESSMENT         PG2     01
                    SKIN                         02
    (NAILS)                   (HAIR)             03
NORMAL      BRITTLE     NORMAL     THIN          04
PALE        THIN        ALOPECIA   THICK         05
CYANOTIC    THICK       HIRSUTE                  06
CLUBBED     RIDGED      SCALY SCALP              07
DYSTROPIC                                        08
(SKIN LESION)  FRECKLE       PUSTULE             09
ABRASION       FISSURE       PURPURA             10
BIRTHMARK      LACERATION    RASH                11
BULLA          LUMP          SCALE               12
CALLOUS        MASS          SCAR                13
CRUST          MOLE          STRIAE              14
ECCHYMOSIS     NEVI          ULCER               15
DECUBITUS      PETECHIAE     VESICLE             16
EROSION        PLAQUE        WHEAL               17
--___               **       *DESCRIPTION        18
                    **       *COLOR,CONS         19
SIZE--___                                        
            *BACK     *NEXT   *ANATOMY           20
--------------------------------------------
   RETURN                       REVIEW
ERR         TYPE        RETRIEVE
```

FIGURE 2–6. Computerized assessment screen. (Courtesy of New York University Medical Center.)

```
                    CliniCom Medical Center - QA        06/12/90 10:39

            PATIENT ADMISSION ASSESSMENT REPORT (pat_adasm)
                 From 06/12/90 00:00  To 06/12/90 10:38
                 ---------------------------------------
```

Admission Assessment

Neurological (normal parameters)
 06/12 10:30 Alert & oriented to person, place and time. Verbalization clear and understandable
             (exclude speech impediments). Able to follow and understand directions. Pupils
             equal & reactive to light. Equal strength and voluntary movement in all
             extremities.. (AMJ)
Respiratory (normal parameters)
 06/12 10:30 Respirations quiet and regular, rate within patient's norm. (AMJ)
       10:30 Respirations appear effortless. Nasal passages appear clear. (AMJ)
Respiratory (OUTSIDE normal parameters)
 06/12 10:30 Breath sounds (by auscultation): scattered fine crackles bilateral base(s). (AMJ)
       10:30 Cough description: intermittent and harsh. Cough can be precipitated by:
             exertion. (AMJ)
       10:30 Description of Sputum: small amount, cloudy and thick. (AMJ)
Cardiovascular (normal parameters)
 06/12 10:30 Regular apical pulse within patient's normal rate. Absence of edema. Neck veins
             flat at 45 degrees. Absence of pain/discomfort in chest, neck, jaw, left arm. Cap
             refill < 3 sec. Peripheral pulses palpable and equal. No calf tenderness. (AMJ)
Gastrointestinal (normal parameters)
 06/12 10:30 Abdomen soft and non-distended. Bowel sounds high-pitched, gurgling and
             active.(5-34/min.) No abdominal pain reported with or without palpation. Tolerates
             prescribed diet without nausea or vomiting. Having BMs within own normal pattern
             and consistency. Stools are normal coloration. Well-nourished appearance. (AMJ)
Renal/Urinary (normal parameters)
 06/12 10:30 Empties bladder without dysuria. Bladder not distended after voiding. Urine clear,
             yellow to amber in color, normal urine odor. Able to void in last 8 hours. Volume
             voided is normal for patient. Frequency of voiding is normal for patient. (AMJ)
Renal/Urinary (OUTSIDE normal parameters)
 06/12 10:30 Patient's control - stress incontinence (cough/sneeze/activity). (AMJ)
Skin/Lymphatic (normal parameters)
 06/12 10:30 Skin color within patient's norm. Skin is warm, dry, smooth, soft, and flexible.
             Good tissue turgor present, no edema noted. Mucous membranes moist. Skin integrity
             is intact. (AMJ)
Musculoskeletal (normal parameters)
 06/12 10:30 Absence of joint swelling, erythema and tenderness. Active and passive ROM of all
             joints is normal. Absence of muscle weakness or atrophy. Normal muscle tone. All
             movement is pain free. Able to participate in normal activity without fatigue.
             (AMJ)
Reproductive/Male (normal parameters)
 06/12 10:30 Genitals are not swollen. Absence of pain with or without palpation. Absence of
             purulent urethral discharge. Absence of erythema or rash. (AMJ)

Psychological/Social (normal parameters)
 06/12 10:30 Mood and affect are expressed appropriately for situation. Thoughts are clear,
             reality-based, and progress logically. Interpretation of reality is appropriate.
             Support system present and adequate to meet patient's needs. Has not recently
             attempted suicide or verbalized a plan for suicide. Absence of recent problems
             with or treatment for drug/alcohol use. (AMJ)
Care Providers:
JONES, ANNE (AMJ) NRN

      0500-A   Name: SMITH, CHARLEY B. MD: SILVER,JOHN
      Sex: M Age: 41Y Adm: 05/21/90 21:18 Patient Id: 456456456 Med Rec No: 654654654
```
---

**SMITH, CHARLEY B.  PATIENT ADMISSION ASSESSMENT REPORT (pat_adasm) –**

**FIGURE 2–7.** Documentation of Computerized Assessment. (Courtesy of Clinicom Inc., Boulder, CO.)
```

SUMMARY

The assessment phase of the nursing process consists of the accumulation and documentation of information about a client. Data collection involves interviewing, observation, and physical examination and concludes with documentation of the information obtained in the client's medical record. Assessment involves interaction between the nurse and the client and requires a broad knowledge base as well as specific interpersonal and technical skills. Assessment is a continuous activity that begins at the time of admission and continues during each client contact. It forms the foundation for subsequent phases of the nursing process—diagnosis, planning, implementation, and evaluation.

REFERENCES

American Nurses' Association: A Social Policy Statement. Kansas City, MO: American Nurses' Association, 1980.

American Nurses' Association: Standards of Nursing Practice. Kansas City, MO: American Nurses' Association, 1973.

Andreoli K, and Musser L: Computers in nursing care: the state of the art. Nursing Outlook 1985; 33(1):16–25.

Bellack J, and Bamford P: Nursing Assessment. Belmont, CA: Wadsworth, 1984.

Gluck J: The computerized medical record system: meeting the challenge for nursing. In Zielstorff R: Computers in Nursing. Rockville, MD: Aspen, 1980.

Tamarisk NK: The computer as a clinical tool. Nursing Management 1982; 13(8):46–49.

BIBLIOGRAPHY

Adams GA: Computer technology: its impact on nursing practice. Nursing Administration Quarterly 1986; 10(2):21.

Barry C, and Gibbons L: Information systems technology: Barriers and challenges to implementation. Journal of Nursing Administration 1990; 20(2):40–42.

Bates B: A Guide to Physical Examination, 4th ed. Philadelphia: JB Lippincott, 1987.

Carnevali D: Nursing Care Planning, 3rd ed. Philadelphia: JB Lippincott, 1983.

Carpenito LJ: Nursing Diagnosis—Application to Clinical Practice, 3rd ed. Philadelphia: JB Lippincott, 1989.

Fiesta J: The Law and Liability—A Guide for Nurses, 2nd ed. New York: John Wiley & Sons, 1988.

Gordon M: Nursing Diagnosis: Process and Application, 2nd ed. New York: McGraw-Hill, 1987.

Grobe S: Computer Primer and Resource Guide for Nurses. Philadelphia: JB Lippincott, 1984.

Guzzetta CE, Bunton S, Prinkey L, et al: Unitary person assessment tool: easing problems with nursing diagnoses. Focus on Critical Care 1988; 15(2):12–24.

Hemelt MD, and Mackert ME: Dynamics of Law in Nursing and Health Care, 2nd ed. Reston, VA: Reston, 1982.

Kozier B, and Erb G: Fundamentals of Nursing, 3rd ed. Menlo Park, CA: Addison-Wesley, 1987.

Luckmann J, and Sorenson K: Medical Surgical Nursing: A Pathophysiologic Approach, 3rd ed. Philadelphia: WB Saunders, 1987.

Morrissey-Ross M: Documentation: if you haven't written it, you haven't done it. Nursing Clinics of North America 1988; 22(4):363–371.

Malasanos L: Health Assessment, 3rd ed. St. Louis: CV Mosby, 1986.

Phipps WJ, Long BC, and Woods NF (eds): Medical-Surgical Nursing: Concepts and Clinical Practice, 3rd ed. St. Louis: CV Mosby, 1987.

Romano C, McCormack KA, and Neely LD: Nursing documentation: a model for computerized data base. Advances in Nursing Science 1982; 4(2):43–45.

Stearns L: Nursing diagnosis: an assessment form. Nursing Management 1988; 19(4):101–102.

Yura H, and Walsh MB: The Nursing Process, 5th ed. New York: Appleton-Century-Crofts, 1988.

3

THE DIAGNOSTIC PROCESS

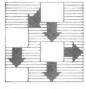

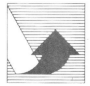

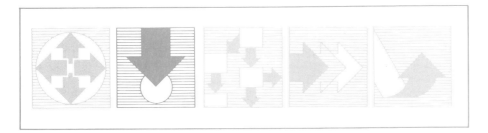

INTRODUCTION

The diagnostic process, the second phase of the nursing process, is a complex intellectual function. There are four steps in this process—data processing, formulation of the nursing diagnostic statement, validation, and documentation. The outcome of the diagnostic process, the nursing diagnostic statement, forms the foundation for the remaining phases of the nursing process—planning, implementation, and evaluation. This chapter will explore the concept and evolution of nursing diagnosis as well as the data processing component of the diagnostic process. Chapter 4 will describe how to write, validate, and document a nursing diagnostic statement.

NURSING DIAGNOSIS

Before attempting to describe the diagnostic process, it may be helpful to define and discuss the concept of nursing diagnosis.

Historical Evolution of Nursing Diagnosis

Chapter 1 described the historical evolution of the nursing process. The term *nursing diagnosis* was first used in the 1950s. In 1960, Faye Abdellah introduced a classification system for identifying 21 client clinical problems. This system was used in the curriculum of nursing schools to assist students to identify client responses to health and illness requiring nursing intervention.

In the 1970s, several nursing leaders recognized the need to develop terminology to describe the health problems diagnosed and treated by nurses. In

1973, the First National Conference on the Classification of Nursing Diagnoses was held at the St. Louis University School of Nursing. The group began to formulate nursing diagnoses and published a tentative list. Since then, the group has continued to work to develop and refine nursing diagnoses.

The American Nurses' Association endorsed and legitimated the use of the term *nursing diagnosis* in 1973 in the published *Standards of Nursing Practice* (ANA, 1973). Standard II states "Nursing diagnoses are derived from the data of the health status of the client." Subsequently, several states began incorporating the concept into their nurse practice acts. This provided nurses with a legal right and professional obligation to make nursing diagnoses. At this time, a nursing diagnosis was viewed as an outcome or label that resulted from the diagnostic process. The development of the nursing diagnosis became the second step of the five phase nursing process.

Throughout the 1970s and into the 1980s, nursing research and literature explained the concept of nursing diagnosis and supported its incorporation into the nursing process. The 1980s also saw the addition of new diagnoses (including the first that were wellness-oriented), refinement of existing diagnoses, and continued research validation. The North American Nursing Diagnosis Association (NANDA) agreed on a method of organizing the diagnoses and the American Nurses' Association adopted the NANDA diagnoses as the official system of nursing diagnosis. The National League for Nursing (NLN), in its approval criteria for schools of nursing, also required that the concept of nursing diagnosis be incorporated into the curriculum as a component of the nursing process. The ability of graduate nurses to use the diagnostic process was also evaluated in the NCLEX examination for licensure of registered nurses.

The expectations for nursing diagnosis in the 1990s include refinement of existing diagnoses, development of additional diagnoses (including expansion of those related to well clients), and continued research and validation. Nursing diagnoses may also be one of the essential components of financial systems designed for direct reimbursement for nursing services.

Definitions of Nursing Diagnosis

A diagnosis is essentially a statement that identifies the existence of an undesirable state. This definition applies whether the diagnostician is a health care worker, lawyer, electrician, or mechanic. The subject matter of the diagnosis is derived from those areas in which the diagnostician possesses a level of expertise. Lawyers write diagnoses pertaining to elements of law, physicians diagnose disease states, and electricians identify electrical system malfunctions.

Nurses, by virtue of their nurse practice acts, are responsible for diagnosing and treating human responses to actual and potential health problems (ANA, 1980). Nursing expertise that is developed as a result of education and experience identifies those nursing functions which can be ordered independently without collaboration with physicians or other health care professionals. These functions may include (1) preventive approaches, such as education, changes in position, and detection of potential complications, or (2) corrective approaches such as forcing fluids, skin care, and counseling. This focus on independent nursing actions not only avoids duplication and overlap with other disciplines but also continues to define and validate the elements of nursing practice.

The literature identifies several definitions of nursing diagnosis. Three of these are listed below.

☐ A nursing diagnosis is a statement of a patient problem that is arrived at by making inferences from the collected data. The problem is one that can be alleviated by nursing (Mundinger and Jauron, 1975).

☐ Nursing diagnoses, or clinical diagnoses made by professional nurses, describe actual or potential problems that nurses, by virtue of their education and experience, are capable and licensed to treat (Gordon, 1976).

☐ A nursing diagnosis is a label for a patient condition (response to health or illness) that nurses are able and legally responsible to treat (Moritz, 1982).

For the purposes of this discussion, the NANDA definition of nursing diagnosis will be used—a nursing diagnosis is a clinical judgment about individual, family, or community responses to actual and potential health problems/life processes. Nursing diagnoses provide the basis for selection of nursing interventions to achieve outcomes for which the nurse is accountable (NANDA, 1990).

Regardless of which definition is used, the experts agree that a nursing diagnosis includes certain essential features, which are identified in Table 3–1.

The remaining information in this chapter will describe the diagnostic process by which the nurse determines correct nursing diagnoses for individual clients.

TABLE 3–1.   A NURSING DIAGNOSIS. . .

☐ is a statement of a client problem
☐ refers to a health state or a potential health problem
☐ is a conclusion resulting from identification of a pattern or a cluster of signs and symptoms
☐ is based on subjective and objective data
☐ is a statement of nursing judgment
☐ is a short, concise statement
☐ consists of a two-part statement that includes the human response and related factors when known
☐ refers to conditions that nurses are licensed to treat
☐ should be validated with the client whenever possible

Adapted from Shoemaker J: Essential features of a nursing diagnosis. In McLane M, McFarland K, and Kim M (eds): Classification of Nursing Diagnoses: Proceedings of the Fifth National Conference. St. Louis: CV Mosby, 1984, 107–108.

STEPS IN THE DIAGNOSTIC PROCESS

As mentioned earlier, there are four steps involved in the diagnostic process—data processing, formulation of the diagnostic statement, validation, and documentation.

Data Processing

The information collected by the nurse about an individual client is vital to the development of the nursing diagnosis and subsequent nursing care planning. Before planning can occur, collected data must be processed—classified, interpreted, and validated. Although data processing will be examined as the first step of the diagnostic phase, it is not so specifically isolated. These types of activities occur continuously throughout the nursing process.

Classification

While assessing a client, the nurse accumulates a large volume of data. The nurse may find it extremely difficult to manage this volume in total. The classification process allows the nurse to develop more manageable categories of information. It also stimulates discrimination between data, which helps the nurse to focus on data that are pertinent to the client's needs.

Classification involves sorting information into specific categories. Examples include body systems, functional health patterns, historical data, or significant symptoms. The classification process is facilitated by assessment tools that are organized into specific categories.

Examples

DATA ⟶	CLASSIFICATION
Appendectomy three years ago	Past medical history
Sleeps during day	Sleep/rest pattern
Full range of motion	Motor ability
Colostomy	Gastrointestinal system
Mother died of cancer	Family history
Chest pain	Significant symptom
Laxatives every other day	Bowel elimination pattern
Church elder	Spiritual history
Vomiting for three days	History of present illness
Sacral redness	Integumentary system

Placing data into categories also helps the nurse to begin to identify missing data that require further discussion, observation, or physical examination.

Example. Barbara Draper is a 35 year old woman who visits the Women's Health Care Center. During the interview she indicates that her mother died of cancer of the breast (family history) and that she had a breast biopsy two years ago (past medical history).

Classification of this information reveals a missing component—current status of breast disease. Therefore, the nurse might (1) question the client regarding the outcome of the biopsy and frequency of breast self-examination, (2) pay particular attention to palpation for breast masses during the physical examination, and (3) assess the client's emotional response to this particular health problem.

Interpretation

The second step in data processing is interpretation, which involves identification of significant data, comparison with standards or norms, and recognition of patterns or trends. Cues and inferences developed from the scientific nursing knowledge base assist the nurse to interpret the data. A cue is a piece of information about an individual client obtained during the assessment process. It is the nurse's perception of what exists based on subjective and objective data obtained from the client and other secondary sources. Cues may include signs which are objective data such as blood pressure and weight or symptoms which are subjective data such as pain and sadness.

Examples of Cues

Temperature 102°F
Grimacing
6 ft, 375 lb
White blood count 24,000/mm (normal 5000 to 9000/mm)

"Inferencing" is the assignment of meaning to a cue. An inference is a judgment made by the nurse on the basis of education and experience. In the examples identified above, the nurse might make the following inferences based on the cues identified during the assessment of a client.

CUES ⟶	INFERENCE
Temperature 102°F	Elevated temperature
Grimacing	Possible pain, anxiety
6 ft, 375 lb	Obesity
White blood count 24,000/mm	Probable infection

Clusters are groups of cues. The potential for making accurate judgments is increased when the nurse bases an inference on a cluster of cues rather than on a single cue. In the case of the client with a temperature elevation, note that two different inferences could be made based on the particular cluster of cues identified during the assessment of a client.

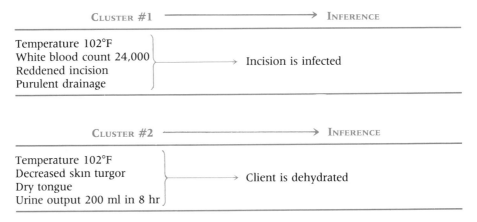

CLUSTER #1 ⟶ INFERENCE

Temperature 102°F
White blood count 24,000
Reddened incision   ⟶ Incision is infected
Purulent drainage

CLUSTER #2 ⟶ INFERENCE

Temperature 102°F
Decreased skin turgor
Dry tongue   ⟶ Client is dehydrated
Urine output 200 ml in 8 hr

The nurse uses theory, knowledge, experience, and data collected about the client to make correct inferences. Some inferences are very clearly based on clinical knowledge. For example, the presence of frequent loose stools, abdominal pain and cramping, and anal irritation suggest a bowel disorder, specifically diarrhea.

Other data may provide fewer concrete cues and clusters and require more interpretation. For example, the client with clenched fists and rigid body posture who is crying may be angry, frightened, or experiencing pain. Here, the nurse may (1) make a preliminary interpretation and validate it with the client, or (2) continue to gather additional cues which may help to clarify the inferences based on the identified cues.

The interpretation of data based on cues and clusters is a complex process. Initially, the beginning practitioner may experience difficulty in identifying cues or correctly clustering related cues. However, as nursing knowledge, skill, and expertise increase, the nurse makes accurate clinical judgments more consistently.

Example. Joan Granberry is a nurse on a 24 bed surgical unit. Her clinical knowledge indicates that pain is a common phenomenon in the postoperative client. Bob Brown is a 38 year old client who returns to the unit two hours after an appendectomy. Mr. Brown denies that he is experiencing pain during his postoperative assessment. However, Joan notes that he is restless, grimaces often, and that his pulse rate and blood pressure are elevated. Based on this cluster of cues, the nurse concludes that the patient may be experiencing pain and continues to gather additional data to support this judgment.

As the nurse becomes more experienced in using the diagnostic process, the ability to anticipate, identify, and interpret specific client responses increases. For example, the experienced postpartum nurse recognizes that most first-time nursing mothers experience anxiety about their ability to breastfeed. On the basis of this knowledge, the nurse assesses for cues that this response might be present and initiates nursing interventions to assist the client to decrease her anxiety.

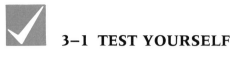

3–1 TEST YOURSELF

IDENTIFICATION OF INFERENCES

Read the cues/clusters in column I and identify possible inferences in column II.

CUE/CLUSTER	INFERENCE
1. Blood pressure 90/50 mm Hg (normally 120/70)	
2. Female, age 25 with bright red vaginal bleeding (one pad in six hours)	
3. Urine glucose 2% (normal = 0)	
4. Dilated pupils in an alert, oriented client without injury and taking medication	
5. Height 5 ft, 1 in; weight 220 lb; pendulous abdomen	
6. Blood pressure 190/104 mm Hg; client states "I wasn't supposed to eat salt."	
7. Whimpering one year old child; restlessness; pulling left ear	
8. Insomnia; heart rate 110 beats/min; irritability; says "I feel nervous."	
9. History of accidents; unsteady gait; impaired vision	
10. Newly diagnosed diabetic; states "I've never tested my blood for sugar before."	

3–1 TEST YOURSELF □ ANSWERS

Cue/Cluster	Inference
1. Blood pressure 90/50 mm Hg (normally 120/70)	Abnormally low for client
2. Female, age 25 with bright red vaginal bleeding (one pad in six hours)	Menstruation
3. Urine glucose 2% (normal = 0)	Abnormal glucose level
4. Dilated pupils in an alert, oriented client without injury and taking medication	Effects of medication
5. Height 5 ft, 1 in; weight 220 lb; pendulous abdomen	Obesity
6. Blood pressure 190/104 mm Hg; client states "I wasn't supposed to eat salt."	Abnormally elevated blood pressure
7. Whimpering one year old child; restlessness; pulling left ear	Pain in left ear
8. Insomnia; heart rate 110 beats/min; irritability; says "I feel nervous."	Anxiety
9. History of accidents; unsteady gait; impaired vision	At risk for injury
10. Newly diagnosed diabetic; states "I've never tested my blood for sugar before."	Lack of knowledge about blood sugar testing

Validation

The final step in data processing is validation. In this phase, the nurse attempts to verify the accuracy of the data interpretation. This is most often accomplished through direct interaction with the client or significant other(s), consultation with other health care professionals, or comparison of data with an authoritative reference.

Validation with the Client or Significant Others. Ideally, the nurse should validate findings with the client. This is generally accomplished through the use of reflective statements.

Example. Barbara Sabotka is a 30 year old client admitted for an elective cesarean section. During the assessment interview, the nurse notices that Barbara is easily distracted, paces intermittently while wringing her hands, and speaks very rapidly. These cues could lead the nurse to infer that this client is nervous about the scheduled surgery.

Nurse: You seem anxious, Mrs. Sabotka.

Client: Yes, I am upset.

Nurse: Upset?

Client: I'm really worried about my four year old. He had a high fever and bad cough so my husband took him to the doctor. He hasn't called me yet to tell me what the doctor found. I'm so afraid he has pneumonia.

In this situation, the nurse validated the presence of anxiety in the client. The use of a reflective statement negated the nurse's interpretation of the source of the client's anxiety. The nurse was able to identify that Mrs. Sabotka's concern was focused on her child. Therefore, nursing interventions would be directed toward assisting the client to acquire information about the child's condition.

There are times when the nurse may find that it is not possible to validate interpretations with the client directly.

Example.   The nurse admitting a comatose client, Danz Blasser, notices a small healed scar approximately $2\frac{1}{2}$ in long just below his left clavicle. There is also a small bulge under the patient's skin. Based on knowledge and past experience, the nurse interprets these findings to indicate the presence of a permanent cardiac pacemaker.

In this situation, the client is unable to confirm the nurse's judgment. Therefore, Mr. Blasser's daughter might be interviewed for confirmation.

Nurse: I noticed that your father has a small scar on his chest.

Daughter: Yes, he had a pacemaker put in six months ago after his heart attack. He has been checked every month, and it's been working fine.

Mr. Blasser's daughter has validated the presence of the pacemaker and in that process has provided additional important information about the client's past medical history as well as his compliance with suggested pacemaker follow-up.

Validation with Other Professionals.   Another method of validation is collaboration with other health professionals. In the case of Danz Blasser described previously, the nurse was able to verify the presence of a cardiac pacemaker through discussion with the client's daughter. In her absence, however, the nurse might have contacted the attending physician, inquired about old charts in the medical records department, or consulted with nurses in the coronary care unit.

Example. Nancy Adels is a 48 year old client with a diagnosis of metastatic cancer of the colon. She is four days postop after surgery for a permanent ileostomy. Based on her observations of the client, the nurse identifies cues indicating that the client is denying her diagnosis. Subsequent discussion with the stomal therapist and the physician validates the nurse's interpretation.

Validation with Reference Sources. The nurse may also use reference sources to substantiate interpretations.

Example. Kathy Prihoda, a nurse in the clinic, is examining Jenny, an eight month old. She notices that the child does not turn over independently, sit unaided, or hold her bottle.

In this situation, the nurse might use a pediatric reference source to verify initial perceptions that Jenny is not at an appropriate developmental level for her age. Reference sources might include texts, journals, or developmental charts.

Validation is an important component of the diagnostic process. The approaches previously described facilitate verification of the accuracy and completeness of the nurse's interpretations. Validation assists the nurse to recognize errors, isolate discrepancies, and identify the need for additional data. This phase in the processing of data forms the link between assessment and formulation of nursing diagnoses.

3–2 TEST YOURSELF

SOURCES OF VALIDATION

Identify methods of validation that might be used by the nurse in the situations described below.

VALIDATION
    A. Directly with the client or significant others
    B. Collaboration with health care professionals
    C. Reference sources

SITUATION
    1. Jeremy Pressman is seen in the outpatient clinic for a well baby visit. He is 18 months old and weighs 18 pounds. His mother asks, "Is he underweight?" How can this be validated?

2. A 17 year old teenager is brought into the emergency department complaining of abdominal pain. Shortly after he is placed on a stretcher, he vomits brown liquid. The nurse realizes that the vomitus could be old blood but knows that certain liquids, such as coffee or hot chocolate, can resemble old blood. What should the nurse do to pursue this?

3. Pat Derby, a 19 year old college sophomore, is seen at the University student health center because he claims that voices are telling him to kill his accounting professor. The nurse practitioner interviews Pat to obtain more information about his thought processes. During the discussion, Pat indicates that Dr. Johnson saw him three weeks ago when he had these same feelings. What would be an appropriate next step?

4. Ann Bodrog is brought to the hospital by her son. You suspect that she is profoundly depressed and she does not respond to your questions regarding her health history. What should you do next?

5. Carol Puca is admitted for anorexia nervosa. You recognize that she was on your unit about two months ago with the same problem. When questioned about her attendance at counseling sessions, Carol says she has gone but she avoids eye contact. You suspect that she has not attended regularly. How might you pursue this?

3–2 TEST YOURSELF □ ANSWERS

1. C—Consult a growth chart (reference source)
2. A—Ask the client or family about intake of coffee or hot chocolate
3. B—Contact Dr. Johnson
4. A—Ask the client's son about symptoms and possible causes of depression
5. B—Call the group facilitator or social worker to verify the client's attendance at counseling sessions

ERRORS IN THE DIAGNOSTIC PROCESS

Introduction

Up to this point, the text has presented information on data collection, classification, interpretation, and validation. These are the components necessary for the diagnostic process to be completed accurately. The nurse gathers data, identifies cues, makes inferences about the health status of the client, and validates these judgments with the client. The outcome of this process is a label—the *nursing diagnosis*. If any of these steps are carried out incorrectly or incompletely, the label may be inaccurate.

There are three major sources of errors in the diagnostic process. They are (1) inaccurate or incomplete data collection, (2) inaccurate interpretation of data, and (3) lack of clinical knowledge.

Inaccurate or Incomplete Data Collection

The nurse's ability to formulate nursing diagnoses is dependent upon an accurate and complete data base. Several factors may interfere with the collection of data. These may include communication problems, withholding information, and distractions/interruptions.

Communication Problems

There are a variety of communication problems that may result in inaccurate or incomplete data collection.

Language Barrier. Either the client or the nurse may have a language barrier that interferes with the collection of data.

Example. When Juan Rivera came to the emergency department, the nurse noted that he was obviously anxious, diaphoretic, grimacing, and holding his abdomen. When the nurse, Jeff Halter, began to question Juan, he determined that the client did not speak English.

The nurse recognized that additional information was necessary to accurately determine the client's problem. If available, family members who understand English or staff who speak the client's language might be utilized to collect additional pertinent data.

Slang or Jargon.   Even when the nurse and client speak the same language, either may use language that confuses the other. The client's age, environment, or cultural background may involve the use of expressions that are foreign to the nurse.

Example

Nurse: Mr. Blass, have you had prostate problems in the past?
Client: No, I haven't, but my "night work" hasn't been too good lately.

Further questioning revealed that Mr. Blass was describing a recent history of sexual dysfunction.

The nurse may also use technical jargon or terminology that is foreign to the client.

Example

Nurse: Mrs. Connor, have you ever had an IVP?
Client: An IV what?

Biased Questions.   This type of question, as described in Chapter 2, tends to intimidate clients and may result in inaccurate or incomplete data. Clients may give the response they believe is expected or choose not to respond at all.

Examples

"You're not frightened, are you?"
"Does being obese interfere with your work?"

Withholding Information

Clients may not share information for a number of reasons. They may be anxious, embarrassed, suspicious, or unaware of the importance of the information.

Example.   Cathy Stevens is admitted to an ambulatory surgery center for an elective breast biopsy. The nurse asks the client if she has any allergies. Assuming that the nurse means allergies to medications, Cathy says "no."

In reality, the client has a shellfish allergy that could predispose her to reactions if iodine-based skin preparations are used to cleanse her skin before surgery.

Distractions

There are a number of distractions that may interfere with the concentration required to collect data. These may include interruptions, a noisy nonprivate environment, or thoughts that are preoccupying the nurse or client.

The nurse who is rushed may not listen carefully to the information provided.

Example. When Steven Samuel was admitted with emphysema, he said he had no family. The nurse, who was rushed, did not pursue this by asking if he had friends who would be visiting him. When Mr. Samuel became progressively more depressed as his hospitalization continued, the nurses assumed that his depression was related to his chronic illness. However, when encouraged to talk about his feelings, Steven revealed that he was upset because no one had visited him. The nurses then realized that his loneliness was the source of his withdrawal. The nurse who admitted the client might have anticipated this problem if inquiries had been made about his support systems.

Frequently, interruptions may also interfere with complete data collection.

Example. Pat Mihalick is interviewing Sam Madeira, a newly admitted client on a medical unit. During the course of the interview, the telephone rings four times with calls from Mr. Madeira's office. When Pat attempts to document her assessment, she realizes that she has not completed a portion of the interview. Perhaps this could have been avoided had she asked the operator to hold the client's calls.

At times, the client's preoccupation with other topics may lead to an incomplete data base.

Example

Client: Oh yes, I've had high blood pressure for years. I stopped watching my diet because it's too much trouble. I don't cook much since I live alone. I used to live with my sister, but she moved to Florida. She just loves it there.

Nurse: Where is she living in Florida?

Client: She lives in Orlando. The city is growing so fast because of the climate and the attractions. Now, that's a wonderful place. Have you ever been there?

Nurse: Yes.

Client: What I like best about it is the weather. I could spend months there. It's nicer than other places I've gone. Of course, I enjoy the Houston area too. . . .

In this situation, the nurse allowed the conversation to be directed away from the client's hypertension, which was the reason for her visit to the physician's office. Clearly, the client was preoccupied with other thoughts, but the nurse lost control of the interview process and did not investigate the client's nonadherence to the diet.

Inaccurate Interpretation of Data

Two different types of errors may lead to inaccurate interpretation of data: (1) using only one cue or observation to reach premature inferences, and (2) allowing personal prejudices or biases to influence the interpretation of data.

Premature Interpretation of Data

A common type of error is the development of a judgment before all the important information is collected or considered. Problems can occur when only one observation is used since clusters of information or patterns of behavior are more significant than single cues or episodes. This type of error occurs in the following situation.

Example. Ann Weaver puts on her call light at 4 PM while she is talking on the phone. The 3–11 nurse who answers her light is not familiar with Anne's pattern of requiring pain medication every three hours for arthritis. When the nurse enters the room, Anne is laughing at something that is being said on the phone. "Oh nurse," she says, "could you bring me my pain medication?" The nurse walks away thinking "How much pain could she be in if she can laugh like that?" When the nurse checks Anne's medication record, it becomes clear that Anne's request for medication represents a pattern of behavior. The telephone conversation has temporarily distracted the client's responses to the pain. The established pattern of behavior is more valid than the nurse's single observation of the client laughing.

Sometimes a nurse reaches a conclusion based on a single cue rather than pursuing further investigation. Therefore, the interpretation of the data and the resulting diagnosis may be faulty, as in the following case.

Example. Pat Banks, a home care nurse, was visiting Mr. Falk after his discharge from the hospital. The client had an indwelling catheter. When Mrs. Falk said that urine was leaking around the catheter, Pat decided that the 5 ml balloon probably wasn't inflated enough to hold the catheter securely in place. She instilled more sterile water into the balloon.

The next day Mrs. Falk called, quite upset, saying that the urine leakage was worse and that Mr. Falk was in great discomfort. When Pat visited him that day, she discovered that the catheter had disloged from Mr. Falk's bladder. The balloon was probably in his urethra. After Pat replaced the catheter, Mr. Falk was more comfortable and the catheter stopped leaking ("Confidentially," 1983b).

Pat took one cue—a leaking catheter—and came to the wrong conclusion because she failed to gather more data before taking action. Her misinterpretation of the cue resulted in additional discomfort for Mr. Falk.

Another type of error is jumping to inaccurate conclusions using the medical diagnosis as a cue. The nurse who expects a diabetic client to have specific responses because of the medical diagnosis may be unable to recognize the individuality of the client's needs.

Example Marge Chapman is a newly diagnosed insulin-dependent diabetic. The nurse initiated a diagnosis that included interventions to instruct Mrs. Chapman in techniques for insulin injection. In reality, Mrs. Chapman was quite familiar with injection technique. Her mother and aunt require insulin injections which Mrs. Chapman has administered for years.

In cases like Mrs. Chapman's, the nurse assumed that because the client's medical diagnosis was diabetes, she would require injection technique instruction. Therefore, diagnoses and interventions may be developed that have no bearing on the client's most pressing problems. To maintain a low rate of diagnostic error, the nurse must take the time to validate interpretations of the client's responses.

Personal Prejudices

Personal prejudices and lack of awareness of cultural practices and beliefs can influence a nurse's interpretation of data. Sometimes the behavior of a client or family can become so annoying that the nurse is tempted to ignore important cues. Consider what could have happened in this situation.

Example. Keith Fishbein was recovering well from gallbladder surgery, but his family hovered around his bed as though he were at death's door. Although Mr. Fishbein himself never complained, his wife and two children had a hundred trivial requests. And they wanted everything done immediately. One evening Mrs. Fishbein excitedly demanded that the nurse check her husband who had pain in his left leg. The nurse thought "What next?" as she went into the room fully expecting another false alarm. To her surprise, she was unable to find a pulse in Mr. Fishbein's leg. He was rushed to surgery for removal of a blood clot ("Confidentially," 1983a).

Example. Susan Smithson arrives on duty to find a group of 40 gypsies in the waiting room of her unit. Her inquiries of other staff reveals that one of the patients on the unit is the gypsy queen. Unaware of the custom that requires their presence, Susan requests that the group leave the unit. This is particularly distressing to the client.

The nurse must be aware of personal values and biases, recognize how these influence perceptions, and attempt to overcome prejudices. When presented with unfamiliar cultural practices or beliefs, the nurse should seek out resources to assist in understanding the client's responses. This will enhance the nurse's ability to interpret cues correctly.

Lack of Clinical Knowledge or Experience

Lack of clinical knowledge or experience may affect the collection and interpretation of data. It can result in any of the following: (1) critical data not being collected, (2) incorrect clustering of cues, or (3) inaccurate interpretation of cues.

The inexperienced nurse may simply overlook important assessment data because of inadequate clinical knowledge. For example an inexperienced nurse may fail to recognize that an elderly client with sacral edema is at risk for skin breakdown.

In other cases, the nurse may focus entirely on one aspect of care and ignore another set of cues.

Example.   Louise Rubino's first nursing position was as a staff nurse in a community health agency in a poor urban area. One of her first clients had diabetes and needed instruction to be able to plan low cost, nutritious meals. Louise asked her supervisor to accompany her to the client's home to see the progress she'd made. The nursing supervisor was very impressed until she asked the client to remove her shoes and stockings. To Louise's dismay, the client's ankles and feet were encrusted with dirt. For the next half hour, Louise bathed the client's feet and explained the importance of foot care ("Confidentially," 1984).

In this case, the nurse focused on dietary instruction and missed other important cues that indicated a deficit in the client's knowledge about foot care. Louise learned an important lesson: never get so involved with one aspect of nursing care that you overlook something equally important.

Example.   An 80 year old woman who had been in the hospital for ten days fell while getting out of bed at midnight to go to the bathroom. The woman had received flurazepam (Dalmane) about an hour before. Although the bedrails at her head were elevated, those by her legs were down. The manufacturer of Dalmane warns that dizziness, drowsiness, lightheadedness, staggering, ataxia, and falls have occurred with its use, particularly in elderly or debilitated persons (Cushing, 1985).

In this example, the nurse did not identify the client's potential for falling associated with the use of the drug. The nurse's lack of experience with the drug and subsequent failure to initiate adequate preventive measures contributed to the client's injury.

Example.   Pat Hendrickson, a new graduate, is making rounds on her patients at the beginning of the night shift. When she approaches Mr. Gray, the client tells her that a large man has been watching him from the hall for the last two hours. Pat looks in the hall and detects only a housekeeping cart. Assuming that his condition was due to his age, the unfamiliar environment, or electrolyte imbalance, she reviews the client's chart and calls the physician to report her findings. Pat did not observe the client's eyeglasses lying on the bedside cabinet. In reality, the client had very poor visual acuity without his glasses and thought that the cleaning cart, which had been left in the hall across from his room, was a human form.

The nurse who lacks adequate clinical knowledge or experience can compensate for these deficits by seeking information and guidance from more experienced nurses or other resources. Careful development of an organized approach for data collection and interpretation is also critical for accurate data analysis and diagnosis.

COMPUTERS AND THE DIAGNOSTIC PROCESS

Computers are being used by nurses during the diagnostic process to organize and interpret data collected during assessment. Computer systems designed to assist in clinical diagnosis and to make recommendations for outcomes and interventions are known as computer-assisted diagnosis (CAD) systems.

Computer-assisted nursing diagnosis involves the use of the computer to process nursing assessment data. Most commonly, data is entered by the nurse at the nurse's station. However, in more sophisticated systems, data may be entered at the client's bedside using a CRT (cathode ray tube) which looks like a television screen, and either a keyboard or a light pen. In other systems, the client can be instructed to use similar equipment either at the bedside or in a central location to respond to assessment questions at the time of admission.

After the data are entered, the computer compares the cues identified during the assessment process to the defining characteristics for each nursing diagnosis in its data base. A list of possible diagnoses is generated and the nurse is able to accept or reject each entry on the list or enter other appropriate diagnoses. Figure 3–1 demonstrates an example of a computer-assisted nursing diagnosis generated from a nursing assessment.

The chief advantages of computer-assisted nursing diagnosis center on the system's ability to identify patterns that might be overlooked by the nurse. These systems use consistent, organized processes to organize, analyze, and interpret data. The computer is not affected by distraction, fatigue, headaches, or any of the other human variables that impact on the processing of data.

However, the ability of any computerized system to generate nursing diagnoses is only as good as the program on which it is based. Lack of clinical knowledge on the part of the developer of the software can result in inaccurate diagnoses. Some nursing diagnoses lack large reliable data bases which may make accurate diagnoses difficult. Additionally, clients can display an infinite

```
DFALT-G981          NYUMC HOSP 4
05/28/85  11:55 AM              PAGE  001

========== ========== ========== ========== ======
DEMONSTRATION DAN-1        1336
 4342877  85464  04/02/40   44  M
 MARKS  CLEMENT  MD
========== ========== ========== ========== ========== ==========
```

```
PRIMARY  DIAGNOSIS:   GI  BLEED...

NURSING  DIAGNOSIS
 05/22  ACTUAL  SKIN  BREAKDOWN R/T....INCONTINENCE  OF  URINE/FECES    JBKA
EXPECTED  OUTCOMES                                   R/P    R/D
 05/22  DECREASE  IN  SIZE  OF  DECUBITUS  ULCER       QD    5/30         JBKA
NURSING  ORDERS
 05/22  TURN  &  POSITION  Q2H                                           JBKA
 05/22  FOLLOW  SCHEDULE--RT-BACK-LT                                     JBKA
 05/22  DO  NOT  ELEVATE  HOB  MORE  THAN  30  DEG                       JBKA
 05/22  USE  APPROPRIATE  PRESSURE-RELIEVING  DEVICE:
        WATER  MATTRESS                                                  JBKA
 05/22  OOB  IN  STRETCHER  CHAIR  TID                                   JBKA
 05/22  PAD  BEDPAN                                                      JBKA
 05/22  PASSIVE  ROM  TO  ALL  EXTREMITIES  Q4H                          JBKA
 05/22  DIETARY  CONSULT  REGARDING  ASSESSMENT  OF
        NUTRITIONAL  STATUS                                              JBKA
 05/22  CHECK  FOR  FECAL/URINARY  INCONTINENCE
        Q1/2H.  (NA  TO  CHECK  Q1H  ON  THE  1/2H  &  RN  TO
        CHECK  Q1H  ON  THE  HOUR)                                       JBKA
 05/22  CLEAN  SKIN  THOROUGHLY  &  PAT  DRY  POST  VOID/BM              JBKA
 05/22  METHOD  OF  TREATMENT:  STAGE  3- STOMA  ADHESIVE
        METHOD                                                           JBKA
 05/22  WEAR  STERILE  GLOVES  WHEN  IN  CONTACT  W/
        WOUND.
        CLEANSE  AREA,  USING  A  STERILE  IRRIG  TRAY  W/
        1/2  STRENGTH  PEROXIDE  &  NS.
        RINSE  THOROUGHLY  W/  NS  &  PAT.  DRY  W/  STERILE
        GAUZE                                                            JBKA
 05/22  APPLY  HEAT  LAMP  X15  MINS  12  INCHES  FROM  SKIN
        &  AT  THE  SIDE  OF  BED  SO  THAT  INADVERTENT  PT
        MOVEMENT  WILL  NOT  CAUSE  LAMP  TO  CONTACT
        SKIN.
        PAT  ANTACID  OVER  THE  AFFECTED  AREA  USING
        STERILE  GAUZE.  ALLOW  TO  DRY  THOROUGHLY                      JBKA
 05/22  APPLY  MYCOSTATIN  POWDER  AS  ORDERED  BY  MD.
        REMOVE  EXCESS  POWDER  BY  BRUSHING  W/  STERILE
        GAUZE.
        APPLY  A  LIGHT  COAT  OF  SKIN  PREP.  ALLOW  AREA
        TO  DRY  THOROUGHLY                                              JBKA
 05/22  APPLY  STOMA  ADHESIVE  TO  COVER  THE  ENTIRE
        AREA  EXTENDING  1  INCH  BEYOND  THE  REDNESS  ON
        ALL  SIDES.  ROUND  THE  CORNERS  W/  A  SCISSOR  TO
        PREVENT  WRINKLING.
        SECURE  THE  EDGES  OF  THE  STOMA  ADHESIVE  W/  1
        INCH  PAPER  TAPE                                                JBKA
 05/22  LEAVE  DSG  IN  PLACE  2-3  DAYS  IF  THE  INTEGRITY
        OF  THE  DSG  REMAINS  INTACT                                    JBKA

========== ========== ========== ========== ========== ==========
DEMONSTRATION  DAN-1                              PATIENT  CARE  PLAN
```

FIGURE 3–1. Computer sample of nursing diagnosis. (Courtesy of New York University Medical Center.)

variety of responses to health problems, making it difficult to anticipate all such responses. Nurses using computers for diagnosis need to exercise professional judgment in evaluating the conclusions developed by the computer system.

SUMMARY

The diagnostic process follows the assessment phase. In this phase data are processed, classified, interpreted, and validated. The outcome of this diagnostic process is a nursing diagnostic statement. The steps of the diagnostic process can be affected by several types of errors, including inaccurate or incomplete data, inaccurate interpretation of data, or lack of knowledge or experience. Errors can result in nursing diagnostic statements that are not appropriate for the client.

Computer-assisted diagnosis systems automate the diagnostic process and facilitate the nurse's ability to make accurate, individualized nursing diagnoses for clients. This chapter has explored the organization and interpretation of data accumulated during the assessment phase. Chapter 4 will address the formulation, validation, and documentation of the diagnostic statement.

REFERENCES

Abdellah F, Martin A, Beland I, and Matheney R: Patient Centered Approaches to Nursing: New York: Macmillan, 1960.

American Nurses' Association: A Social Policy Statement. Kansas City, MO: American Nurses' Association, 1980.

American Nurses' Association: Standards of Nursing Practice. Kansas City, MO: American Nurses' Association, 1973.

Confidentially. Nursing '83, 70, January, 1983a.

Confidentially. Nursing '83, 94, April, 1983b.

Confidentially. Nursing '84, 72, December, 1984.

Cushing M: First, anticipate the harm. . . . American Journal of Nursing 1985 Feb; 85(2):137–138.

Gordon M: Nursing diagnosis and the diagnostic process. American Journal of Nursing 1976 Aug; 76(8):1298–1300.

Moritz D: Nursing diagnosis in relation to the nursing process. In Moritz D and Kim M (eds): Classification of Nursing Diagnoses: Proceedings of the Third and Fourth National Conferences. New York: McGraw-Hill, 1982.

Mundinger M and Jauron G: Developing a nursing diagnosis. Nursing Outlook 23:94–98, 1975.

North American Nursing Diagnosis Association. Nursing Diagnosis Newsletter. Spring, 1990.

Shoemaker J: Essential features of a nursing diagnosis. In McLane M, McFarland K, and Kim M (eds): Classification of Nursing Diagnoses: Proceedings of the Fifth National Conference. St. Louis: CV Mosby, 1984.

BIBLIOGRAPHY

Allen CJ: Incorporating a wellness perspective for nursing diagnosis in practice. In Carroll-Johnson, RM (ed): Classification of Nursing Diagnoses: Proceedings of the Eighth Conference. Philadelphia: JB Lippincott, 1989, pp 37–42.

Andreoli K, and Musser L: Computers in nursing care: the state of the art. Nursing Outlook 1985; 33(1):16–25.

Duesphol A: Nursing Diagnosis Handbook. Philadelphia: WB Saunders, 1986.

Fredetta SL: Common diagnostic errors. Nurse Educator 1988; 13(3):31–35.

Gordon M: Nursing Diagnosis—Process and Application, 2nd ed. New York: McGraw-Hill, 1987.

Kim M, and McFarland G: Analysis and views on issues and trends related to nursing diagnoses and the national conference. In McLane A, McFarland K, and Kim M (eds): Classification of Nursing Diagnoses: Proceedings of the Fifth National Conference. St. Louis: CV Mosby, 1984, pp 556–570.

McLane AM: Measurement and validation of diagnostic concepts: a decade of progress. Heart Lung 1987; 16(6):616–624.

Tribulski J: Nursing diagnosis: waste of time or valued tool. RN 1988; 51(12):30–34.

Whitley G, and Dillon A: Nursing curricula in the 80s—the impact of nursing diagnosis. Journal of Nursing Education 1988; 27(5):233–235.

4 WRITING A NURSING DIAGNOSIS

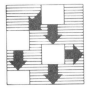

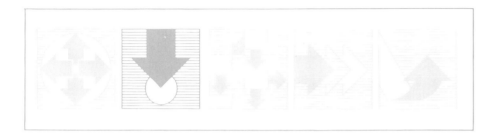

INTRODUCTION

The assessment phase of the nursing process provides the basis for the diagnostic process. As described in Chapter 3, collected data are organized, analyzed, interpreted, and validated by the nurse. The outcome of the diagnostic process is the diagnostic statement, which becomes the framework for subsequent phases of planning, implementation, and evaluation. This chapter focuses on how to write, validate, and document the nursing diagnostic statement.

THE NORTH AMERICAN NURSING DIAGNOSIS SYSTEM

There are several ways to state nursing diagnoses using a number of diagnostic systems. The most commonly used system was developed by the North American Nursing Diagnosis Association (NANDA). The NANDA system of diagnosis was adopted by the American Nurses' Association as the official system of diagnosis for the United States in 1988, and it is the system that will be utilized throughout this text. Before exploring how to write a diagnosis, it might be helpful to discuss the NANDA organization and the system as it has evolved.

The First National Conference on Classification of Nursing Diagnosis was held in 1973 and resulted in publication of the first list of approved diagnoses. The North American Nursing Diagnosis Association evolved from the group formed at the First National Conference and has been in existence in its current form since 1982. Conferences have been held approximately every two years since that time. The members of the organization have continued to develop and refine the list of approved diagnoses.

The process by which new diagnoses are submitted and approved by NANDA is both organized and systematic. First, the proposed diagnosis is submitted to NANDA and placed into the diagnosis review cycle. In order to enter the cycle, each proposed diagnosis must include certain essential elements including label, definition, defining characteristics and related factors. The proposed diagnosis must be consistent with the NANDA definition of a nursing diagnosis, as presented in Chapter 3. The label provides a name for the diagnosis. The definition provides a clear, precise description of the diagnosis, delineates its meaning and differentiates it from other diagnoses. Defining characteristics are clinical criteria that cluster as manifestations of the diagnosis—the critical behaviors or major signs/symptoms that represent a diagnostic label. Related factors are conditions or circumstances that can cause or contribute to the development of the diagnosis. Proposed diagnoses must also include validation documentation such as references from the literature or research studies to support the rationale for the diagnostic label, defining characteristics and related factors. A sample nursing diagnostic statement with related outcome criteria and nursing interventions must also be included. Table 4–1 is a sample of a NANDA-approved diagnosis with its name, definition, defining characteristics, and related factors.

TABLE 4–1. SAMPLE OF NANDA APPROVED NURSING DIAGNOSIS

DIAGNOSIS NAME: FATIGUE

Definition:
The state in which an individual experiences an overwhelming sense of exhaustion and decreased capacity for physical and mental work

Defining Characteristics:
Major:
 Verbalization of an unremitting and overwhelming lack of energy
 Inability to maintain usual routines
Minor:
 Perceived need for additional energy to accomplish routine tasks
 Increase in physical complaints
 Impaired ability to concentrate
 Decreased performance
 Lethargy or listlessness
 Disinterest in surroundings/introspection
 Decreased libido
 Accident prone

Related Factors:
Decreased/increased metabolic energy production
Increased energy requirements to perform activities of daily living
Overwhelming psychological or emotional demands
Excessive social and/or role demands
States of discomfort
Altered body chemistry
 Medications
 Drug withdrawal
 Chemotherapy

Modified from Taptich BJ, Iyer P, Bernocchi-Losey D: Nursing Diagnosis and Care Planning. Philadelphia: WB Saunders, 1989.

TABLE 4–2. ALPHABETICAL LISTING OF APPROVED NURSING DIAGNOSES, NORTH AMERICAN NURSING DIAGNOSIS ASSOCIATION

Activity intolerance
Activity intolerance, potential
Adjustment, impaired
Airway clearance, ineffective
Anxiety
Aspiration, potential for
Body image disturbance
Body temperature, potential altered
Breastfeeding, effective
Breastfeeding, ineffective
Breathing pattern, ineffective
Cardiac output, decreased
Communication, impaired verbal
Conflict, decisional
Conflict, parental role
Constipation
Constipation, colonic
Constipation, perceived
Coping, defensive
Coping, family-ineffective: compromised
Coping, family-ineffective: disabling
Coping, family: potential for growth
Coping, individual ineffective
Denial, ineffective
Diarrhea
Disuse syndrome, potential for
Diversional activity deficit
Dysreflexia
Family processes, altered
Fatigue
Fear
Fluid volume deficit (1, 2)
Fluid volume deficit, potential
Fluid volume excess
Gas exchange, impaired
Grieving, anticipatory
Grieving, dysfunctional
Growth and development, altered
Health maintenance, altered
Health seeking behaviors (specify)
Home maintenance management, impaired
Hopelessness
Hyperthermia
Hypothermia
Incontinence, bowel
Incontinence, functional
Incontinence, reflex
Incontinence, stress
Incontinence, total
Incontinence, urge
Infection, potential for
Injury, potential for
Knowledge deficit (specify)

Mobility, impaired physical
Noncompliance
Nutrition, altered: less than body requirements
Nutrition, altered: more than body requirements
Nutrition, altered: potential for more than body requirements
Oral mucous membrane, altered
Pain
Pain, chronic
Parenting, altered
Parenting, altered: potential
Personal identity disturbance
Poisoning, potential for
Post trauma response
Powerlessness
Protection, altered
Rape-trauma response
Rape-trauma syndrome: compound reaction
Rape-trauma syndrome: silent reaction
Role performance, altered
Self-care deficit: bathing/hygiene
    dressing/grooming
    feeding
    toileting
Self-esteem, chronic low
Self-esteem disturbance
Self-esteem, situational low
Sensory/perceptual alteration (specify)
    (visual, auditory, kinesthetic, gustatory, tactile, olfactory)
Sexual dysfunction
Sexuality patterns, altered
Skin integrity, impaired
Skin integrity, potential impaired
Sleep pattern disturbance
Social interaction, impaired
Social isolation
Spiritual distress
Suffocation, potential for
Swallowing, impaired
Thermoregulation, ineffective
Thought processes, altered
Tissue integrity, impaired
Tissue perfusion, altered (specify type)
    (cardiopulmonary, cerebral, gastrointestinal, peripheral, renal)
Trauma, potential for
Unilateral neglect
Urinary elimination, altered patterns of
Urinary retention
Violence, potential for: self-directed or directed at others

The second step in the diagnosis review cycle is publication in the Nursing Diagnosis Journal which places the proposed diagnosis in the public domain. Next, it is forwarded for review by a clinical/technical task force with expertise related to the proposed diagnosis. It is then reviewed by the diagnosis review commitee, which recommends acceptance, modification, or rejection. Next, the proposed diagnosis is reviewed by the NANDA board of directors who forward accepted diagnoses to the general assembly for review and discussion at the biannual National Conference. The final step is a mail ballot to NANDA members. Approved diagnoses are then included on the official NANDA list shown in Table 4–2 (Carroll-Johnson, 1989).

The NANDA-approved diagnoses are classified according to Taxonomy I, which was proposed by the Nurse Theorist Group convened by NANDA in 1978. These 14 nursing theorists, through a democratic process, agreed upon some basic conclusions and proposed that the nine human response patterns of the "Unitary Person" should form the framework for organizing the diagnoses. These nine patterns reflect how individuals interact with the environment that surrounds them. The nursing diagnoses categorized under each pattern describe how they respond to particular states of health or illness. The patterns include exchanging, valuing, perceiving, feeling, relating, communicating, moving, knowing, and choosing. Table 4–3 identifies the patterns, their definitions, and gives an example of a nursing diagnosis that is included in the pattern. Each of the existing NANDA-approved diagnoses have been placed under these nine categories (Table 4–4). Subcategories are used when diagnoses require more specificity. For example, in the exchanging pattern fluid volume includes two subcategories—fluid volume deficit and fluid volume excess. The list of diagnoses continues to expand as nurses identify and validate labels that describe the realm of nursing practice. Taxonomy I can also be expected to change as nurses continue to clarify the concept of nursing diagnosis and to develop effective methods of organization.

TABLE 4–3. NANDA TAXONOMY I—HUMAN RESPONSE PATTERNS

PATTERN AND DEFINITION	EXAMPLE
Exchanging A human response pattern involving mutual giving and receiving	Fluid volume excess may occur as a result of the *exchange* of fluid and electrolytes at the cellular level when the client consumes excessive fluid or sodium
Communicating A human response pattern involving sending messages	Impaired verbal *communication* may occur when the client does not speak the dominant language
Relating A human response pattern involving establishing bonds	Altered parenting may result when a new mother is unable to *bond* with her premature infant

TABLE 4–3.   NANDA TAXONOMY I—HUMAN RESPONSE PATTERNS
continued

PATTERN AND DEFINITION	EXAMPLE
Valuing A human response pattern involving the assigning of relative worth	Spiritual distress may be found in individuals who are unable to attend *valued* religious services
Choosing A human response pattern involving the selection of alternatives	Decisional conflict may occur when clients are given numerous treatment options and are expected to *choose* one
Moving A human response pattern involving activity	Impaired physical mobility may result when a child is unable to *move* normally because of traction
Perceiving A human response pattern involving the reception of information	Visual sensory *perceptual* alterations may occur when the client doesn't wear or loses corrective lenses or glasses
Knowing A human response pattern involving the meaning associated with information	*Knowledge* deficit exists when a client cannot identify the factors that precipitate angina
Feeling A human response pattern involving the subjective awareness of information	Anxiety may occur when a client *feels* uneasy when preparing for a first hospital experience

TABLE 4–4.   NANDA TAXONOMY OF NURSING DIAGNOSES

PATTERN 1:	EXCHANGING	PATTERN 1:	EXCHANGING
1.1.2.1	Altered Nutrition: More than body requirements	1.3.1.1	Constipation
		1.3.1.1.1	Perceived Constipation
1.1.2.2	Altered Nutrition: Less than body requirements	1.3.1.1.2	Colonic Constipation
		1.3.1.2	Diarrhea
1.1.2.3	Altered Nutrition: Potential for more than body requirements	1.3.1.3	Bowel Incontinence
		1.3.2	Altered Patterns of Urinary Elimination
1.2.1.1	Potential for Infection	1.3.2.1.1	Stress Incontinence
1.2.2.1	Potential Altered Body Temperature	1.3.2.1.2	Reflex Incontinence
1.2.2.2	Hypothermia	1.3.2.1.3	Urge Incontinence
1.2.2.3	Hyperthermia	1.3.2.1.4	Functional Incontinence
1.2.2.4	Ineffective Thermoregulation	1.3.2.1.5	Total Incontinence
1.2.3.1	Dysreflexia	1.3.2.2	Urinary Retention

Table continued on following page

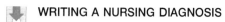

TABLE 4–4. NANDA TAXONOMY OF NURSING DIAGNOSES *Continued*

PATTERN 1:	EXCHANGING	PATTERN 6:	MOVING
1.4.1.1	Altered (Specify Type) Tissue Perfusion (Renal, Cerebral, Cardiopulmonary, Gastrointestinal, Peripheral)	6.1.1.1	Impaired Physical Mobility
		6.1.1.2	Activity Intolerance
		6.1.1.2.1	Fatigue
1.4.1.2.1	Fluid Volume Excess	6.1.1.3	Potential Activity Intolerance
1.4.1.2.2.1	Fluid Volume Deficit (1)	6.2.1	Sleep Pattern Disturbance
1.4.1.2.2.1	Fluid Volume Deficit (2)	6.3.1.1	Diversional Activity Deficit
1.4.1.2.2.2	Potential Fluid Volume Deficit	6.4.1.1	Impaired Home Maintenance Management
1.4.2.1	Decreased Cardiac Output	6.4.2	Altered Health Maintenance
1.5.1.1	Impaired Gas Exchange	6.5.1	Feeding Self-Care Deficit
1.5.1.2	Ineffective Airway Clearance	6.5.1.1	Impaired Swallowing
1.5.1.3	Ineffective Breathing Pattern	6.5.1.2	Ineffective Breastfeeding
1.6.1	Potential for Injury	6.5.1.2.3	Effective Breastfeeding
1.6.1.1	Potential for Suffocation	6.5.2	Bathing/Hygiene Self-Care Deficit
1.6.1.2	Potential for Poisoning	6.5.3	Dressing/Grooming Self-Care Deficit
1.6.1.3	Potential for Trauma	6.5.4	Toileting Self-Care Deficit
1.6.1.4	Potential for Aspiration	6.6	Altered Growth and Development
1.6.1.5	Potential for Disuse Syndrome		
1.6.2	Altered Protection	PATTERN 7:	PERCEIVING
1.6.2.1	Impaired Tissue Integrity	7.1.1	Body Image Disturbance
1.6.2.1.1	Altered Oral Mucous Membrane	7.1.2	Self-Esteem Disturbance
1.6.2.1.2.1	Impaired Skin Integrity	7.1.2.1	Chronic Low Self-Esteem
1.6.2.1.2.2	Potential Impaired Skin Integrity	7.1.2.2	Situational Low Self-Esteem
PATTERN 2:	COMMUNICATING	7.1.3	Personal Identity Disturbance
2.1.1.1	Impaired Verbal Communication	7.2	Sensory/Perceptual Alterations (Specify) (Visual, Auditory, Kinesthetic, Gustatory, Tactile, Olfactory)
PATTERN 3:	RELATING		
3.1.1	Impaired Social Interaction	7.2.1.1	Unilateral Neglect
3.1.2	Social Isolation	7.3.1	Hopelessness
3.2.1	Altered Role Performance	7.3.2	Powerlessness
3.2.1.1.1	Altered Parenting		
3.2.1.1.2	Potential Altered Parenting	PATTERN 8:	KNOWING
3.2.1.2.1	Sexual Dysfunction	8.1.1	Knowledge Deficit (Specify)
3.2.2	Altered Family Processes	8.2	Altered Thought Processes
3.2.3.1	Parental Role Conflict		
3.3	Altered Sexuality Patterns	PATTERN 9:	FEELING
PATTERN 4:	VALUING	9.1.1	Pain
4.1.1	Spiritual Distress (distress of the human spirit)	9.1.1.1	Chronic Pain
		9.2.1.1	Dysfunctional Grieving
PATTERN 5:	CHOOSING	9.2.1.2	Anticipatory Grieving
5.1.1.1	Ineffective Individual Coping	9.2.2	Potential for Violence: Self-directed or directed at others
5.1.1.1.1	Impaired Adjustment		
5.1.1.1.2	Defensive Coping	9.2.3	Post-Trauma Response
5.1.1.1.3	Ineffective Denial	9.2.3.1	Rape-Trauma Syndrome
5.1.2.1.1	Ineffective Family Coping: Disabling	9.2.3.1.1	Rape-Trauma Syndrome: Compound Reaction
5.1.2.1.2	Ineffective Family Coping: Compromised	9.2.3.1.2	Rape-Trauma Syndrome: Silent Reaction
5.1.2.2	Family Coping: Potential for Growth		
5.2.1.1.	Noncompliance (Specify)	9.3.1	Anxiety
5.3.1.1	Decisional Conflict (Specify)	9.3.2	Fear
5.4	Health Seeking Behaviors (Specify)		

COMPONENTS OF THE DIAGNOSTIC STATEMENT

A nursing diagnostic statement consists of two parts joined by the phrase "related to." The diagnostic statement begins with a determination of the human response of concern in the client (Part I) and identifies the related factors (Part II).

Part I—The Human Response

A human response, in the context of nursing diagnosis, identifies how the client responds to a state of health or illness. The first part of the diagnostic statement specifies a particular human response of concern identified by the nurse during the assessment phase. This clause indicates for nurses what needs to change in an individual client as a result of nursing intervention. For example, if the nurse determines that the client is experiencing difficulties in deciding among a number of ways to treat a medical problem, the human response might be termed "decisional conflict." The first part of the statement also determines the client-centered outcomes that will measure the change.

When writing the first part of the diagnostic statement, the nurse should consider the following.

1. What is the human response suggested by the assessment data?
2. To what degree is the human response problematic?

The human response can be selected from the list of accepted nursing diagnoses approved by NANDA (see Table 4–2). The degree to which the human response is present or the type of response identified may be clarified by the use of modifiers or qualifying statements (Table 4–5). Punctuation marks such as commas, colons, and parentheses are often used in the first part of the diagnostic statement to separate or clarify the diagnosis.

Example.   Mrs. James is a 72 year old client who had a total hip replacement this morning as a result of chronic arthritic changes in her hip. During your assessment, she complains of postoperative incisional pain and indicates that she would like a laxative since she will be in bed for a while. She states that she has become constipated in the past when she wasn't "up and around."

This information suggests two nursing diagnoses that reflect the presence of human responses of concern in this client. The first parts would be written:

1. Pain   indicates that the client is
                                       experiencing pain

2. Potential for constipation   identifies the possibility that the
                                       client will become constipated

TABLE 4–5. NURSING DIAGNOSIS MODIFIERS

MODIFIER	DEFINITION	EXAMPLE
Altered	A change from the usual optimum for a particular client	Altered body temperature
Potential	The individual is at risk for a problem	Potential for infection
Ineffective	Not producing the desired effect; not capable of performing satisfactorily	Ineffective thermoregulation
Decreased	Smaller; lessened; diminished; lesser in size, amount, or degree	Decreased cardiac output
Impaired	Made worse, weakened; damaged, reduced; deteriorated	Impaired swallowing
Deficit	Amount or quantity that is less than is necessary, desirable, or usable	Diversional activity deficit
Excess	Amount or quantity that is more than is necessary, desirable, or usable	Fluid volume excess
Dysfunctional	Abnormal; impaired or incompletely functioning	Sexual dysfunction
Disturbance	The state of being agitated, interrupted, or interfered with	Sleep pattern disturbance
Acute	Severe, but of short duration	Acute urinary retention
Chronic	Lasting a long time; recurring; habitual; constant	Chronic pain
Less than	A smaller amount	Altered nutrition: less than body requirements
More than	A larger amount	Altered nutrition: more than body requirements
Anticipatory	Occurring in advance	Anticipatory grieving
Compromised	To lay open to danger; to endanger the interests of	Ineffective family coping: compromised

Source: Webster's New World Dictionary, College Edition. Cleveland: The World Publishing Company, 1959. Modified from North American Nursing Diagnosis Association Taxonomy Committee, Diagnosis Qualifiers, North American Nursing Diagnosis Association, St. Louis, 1986.

Part II—The Related Factors

The related factors (etiology) are identified in the second part of the diagnostic statement. In order to prevent, minimize, or alleviate a response in the client, the nurse must know why it is occurring. The related factors identify the physiological, psychological, sociocultural, environmental, or spiritual factors believed to be causing or contributing to the response seen in the client.

Examples of Related Factors

PHYSIOLOGICAL	PSYCHOLOGICAL
Immobility	Fear of death
Effects of sensory deficit	Feelings of loneliness
Side effects of medications	Separation from family

SOCIOCULTURAL	ENVIRONMENTAL
Decreased ability to procure food	Excessive noise
Language barrier	Noxious odors
Lack of support systems	Sensitivity to light

SPIRITUAL

Inability to practice religious beliefs
Challenged beliefs about God
Conflict between religious beliefs and prescribed health regimen

In the preceding case of Mrs. James, two responses were identified. The second parts of the diagnostic statements could be written as follows:

HUMAN RESPONSE		RELATED FACTOR
1. Pain	related to	effects of surgery
2. Potential for constipation	related to	prolonged immobility

Remember that the related factors help to identify the variables that contribute to the presence of the human response. They also suggest specific nursing interventions that will prevent, correct, or alleviate the response. For example, the following nursing diagnoses identify the same human response but reflect quite different related factors.

HUMAN RESPONSE		RELATED FACTORS
1. Altered nutrition: less than body requirements	related to	difficulty in swallowing
2. Altered nutrition: less than body requirements	related to	decreased appetite
3. Altered nutrition: less than body requirements	related to	feelings of loneliness

Because the nursing interventions are dependent upon the related factors, those suggested by each of the diagnostic statements listed above are also quite different. The nursing interventions that might be initiated in the presence of swallowing difficulties might include the following:

1. Sit the client in an upright position, 60 to 90 degrees.
2. Encourage the client to:

   ☐ take small amounts of semisolid food

   ☐ place food at the back of the mouth

   ☐ think about swallowing.

If the client is experiencing decreased appetite, the following interventions may help:

1. Determine food preferences.
2. Serve food in an appealing manner.
3. Provide small, frequent feedings.

For the client who does not eat because she is lonely following her husband's death, the nurse may include these interventions:

1. Encourage the client to verbalize feelings about the death of her husband.
2. Explain the hazards of continued decreased intake.
3. Arrange consultation with a psychiatric clinical specialist.
4. Provide information about support groups—Widows and Widowers; I Can Cope.

Summary of Components of the Diagnostic Statement

The nursing diagnostic statement consists of two parts joined by the words "related to." Part I includes the human response identified by the nurse during the assessment phase of the nursing process. It determines the outcomes that will measure progress in preventing, minimizing, or alleviating the client's health problem. Part II consists of the related factors that contribute to the response.

TABLE 4–6. EXAMPLES OF NURSING DIAGNOSTIC STATEMENTS

☐ Impaired verbal communication related to language barrier
☐ Potential for injury related to impaired visual perception
☐ Sexual dysfunction related to fear of rejection
☐ Diversional activity deficit related to inability to participate in usual activities
☐ Impaired skin integrity related to irritating wound drainage
☐ Potential for aspiration related to decreased level of consciousness
☐ Altered growth and development related to effects of prolonged hospitalization
☐ Impaired adjustment related to effects of recent relocation

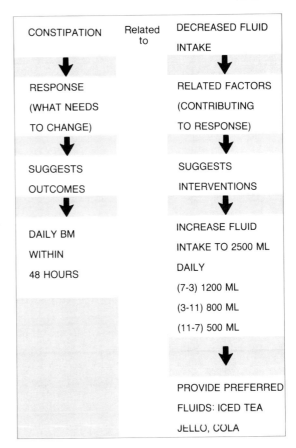

FIGURE 4–1. Flowchart of a sample nursing diagnosis illustrating the relationship of its components.

This part suggests the interventions that may be appropriate in the management of the client's care. Modifiers and punctuation marks may be used to increase the clarity of a nursing diagnosis. Figure 4–1 illustrates the relationship between the components of a nursing diagnostic statement. Sample nursing diagnostic statements are listed in Table 4–6.

GUIDELINES FOR WRITING A NURSING DIAGNOSTIC STATEMENT

Formulating a nursing diagnosis may be considered a new skill. As with any other new skill, it takes practice. The nurse will, with practice, find that the process of writing nursing diagnostic statements becomes easier. The following guidelines have been included to assist you in developing correctly written diagnoses.

1. Write the Diagnosis in Terms of the Client's Response Rather than Nursing Need

The first part of the diagnostic statement identifies the client's response to health or illness. Therapeutic or functional needs, such as "needs frequent turning" or "needs coughing and deep breathing," describe nursing interventions rather than client responses and should not be included in the diagnostic statement.

Example. Stella Blackwell is a 45 year old client who has a nasogastric tube following surgery. She tells her nurse that she is thirsty and that her mouth and lips are dry. The nurse recognizes that the client "needs additional fluids" and communicates this response in the diagnostic statement "fluid volume deficit related to decreased oral intake."

Examples

INCORRECT	CORRECT
Needs suctioning because she has many secretions	Potential for aspiration related to excessive oral secretions
Needs frequent rest periods because of shortness of breath	Fatigue related to persistent shortness of breath

2. Use "Related to" Rather than "Due to" or "Caused by" to Connect the Two Parts of the Statement

Part I and Part II of the diagnostic statement should always be linked by the words "related to." This identifies a relationship between the human response and the related factors, implying that if one part of the diagnosis changes, the other part may change also.

Example

INCORRECT	CORRECT
Potential for injury caused by change in mental status	Potential for injury related to change in mental status

3. Write the Diagnosis in Legally Advisable Terms

A diagnostic statement such as "impaired skin integrity related to infrequent turning" is not legally advisable. This statement implies negligence or blame that may not be accurate and can create potential legal problems for the personnel caring for the client. This statement could be better phrased as "impaired skin integrity related to prolonged immobility." The therapeutic nursing orders would be similar in both instances, but the second statement is factual and does not imply fault.

Examples

INCORRECT	CORRECT
Potential for injury related to inadequately maintained skin traction	Potential for injury related to hazards of skin traction
Ineffective airway clearance related to excessive sedation	Ineffective airway clearance related to effects of sedation

4. Write Diagnoses Without Value Judgments

Nursing diagnoses should be based on objective and subjective data collected and validated in conjunction with the client or significant other. The behavior of the client should not be judged by the nurse's personal values and standards. Use of words such as inadequate, poor, and unhealthy in diagnostic statements frequently imply value judgments.

Examples

INCORRECT	CORRECT
Altered parenting related to poor bonding with child	Altered parenting related to prolonged separation from child
Impaired home maintenance management related to poor housekeeping habits	Impaired home maintenance management related to lack of knowledge regarding home safety measures

5. Avoid Reversing the Parts of the Statement

Remember that the first part of the diagnostic statement identifies the human response and suggests outcomes. The second part of the statement defines the related factors and suggests nursing interventions. Reversing the clauses may result in unclear communication about the client's response and its contributing factors, which makes the writing of appropriate outcomes and nursing interventions difficult.

Examples

INCORRECT	CORRECT
Sensory overload related to sleep pattern disturbance	Sleep pattern disturbance related to sensory overload
Decreased caloric intake related to altered nutrition: less than body requirements	Altered nutrition: less than body requirements related to decreased caloric intake

6. Avoid Using Single Cues in the First Part of the Statement

The first part of the diagnostic statement is derived from a cluster of signs and symptoms observed by the nurse during the assessment of the client. An isolated cue is not a nursing diagnosis, but it may provide information to help define the response. Inaccurate diagnoses may occur if the nurse focuses on an isolated sign or symptom rather than on the entire clinical picture.

Example. William Ward, an elderly client admitted to a nursing home, has a history of lung problems. The nurse observes that he is restless. Writing the diagnosis as "restlessness related to change in environment" suggests that restlessness is the response. In fact, the presence of restlessness may be a cue to other responses, such as ineffective airway clearance, altered coping, or fear.

A number of the approved diagnoses may appear to be isolated cues because of their one word titles (pain, fear, anxiety). Remember that these are diagnostic terms that refer to a phenomenon that has a number of defining characteristics. For example, some of the characteristics for the diagnosis of pain include increased blood pressure, pulse, and respiratory rate, reports of pain, clutching of painful area, and facial mask of pain.

7. The Two Parts of the Statement Should not Mean the Same Thing

In some instances, diagnostic statements are written in which the two parts are almost identical. Examine this statement: "ineffective airway clearance related to inability to clear airway." Both parts of the statement have the same meaning. This is confusing for the nurse and may result in difficulties when attempting to determine appropriate nursing interventions for the related factor. The diagnosis should be written as "ineffective airway clearance related to retained secretions."

Examples

Incorrect	Correct
Inability to feed self related to feeding problems	Feeding self-care deficit related to pain in fingers
Ineffective family coping: disabling related to inability to handle client's illness	Ineffective family coping: disabling related to lack of support systems

8. Express the Related Factor in Terms that can be Changed

Keep in mind that the diagnostic statement identifies actual or potential client responses. These responses and the factors that contribute to their existence should be changeable by interventions that are within the realm of nursing practice.

Example. Shelby Donovan is a six year old who is two days postoperative after an appendectomy. She is crying and points to the incisional area and says, "My tummy hurts." The diagnosis "pain related to surgical incision" is not accurate because nursing intervention cannot change the presence of a surgical incision. This can be restated as "pain related to the effects of surgery." Nursing interventions may relieve the effects of surgery—pain, immobility, anxiety, nausea.

Examples

INCORRECT	CORRECT
Knowledge deficit (pregnancy)	Knowledge deficit (prenatal diet)
Dysfunctional grieving related to death of spouse	Dysfunctional grieving related to perceived loss of security

9. Do Not Include Medical Diagnoses in the Nursing Diagnostic Statement

The nursing diagnostic statement differs from the medical diagnosis, since it reflects the essence of nursing rather than medical practice. The following outline demonstrates the primary differences between medical and nursing diagnoses.

MEDICAL	NURSING
Identifies a specific illness	Identifies an actual or potential response to the illness
Clinical manifestations suggest medical need	Responses suggest a nursing need
Implies associated medical interventions	Implies associated nursing interventions

The following examples compare medical and nursing diagnoses that might be found in the same client.

MEDICAL DIAGNOSIS	NURSING DIAGNOSIS
Hepatitis	Ineffective individual coping related to prolonged isolation
Diabetes Mellitus	Knowledge deficit (foot care) related to inability to retain information
Cancer	Altered oral mucous membranes related to effects of chemotherapy
Myocardial Infarction	Ineffective denial related to fear of disability

As identified previously, the medical diagnosis suggests medical interventions; therefore, its use is inappropriate in either of the two parts of the nursing diagnostic statement.

Examples

INCORRECT	CORRECT
Ineffective breathing pattern related to emphysema	Ineffective breathing pattern related to retained secretions
Congestive heart failure related to failure to take medications	Noncompliance (cardiac medications) related to lack of knowledge about action and correct dosage

10. State the Diagnosis Clearly and Concisely

Nursing diagnostic statements should be clear and concise; confusing and wordy statements tend to obscure the nurse's focus.

Example. Kathleen Inman, the mother of a premature infant, reveals that she feels that *she* caused her premature labor. "I wouldn't be in this mess if I hadn't lifted that heavy can of paint—that's why my labor started." The client states that she is concerned about her two year old son, since she spends a great deal of time at the hospital. She also indicates that she sees very little of her husband, which has created tension in their marriage.

The following are examples of diagnostic statements that could be written for this client.

INCORRECT	CORRECT
Altered interactions between husband and wife and mother and two year old son related to mother's hospital visiting patterns	Altered family processes related to mother's hospital visiting patterns
Ineffective individual coping related to belief that she caused the onset of premature labor by lifting heavy paint can on day of delivery	Ineffective individual coping related to feelings of guilt

Neither of the incorrect examples shown is clear or concise. Although the client's comments are cues that suggest disrupted family interactions and feelings of guilt, it is not necessary to include her entire statements in the nursing diagnoses.

Clear and concise diagnostic statements facilitate communication and allow the nurse to concentrate on the client's response and the related factors. This approach promotes quality, individualized nursing care.

VARIATIONS OF THE DIAGNOSTIC STATEMENT

There are three common variations of the diagnostic statement including many related factors, unknown related factors, and one-part statements.

Many Related Factors

Clients' health care problems are rarely simple. The responses seen in clients frequently have a number of related factors that contribute to their existence. For example, fluid volume excess may be related to excessive salt intake, increased fluid intake, or failure to take a diuretic.

Example.   Although Jose Esposito is hypertensive, when admitted to the hospital he tells the nurse that he has discontinued his medication because it was interfering with his sex life. He is 5 ft 4 in and weighs 190 lb. In reviewing the client's typical eating habits, the nurse determines that his caloric intake is excessive. Jose also indicates that his favorite leisure activities are watching TV and drinking beer. He also smokes three packs of cigarettes daily.

In Jose's case, obesity, smoking, and discontinuance of the antihypertensive medication are all contributing to his hypertension. This illustrates the complex nature of his illness. Imagine how redundant the client's plan of care would be if each of the related factors were identified in a separate nursing diagnosis.

"Altered health maintenance related to lack of knowledge of effects of medication on hypertension."
"Altered health maintenance related to lack of knowledge of effects of smoking on hypertension."
"Altered health maintenance related to lack of knowledge of effects of obesity on hypertension."

Combination of all of the factors related to Jose's hypertension allows the nurse to develop one comprehensive diagnosis. This will encourage the implementation of a number of nursing interventions to effectively manage this client's response to his illness. Jose's diagnosis should be written as:

"Altered health related to lack of knowledge of effects of medication, smoking, and obesity on hypertension."

At times, the second part of the diagnostic statement, the related factors may be divided into two parts to provide additional information. When this is done, the words "secondary to" or the abbreviation "2°" are used.

Examples

Fluid volume deficit related to decreased intake of oral fluids secondary to weakness.
Altered nutrition: less than body requirements related to decreased appetite 2° to effects of medication.

Unknown Related Factors

At times the factors related to the existence of a particular client response may be unclear or unknown. It is acceptable to include the words "related to unknown factors" while continuing to identify or define the causative factors.

Examples

Pain related to unknown factors
Chronic low self-esteem related to unknown factors

One-Part Statements

Usually nursing diagnoses are two-part statements joined by the words "related to." A few nursing diagnoses may be written as one-part statements without the words "related to" or identified related factors. This usually occurs when the related factors are obvious or implied.

Examples

Rape-trauma syndrome
Post-trauma response

In the case of a person who is experiencing the signs of a traumatic response to being raped, it is usually clearly evident that the difficulties expressed by the client are the result of the rape. In this situation, it may not be necessary to identify rape as the related factor. Similarly, in the case of "post-trauma response," even though there may be numerous events that could precipitate this response, if the factor is known to all nurses caring for the client, it may not be necessary to identify it in the diagnostic statement. When there is any question about identification of the related factor, it should be included.

VALIDATION OF THE DIAGNOSIS

The third step in the diagnostic process is validation. Before committing the diagnosis to paper, it is helpful to verify its accuracy. This can be accomplished by asking the following questions:

☐ Is the data base sufficient and accurate?

☐ Is there a pattern of cues that suggest the selected diagnosis?

☐ Are the cues used to determine the existence of the human response consistent with its defining characteristics?

☐ Have related factors been identified that contribute to the existence of the response?

☐ Can the nursing diagnosis be altered by nursing interventions?

☐ Would other nurses formulate the same nursing diagnosis based on the data?

After asking these questions, the nurse should validate the diagnosis with the client by describing what the nurse perceives the responses to be. The client should be asked if these are things of concern. If the concerns of the nurse and the client are not in agreement, the dialogue should continue until some consensus is reached.

DOCUMENTATION

After developing and verifying the nursing diagnostic statement, it is documented in the client's medical record by the nurse. The location may vary according to the agency, and institutional policies or guidelines should be followed. Most commonly, the nursing diagnosis is documented on the care plan, nurses' notes, progress notes, discharge summaries, and interagency referral forms. Diagnostic statements should be reviewed at intervals and revised or eliminated as necessary.

SUMMARY

To summarize, nursing diagnostic statements are the outcome of the diagnostic process and consist of two parts joined by the words "related to." The first part identifies the human responses to health or illness which may be prevented, altered, or alleviated by nursing intervention. This part is the basis for client-centered outcomes by which progress can be measured.

The second part of the diagnostic statement includes the related factors that contribute to the existence of the client's response. This part suggests nursing interventions that may be utilized to manage the client's care. Writing diagnostic statements is a skill that requires practice and may be facilitated by the use of consistent guidelines. A variety of resources are available to assist the nurse in acquiring these skills.

The Nursing Diagnosis Journal, published by the Clearinghouse for Nursing Diagnoses at St. Louis University, assists NANDA to share information about nursing diagnoses. The journal encourages nurses to ask questions, exchange views, submit articles, and share experiences on the impact of diagnoses in practice, research, and education. Nurses may subscribe to the journal by contacting North American Nursing Diagnosis Association, St. Louis University Department of Nursing, 3525 Caroline Street, St. Louis, MO 63104.

A number of handbooks have been developed—Taptich (1989), Gordon (1989), and Kim (1989)—that are helpful in formulating nursing diagnoses according to the NANDA system. Each of these sources include the approved diagnoses, definitions, defining characteristics, and related factors.

Completed diagnostic statements should be validated with the client whenever possible and documented in the medical record.

In review, here are the guidelines for writing a nursing diagnostic statement.

1. Write the diagnosis in terms of the client's response rather than nursing need.

2. Use "related to" rather than "due to" or "caused by" to connect the two parts of the statement.

3. Write the diagnosis in legally advisable terms.

4. Write diagnoses without value judgments.

5. Avoid reversing the parts of the statement.

6. Avoid using single cues in the first part of the statement.

7. The two parts of the statement should not mean the same thing.

8. Express the related factor in terms that can be changed.

9. Do not include medical diagnoses in the diagnostic statement.

10. State the diagnosis clearly and concisely.

The following three exercises provide the opportunity to apply the concepts discussed in this chapter. Additional exercises may be found in Appendix G.

4–1 TEST YOURSELF

IDENTIFICATION OF CORRECTLY AND INCORRECTLY WRITTEN DIAGNOSES

The following is a list of nursing diagnostic statements. Decide whether each statement is correctly or incorrectly written. If incorrectly stated, identify the rule(s) violated, by number, from the preceding list.

	Correct	Incorrect	Rule
1. Knowledge deficit related to lack of knowledge of antihypertensive medications			
2. Needs skin care			
3. Fluid volume deficit related to decreased oral intake			
4. Situational low self-esteem caused by effects of relocation			
5. Altered nutrition: more than body requirements related to poor eating habits			
6. Potential for violence related to spouse's continuous verbal threats, arguing, belittling remarks, and physical beatings			

	Correct	Incorrect	Rule
7. Spiritual distress related to separation from religious ties			
8. Chronic pain related to arthritis			
9. Dysfunctional grieving related to death of spouse			
10. Decreased level of consciousness related to potential for aspiration			
11. Fear related to perceived threat of death			
12. Potential for trauma due to cataract surgery and corneal transplant			
13. Dribbling and diminished force of urinary stream related to urinary retention			
14. Altered role performance related to effects of change in health status			
15. Altered thought processes related to impaired thinking			
16. Poor hygiene related to laziness			
17. Potential for infection related to poor use of aseptic technique by staff			
18. Altered protection related to ineffective protective mechanisms			
19. Effective breastfeeding related to previous positive experiences			
20. Constipation related to effects of codeine			

4–1 TEST YOURSELF □ ANSWERS

GUIDELINES FOR WRITING NURSING DIAGNOSES

1. Write the diagnosis in terms of the client's response rather than nursing need.
2. Use "related to" rather than "due to" or "caused by" to connect the two parts of the statement.
3. Write the diagnosis in legally advisable terms.
4. Write diagnoses without value judgments.
5. Avoid reversing the two parts of the statement.
6. Avoid using single cues in the first part of the statement.
7. Be sure that the two parts of the statement do not mean the same thing.
8. Express the related factor in terms that can be changed.
9. Do not include medical diagnoses in the diagnostic statement.
10. State the diagnosis clearly and concisely.

	Correct	Incorrect	Rule
1. Knowledge deficit related to lack of knowledge of antihypertensive medications		✔	7
2. Needs skin care		✔	1
3. Fluid volume deficit related to decreased oral intake	✔		
4. Situational low self-esteem caused by effects of relocation		✔	2
5. Altered nutrition: more than body requirements related to poor eating habits		✔	4
6. Potential for violence related to spouse's continuous verbal threats, arguing, belittling remarks, and physical beatings		✔	10
7. Spiritual distress related to separation from religious ties	✔		
8. Chronic pain related to arthritis		✔	9
9. Dysfunctional grieving related to death of spouse		✔	8
10. Decreased level of consciousness related to potential for aspiration		✔	5
11. Fear related to perceived threat of death	✔		
12. Potential for trauma due to cataract surgery and corneal transplant		✔	2,8
13. Dribbling and diminished force of urinary stream related to urinary retention		✔	5,6

14. Altered role performance   ✔
    related to effects of change
    in health status
15. Altered thought processes   ✔   7
    related to impaired thinking
16. Poor hygiene related to   ✔   4
    laziness
17. Potential for infection   ✔   3
    related to poor use of
    aseptic technique by staff
18. Altered protection related to   ✔
    ineffective protective
    mechanisms
19. Effective breastfeeding   ✔
    related to previous posture
    experiences
20. Constipation related to   ✔
    effects of codeine

4–2 TEST YOURSELF

REVISION OF INCORRECTLY WRITTEN DIAGNOSES

The nursing diagnoses that were incorrectly written in the previous exercise are listed below. Revise each statement to make it correct.

STATEMENT   REVISION

1. Knowledge deficit related to lack of
   knowledge of antihypertensive
   medications
2. Needs skin care
3. Situational low self-esteem caused by
   effects of relocation
4. Altered nutrition: more than body
   requirements related to poor eating
   habits
5. Potential for violence related to spouse's
   continuous verbal threats, arguing,
   belittling remarks, and physical beatings
6. Chronic pain related to arthritis
7. Dysfunctional grieving related to death
   of spouse
8. Decreased level of consciousness related
   to potential for aspiration
9. Potential for trauma due to cataract
   surgery and corneal transplant
10. Dribbling and diminished force of
    urinary stream related to urinary
    retention
11. Altered thought processes related to
    impaired thinking
12. Poor hygiene related to laziness
13. Potential for infection related to poor use
    of aseptic technique by staff
14. Altered protection related to ineffective
    protective mechanisms

107

4–2 TEST YOURSELF □ ANSWERS

There are a number of ways to revise the nursing diagnoses listed in this exercise. One example of a corrected revision for each diagnostic statement is provided below.

STATEMENT	REVISION
1. Knowledge deficit related to lack of knowledge of antihypertensive medications	Knowledge deficit (antihypertensive medications) related to language barrier
2. Needs skin care	Impaired skin integrity related to immobility
3. Situational low self-esteem caused by effects of relocation	Situational low self-esteem related to effects of relocation
4. Altered nutrition: more than body requirements related to poor eating habits	Altered nutrition: more than body requirements related to excessive caloric intake
5. Potential for violence related to spouse's continuous verbal threats, arguing, belittling remarks, and physical beatings	Potential for violence related to recurrent physical and emotional abuse
6. Chronic pain related to arthritis	Chronic pain related to effects of inflammatory process
7. Dysfunctional grieving related to death of spouse	Dysfunctional grieving related to lack of support systems
8. Decreased level of consciousness related to potential for aspiration	Potential for aspiration related to decreased level of consciousness
9. Potential for trauma due to cataract surgery and corneal transplant	Potential for trauma related to impaired perception
10. Dribbling and diminished force of urinary stream related to urinary retention	Urinary retention related to effects of anesthesia
11. Altered thought processes related to impaired thinking	Altered thought processes related to sensory overload
12. Poor hygiene related to laziness	Bathing/hygiene self-care deficit related to lack of access to running water
13. Potential for infection related to poor use of aseptic technique by staff	Potential for infection related to hazards associated with invasive monitoring
14. Altered protection related to ineffective protective mechanisms	Altered protection related to side effects of chemotherapy

 4–3 TEST YOURSELF

Develop correctly written nursing diagnoses for each of the case studies presented below by identifying significant cues/clusters and comparing them with the defining characteristics if possible. Use the guidelines listed previously to correctly phrase the diagnosis. Refer to Appendix F for definitions of the NANDA diagnoses.

#1 Cassie Tilton is an 88 year old woman transferred to your unit from a skilled nursing facility. Her history reveals that she had a "flu-like" syndrome for the past five days with persistent vomiting and diarrhea. Her vital signs are: B/P 108/56, pulse 112, respirations 28, and temperature 101.4°F. Her mucous membranes are dry and her skin turgor is decreased. She indicates that she feels weak, tired, and thirsty.

CUES/CLUSTERS

NURSING DIAGNOSIS:

#2 Chip Ireland is a 35 year old businessman admitted to the outpatient surgicenter for a tonsillectomy. He indicates that he has had recurrent tonsillitis for the last three years. Postoperatively, he complains of being thirsty and requests a cold drink. You observe that he has difficulty swallowing and coughs up the water. He states "my throat is too sore; it feels like it is swollen." Upon examination, you note the presence of redness and edema in the operative area.

CUES/CLUSTERS

NURSING DIAGNOSIS:

#3 Dave Davis, a 54 year old self-employed mechanic, is admitted to your unit at 6:00 AM for an elective cholecystectomy. During your assessment, you observe that he is unusually apprehensive, moderately diaphoretic, restless, and pacing around the room. His voice trembles as he tells you that he has never had surgery before and states "my brother had a simple appendectomy when he was 18 and died on the table; nothing they did could save him."

CUES/CLUSTERS

NURSING DIAGNOSIS:

#4 Emily Fantin is an 86 year old woman who calls the office nurse and requests free samples of laxatives. She complains "I've spent so much money on laxatives at the drug store. I take them twice a day so that my bowels will move three times a day. My mother always told me to take laxatives to keep myself regular. By the way, do you have any sample enemas?"

CUES/CLUSTERS

NURSING DIAGNOSIS:

4–3 TEST YOURSELF □ ANSWERS

#1 Cassie Tilton is an 88 year old woman transferred to your unit from a skilled nursing facility. Her history reveals that she had a "flu-like" syndrome for the past five days with persistent vomiting and diarrhea. Her vital signs are: B/P 108/56, pulse 112, respirations 28, and temperature 101.4°F. Her mucous membranes are dry and her skin turgor is decreased. She indicates that she feels weak, tired, and thirsty.

CUES/CLUSTERS
Weakness
Tired
Thirst
Dry mucous membranes
Decreased skin turgor
Temperature 101.4°F
Low B/P 108/56
Pulse 112
Respirations 28
History of vomiting/diarrhea for five days

NURSING DIAGNOSIS: Fluid volume deficit related to vomiting and diarrhea

#2 Chip Ireland is a 35 year old businessman admitted to the outpatient surgicenter for a tonsillectomy. He indicates that he has had recurrent tonsillitis for the last three years. Postoperative, he complains of being thirsty and requests a cold drink. You observe that he has difficulty swallowing and coughs up the water. He states "my throat is too sore; it feels like it is swollen." Upon examination, you note the presence of redness and edema in the operative area.

CUES/CLUSTERS
Observed difficulty in swallowing
Cough
Complaints of sore throat
States "feels swollen"

NURSING DIAGNOSIS: Impaired swallowing related to edema, effects of surgery

#3 Dave Davis, a 54 year old self-employed mechanic, is admitted to your unit at 6:00 AM for an elective cholecystectomy. During your assessment, you observe that he is unusually apprehensive, moderately diaphoretic, restless, and pacing around the room. His vital signs are: B/P 156/88, pulse 108, respirations 28. His voice trembles as he tells you that he has never had surgery before and states "my brother has a simple appendectomy when he was 18 and died on the table; nothing they did could save him."

CUES/CLUSTERS
Apprehension
B/P 156/88
Pulse 108

Respirations 28
Diaphoresis
Pacing
Voice tremors
Increased verbalization

NURSING DIAGNOSIS: Fear related to perceived threat of death

#4 Emily Fantin is an 86 year old woman who calls the office nurse and requests free samples of laxatives. She complains "I've spent so much money on laxatives at the drug store. I take them twice a day so that my bowels will move three times a day. My mothers always told me to take laxatives to keep myself regular. By the way, do you have any sample enemas?" Upon further questioning you find out that Emily lives alone and does her own cooking. She eats mostly frozen dinners or prepared foods with few fruits and vegetables. In addition, she shops at a local convenience store with a limited supply of fresh produce. She relies on Metamucil daily, and Ex Lax and Milk of Magnesia approximately four times a week. She states that she gets very little exercise.

CUES/CLUSTERS
Expectation of bowel movement three times daily
Takes over-the-counter laxatives
Requesting enemas

NURSING DIAGNOSIS: Perceived constipation related to long-standing family health beliefs

REFERENCES

Carroll-Johnson RM (ed): Classification of Nursing Diagnoses: Proceedings of the Eighth Conference. Philadelphia: JB Lippincott, 1989.

Gordon M: Manual of Nursing Diagnosis. New York: McGraw-Hill, 1989.

Kim MJ, McFarland GK, and McLane AM: Pocket Guide to Nursing Diagnosis, 3rd ed. St. Louis: CV Mosby, 1989.

Taptich BJ, Iyer P, and Bernocchi-Losey D: Nursing Diagnosis and Care Planning. Philadelphia: WB Saunders, 1989.

BIBLIOGRAPHY

Creason N: How do we define our diagnoses? American Journal of Nursing 1987; 87(2):230–231.

Fehring RJ: Methods to validate nursing diagnoses. Heart Lung 16(6):625–629.

Mundinger M, and Jauron G: Developing a Nursing Diagnosis. Nursing Outlook 23(2):94–98.

Neel C: Making nursing diagnosis work for you . . . every day. Nursing 1986; 86(5):56–57.

Porter EJ: Critical analysis of NANDA Nursing Diagnosis Taxonomy. Image Journal of Nursing Scholarship 18(4):136–139.

Price M: Nursing diagnosis: making a concept come alive. American Journal of Nursing 80(4):668–671.

Woodtli AO: Validation of defining characteristics: clinical design. Journal of Neuroscience Nursing 20(5):324–326.

5

PLANNING—Priority Setting and Developing Outcomes

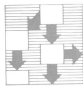

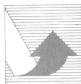

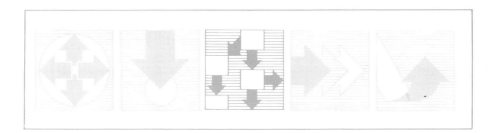

INTRODUCTION

Planning involves the development of strategies designed to reinforce healthy client responses or to prevent, minimize, or correct unhealthy client responses identified in the nursing diagnosis. This phase begins after the formulation of the diagnostic statement and concludes with the actual documentation of the plan of care.

During the planning phase, outcomes and nursing interventions are developed. The outcomes indicate what the client will be able to do as a result of the nursing actions. The nursing interventions describe how the nurse can assist the client to achieve the outcomes.

The planning component of the nursing process consists of four stages:

1. Setting priorities
2. Developing outcomes
3. Developing nursing interventions
4. Documenting the plan

This chapter will address the first two stages—priority-setting and developing outcomes. Chapter 6 will discuss nursing interventions and documentation.

STAGE 1—SETTING PRIORITIES

A thorough nursing assessment may identify many actual or potential responses that require nursing intervention, as shown in Chapter 4. The development of a plan incorporating all of these may be unrealistic or unmanageable. Therefore, a system must be established to determine which diagnosis or diagnoses will be addressed first. One such mechanism is the human needs hierarchy.

Maslow's Hierarchy

Abraham Maslow (1943) described human needs on five levels—physiological, safety or security, social, esteem, and self-actualization (Fig. 5–1). He suggested that the client progresses up the hierarchy when attempting to satisfy needs. In other words, physiological needs are generally of greater priority to the client than the others. Therefore, when these basic needs are unsatisfied, the client may be unwilling or unable to deal with higher level needs.

Kalish's Hierarchy

Richard Kalish (1983) further refined Maslow's system by dividing physiological needs into survival needs and stimulation needs (Fig. 5–2). This division is particularly useful in assisting the nurse to prioritize client needs.

FIGURE 5–1. Maslow's model. (From Maslow A: A theory of human motivation. Psychol Rev 50:370, 1943.)

FIGURE 5–2. Kalish's refinement of Maslow's model. (From Kalish R: The Psychology of Human Behavior, 5th ed. Copyright 1983, 1977, 1973, 1970, 1966 by Wadsworth, Inc. Reprinted by permission of Brooks/Cole Monterey, CA.)

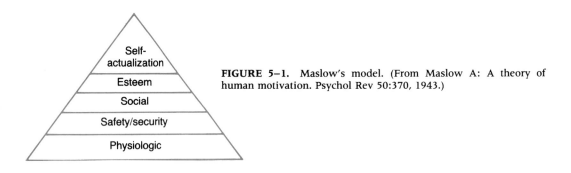

Physiological
Survival Needs

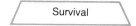

Kalish identified survival needs as those for food, air, water, manageable temperature, elimination, rest, and pain avoidance. When a deficit occurs in any of these areas, the client tends to utilize all available resources to satisfy that particular need. Only then is it possible to be concerned about higher level needs, such as security or esteem.

For this reason, the confused client with an oxygen (air) deficit may continuously climb out of bed to open the window in a hospital room. The basic need for oxygen supersedes concerns about safety. Likewise, the individual who has not slept for three days because of anxiety may not be able to focus on preoperative teaching, even though such information is particularly important for safety in the postoperative period.

Examples of survival needs in nursing diagnostic statements include

Food	Altered nutrition: less than body requirements related to decreased appetite
Air	Impaired gas exchange related to retained secretions
Water	Fluid volume deficit related to persistent vomiting
Temperature	Hyperthermia related to effects of prolonged exposure to heat
Elimination	Diarrhea related to effects of antibiotic therapy
Rest	Sleep pattern disturbance related to excessive noise
Pain	Pain related to muscle spasms

Stimulation Needs

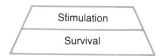

Kalish suggests that stimulation needs include those related to sex, activity, exploration, manipulation, and novelty. When survival needs are met, the client will attempt to satisfy stimulation needs before moving up the hierarchy. For this reason, the younger client who is hospitalized for a prolonged period of time in a psychiatric setting may be unable to focus on therapy when strong sexual urges remain unsatisfied. Similarly, the client who is required to maintain prolonged bedrest at home may require frequent diversionary activities to suppress the desire to get out of bed.

Examples of stimulation needs in nursing diagnostic statements include

Sex	Sexual dysfunction related to discomfort secondary to decreased vaginal secretions

Activity	Diversional activity deficit related to effects of hospitalization
Exploration	Impaired physical mobility related to effects of right-sided weakness
Manipulation	Self-care deficit related to early morning pain secondary to inflammatory process
Novelty	Altered sensory perception related to stimulus deprivation secondary to isolation

Case Study

Mr. Ted Alexander, a 50 year old white divorced salesman from Las Vegas, was on a business trip to Atlantic City when he developed pain in the right lower abdominal quadrant. He took Alka-Seltzer with little relief, and the pain persisted for the next two days. He was busy with appointments during the day and evening and was able to ignore the pain. He ate very little and took two sleeping pills at night. On the afternoon of the third day, the pain became much more intense, and when it continued for several hours and he began to vomit repeatedly, he went to the emergency department.

Physical examination and laboratory data at this time revealed an alert, well-groomed male with generalized abdominal tenderness, rigidity of the abdominal wall, presence of a palpable mass in the right inguinal area, absent bowel sounds, and a white blood count (WBC) of $20,000/mm^3$ (normal = $5000-9000/mm^3$). The diagnosis of ruptured appendix was made. He was admitted to the hospital for initial medical management, with surgery anticipated at a later date.

Your examination of the patient reveals the following: B/P = 140/80 mm Hg, P = 116 beats/minute, R = 26 breaths/minute, T = 101.2° F. The patient indicates that he is 6 ft, 2 in tall and weighs 196 lb. He is alert and oriented and states, "My gut is killing me." His skin is warm to the touch and slightly diaphoretic. The patient states that he had been a heavy drinker for 15 years and was admitted to the hospital with cirrhosis two years ago by his family doctor, Dr. Martland, but has never had surgery. He denies drinking for the past two years but smokes two packs of cigarettes daily.

Mr. Alexander is tense throughout your conversation but shares a number of concerns with you, including his separation from his two teenage children who live with him. He is also anxious about being cared for by an unfamiliar physician. The ED nurse indicates that he wears contact lenses and is concerned because he has left his case and supplies as well as his glasses in his hotel. He gives you $750.00 in cash and traveler's checks to deposit in the hospital safe. He has a partial lower plate of dentures and caps on his four front teeth. Further inquiry reveals that the patient prefers a low-fat diet, occasionally uses laxatives, and has had several occurrences of urinary urgency and nocturia in the last six months.

> The physician states that his treatment plan includes gastric suction, antibiotics, and IV fluid therapy with electrolytes and vitamins until the patient is stabilized enough for exploratory surgery. Mr. Alexander agrees to this plan but is concerned about his job demands and wonders how he will deal with "getting back home when all of this is over."

In this example, the primary physiological need is pain management. The client who experiences pain is frequently unable to deal with higher level concerns. Note that the client verbalized this need in very concrete terms ("My gut is killing me") early in the interviewing process. This is frequently the case, since the physiological need is the most important reason for the client's visit to the physician's office or to the hospital. *Nursing diagnosis: "pain related to inflammatory process."*

Safety

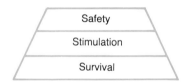

The next levels in the hierarchy are the needs for safety, security, and protection. These become of particular concern to the client when physiological needs have been satisfied. Safety needs are particularly evident in the elderly or very young when they are placed in an unfamiliar environment. Children frequently require the presence of a favorite toy or blanket for security. The elderly client may be at risk for falls, bruises, and the like while trying to adapt to the strangeness of a nursing home environment.

Some examples of diagnostic statements incorporating safety needs include

Security	Impaired home maintenance management related to insufficient finances
Safety	Potential for trauma related to lack of awareness of environmental hazards
Protection	Potential for violence: self-directed related to feelings of hopelessness

Mr. Alexander's concern about being managed by an unfamiliar physician reflects a security need. He has verbalized confidence in his family physician who is 3000 miles away but faces major surgery by a surgeon who is basically unknown to him. Additionally, Mr. Alexander has never had surgery and may be concerned about his safety during the surgical experience. *Nursing diagnoses: "potential for ineffective individual coping related to separation from support systems"; "knowledge deficit (surgical experience)."*

Love and Belonging

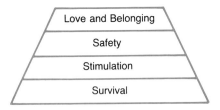

Maslow's social needs are described by Kalish as the necessity for love and a sense of belonging or closeness. These needs reflect a person's ability to affiliate or interact with others in the environment and are met through involvement with family, friends, and coworkers. The nurse frequently identifies social deficits in clients requiring prolonged hospitalization, those isolated for protection or because of infection, and those placed in such areas as critical care units, where visiting privileges may be restricted.

Examples of nursing diagnoses reflecting love and belonging needs include

Love	Altered parenting related to impaired maternal-infant bonding
Belonging	Altered family processes related to effects of terminal illness
Closeness	Social isolation related to prolonged hospitalization

Mr. Alexander has verbalized his concern about being separated from his children during hospitalization. This reflects his parental role and the need for interaction with his children. Fulfillment of this need may be particularly difficult because of the children's location. *Nursing diagnosis: "potential altered in parenting related to separation from children."*

Esteem

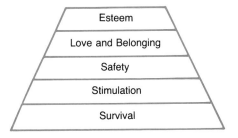

The need for the respect of oneself and others is reflected in this level of the hierarchy. The individual strives for recognition, usefulness, independence, dignity, and freedom. The client's position in the health care system frequently leads to deficits in these areas. Clients may unnecessarily surrender responsibility for elements of daily care to the nurse. Examples might include those who expect the nurse to pour their water, comb their hair, or shave them because they are in a hospital when, in fact, they are capable of self-care.

Examples of nursing diagnoses reflecting esteem needs include "powerlessness related to perceived lack of support systems"; "dysfunctional grieving related to change in body image secondary to mastectomy"; and "personal identity disturbance related to persistent peer pressure."

In Mr. Alexander's case, the need for esteem is demonstrated by his concern about his job demands. *Nursing diagnosis: "situational low self-esteem related to fear of prolonged disability."*

Self-Actualization

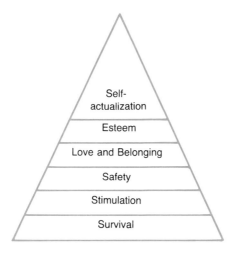

The highest level need is self-actualization, or the need "to make the most of your physical, mental, emotional and social competencies in order to feel that you are being the sort of person you wish to be" (Kalish, 1983). Clients wish to function according to a lifestyle that utilizes their individual knowledge, talents, and skills. Clients in a hospital setting are frequently not concerned with self-actualization needs, since they are preoccupied with fulfilling lower level needs. However, clients may demonstrate concerns about their ability to achieve self-actualization as a result of changes that may have occurred during hospitalization. Nurses who work with clients in other settings, such as in clients' homes, physicians' offices, and health maintenance organizations, may see clients who are focusing on self-fulfillment. This is possible because their needs for survival, stimulation, and safety are being satisfied. Therefore, they are able to focus on esteem and self-actualization.

Examples of nursing diagnoses that relate to self-actualization include "altered thought processes related to effects of alcohol consumption"; "impaired verbal communication related to effects of expressive aphasia"; "potential for violence directed at others related to inability to control behavior"; and "family coping: potential for growth related to successful development of coping skills."

Mr. Alexander has verbalized concern about the effects of the impending surgery on his role as salesman. This reflects a need for self-actualization. *Nursing diagnosis: "potential ineffective individual coping related to possible role changes."*

Maslow's hierarchy provides a constructive resource for the nurse to utilize in setting priorities. Kalish's expansion of Maslow's model assists the nurse in differentiating more clearly between levels of physiological needs. Ordinarily, clients progress up the hierarchy of needs. For example, they attempt to satisfy survival needs before focusing on security or esteem. However, it is important to note that clients may have unsatisfied needs on more than one level at the same time. Lower level needs do not have to be completely resolved before the client begins to address higher level needs.

Example. Victor Klein, a 48 year old man, is admitted to the hospital with a diagnosis of pneumonia. He exhibits an elevated temperature and is dehydrated. He verbalizes concern about his disabled wife who is confined to bed at home. Additionally, he is self-employed.

In this example, the client has simultaneous survival, security, and love or belonging needs. Mr. Klein's immediate concerns relate to his temperature and fluid problems (survival needs). However, these do not have to be completely resolved before he begins to develop strategies to deal with his anxieties about his job (security) and his disabled wife (love and belonging).

5–1 TEST YOURSELF

IDENTIFICATION OF NEEDS

Utilizing Maslow's Hierarchy, identify the type of need being addressed in each of the following nursing diagnostic statements.

NURSING DIAGNOSIS	NEED
1. Potential for violence directed at others related to effects of hallucinations	
2. Role performance disturbance related to effects of chronic pain	
3. Ineffective family coping: disabling related to recurrent marital discord	
4. Sleep pattern disturbance related to sensory overload	
5. Diversional activity deficit related to long-term confinement to home	
6. Spiritual distress related to inability to practice spiritual rituals	
7. Knowledge deficit (signs of hypoglycemia)	
8. Chronic low self-esteem related to obesity	
9. Social isolation related to lack of transportation	

5–1 TEST YOURSELF □ ANSWERS

NURSING DIAGNOSIS	NEED
1. Potential for violence directed at others related to effects of hallucinations	Safety/security
2. Role performance disturbance related to effects of chronic pain	Esteem
3. Ineffective family coping: disabling related to recurrent marital discord	Love and belonging
4. Sleep pattern disturbance related to sensory overload	Physiological (survival)
5. Diversional activity deficit related to long-term confinement to home	Physiological (stimulation)
6. Spiritual distress related to inability to practice spiritual rituals	Self-actualization
7. Knowledge deficit (signs of hypoglycemia)	Safety/security
8. Chronic low self-esteem related to obesity	Esteem
9. Social isolation related to lack of transportation	Love and belonging

STAGE 2—GUIDELINES FOR WRITING OUTCOMES

Outcomes are an important component of the planning phase of the nursing process. Outcomes are also referred to as goals or behavioral objectives. Regardless of what they are called, their purpose is the same—they define how the nurse and the client know that the human response identified in the diagnostic statement has been prevented, modified, or corrected. Therefore, outcomes also serve as a blueprint for the evaluation component of the process because well-written outcomes make it possible to determine the effectiveness of nursing interventions.

The following guidelines will help to develop well-written outcomes.

1. Outcomes Should be Related to the Human Response

Nursing diagnostic statements identify actual or potential responses that are considered to be problematic for the client. This implies that alternative responses are required or preferred. For example, the nursing diagnosis "altered nutrition: less than body requirements related to chewing difficulties" suggests that the nutritional status of the client is less than optimal. This diagnosis indicates that improved nutrition is required. Similarly, the nursing diagnosis "potential for infection related to prolonged weakness and immobility" suggests that the client is at risk for infection and requires nursing intervention or assistance to prevent its occurrence.

Outcomes should reflect the first half of the diagnostic statement by identifying alternative healthful responses that are desirable for the client. Outcomes also help to define specific behaviors that demonstrate that the problem has been prevented, minimized, or corrected. Answering the question "How will I know that the response has been changed? The client will be able to . . ." will help to determine appropriate outcomes.

Examples

Nursing Diagnosis: Altered nutrition: less than body requirements related to chewing difficulties (broken dentures)

OUTCOME:

Incorrect	Correct
No evidence of skin breakdown throughout hospitalization	Consumes 1800 calories of pureed and liquid foods each 24 hour period

Nursing Diagnosis: Potential for infection related to prolonged weakness and immobility

OUTCOME:

Incorrect	Correct
Verbalizes decreased weakness within 24 hours	No evidence of infection throughout hospitalization

In the first example above, the incorrectly stated outcome refers to skin integrity rather than to nutritional status. Certainly, there is a relationship between decreased nutritional status and the potential for skin breakdown. However, the correctly written outcome more appropriately answers the question "How will I know that the client's nutritional status is improved?" This outcome not only identifies the desirable limits of caloric intake for the client but also specifies that this intake be accomplished within each 24 hour period. In the second example, the outcome is related to the second part of the diagnostic statement, referring to "weakness" rather than to the potential for infection. The correctly written outcome also demonstrates a broader, more long-term outcome than in the 24 hour period seen in the previous example.

2. Outcomes Should be Client-Centered

Generally, outcomes are written to focus on the behavior of the client. The outcome should address what the client will do and when and to what extent it will be accomplished.

Examples

Consider the case of an 82 year old woman who falls and fractures her hip. Because she will be on bedrest and unable to ambulate and move in her usual patterns, she is at risk for skin breakdown.

Nursing Diagnosis: Potential impaired skin integrity related to decreased mobility.

OUTCOME:

Incorrect	Correct
Prevent skin breakdown	No evidence of skin breakdown over bony prominences throughout hospitalization

The incorrectly written outcome is nurse-focused rather than client-centered. The correctly written outcome clearly identifies the criterion that will be used to determine whether or not the client's skin integrity has been maintained.

Occasionally, outcomes are written for others when the client is unable to participate. In the case of five year old David, a newly diagnosed insulin-dependent diabetic, his mother was identified as the person who will administer David's insulin until he is old enough to be taught to self-inject.

NURSING DIAGNOSIS	OUTCOME
Knowledge deficit (insulin injection technique)	Prior to discharge, David's mother will demonstrate correct insulin injection technique

3. Outcomes Should be Clear and Concise

A clearly written outcome enhances communication among caregivers and promotes continuity of care. Ambiguous or abstract wording should be avoided because it will tend to confuse rather than help the staff caring for a client. Simple terms and standard terminology will also help.

Examples

Nursing Diagnosis: Ineffective airway clearance related to retained secretions.

OUTCOME:

Incorrect	Correct
CDBPD indep q2	Coughs, deep breathes, and performs postural drainage independently q2h

Outcomes should have as few words as possible yet still be clear. Long, involved outcomes can frequently be stated in fewer words. Compare the following outcomes. Which meets the criteria for being clear and concise?

Nursing Diagnosis: Knowledge deficit (hospitalization and surgical experience)

OUTCOME:

Incorrect	Correct
The client will discuss expectations of this hospitalization and previous hospital admissions and will discuss impending surgery with a basic knowledge of pre and postop care	Prior to surgery, discusses expectations of hospitalization and surgery

When writing outcomes, it is possible to eliminate the words "the client will . . ." at the beginning. It should be obvious from the way the outcome is stated that it is referring to the behaviors that the client will exhibit. Again, the outcome may include family members or others instead of or in addition to the client's behavior.

Nursing Diagnosis	Outcome
Ineffective family coping: compromised related to effects of child's chronic illness	Prior to discharge, Manuel's mother discusses her feelings of inadequacy

4. Outcomes Should Describe Behavior that is Measurable and Observable

Outcomes should address what the client will do, when it will be accomplished, and to what extent. Observable and measurable outcomes define the "what" and "to what extent."

Examples

Nursing Diagnosis: Noncompliance (1800 calorie ADA diet)

OUTCOME:

Incorrect	Correct
Appreciates importance of adhering to 1800 calorie ADA diet	Prior to discharge, states importance of adhering to 1800 calorie ADA diet

It is difficult to evaluate an individual's appreciation of an activity. The client's recognition and acceptance of the behavior can be measured by statements or other similar responses.

When outcomes are measurable, observations can be made to determine whether they have been achieved. Compare the following and note that the second example is both measurable and observable.

Nursing Diagnosis: Fluid volume deficit related to excessive diaphoresis

OUTCOME:

Incorrect	Correct
Drinks adequate amounts of fluids	Drinks 2000 ml in 24 hours

Sometimes nurses write outcomes that are too broad or vague, that may need to be broken down into more specific components.

Nursing Diagnosis: Knowledge deficit (disease process)

OUTCOME:

Incorrect	Correct
After the third teaching session:	After the third teaching session:
Knows about condition (angina)	Lists the cause of angina
	Identifies steps to alleviate pain
	Describes three activities that reduce anginal episodes

5. Outcomes Should be Realistic

The outcomes developed by the nurse should be achievable considering the resources of the client, nursing staff, and the setting. The client's ability to achieve outcomes may be affected by many factors including finances, level of intelligence, and emotional or physical condition.

Example. A diabetic hindered by a low income may be unable to purchase a home glucose monitoring system. Therefore, it may be unrealistic to write an outcome and develop a teaching plan encouraging the use of this system.

The strengths and weaknesses of the nursing staff should be considered when formulating outcomes. Factors to evaluate may include the nurses' level of knowledge, autonomy, and availability.

Example.   A woman who is pregnant with triplets is admitted to an obstetrical unit. None of the nurses working in the department have cared for a similar client. The perinatal clinical specialist has knowledge of the special care required in this situation. The specialist provides the information and assists the staff to formulate realistic client outcomes.

Finally, the resources of the setting must be considered when formulating realistic outcomes. Factors to take into account include the availability of equipment, facilities, and personnel.

Examples

THE IDEAL	THE REAL
Spends four hours a day in a wheelchair	There are two wheelchairs and five clients who need them
Showers every day by 9:00 AM	There are ten clients in a group home who need to use one shower by 9:00 AM each day

Clearly, the outcomes must be realistic for the setting in which they are written. Additionally, the nurse must be able to identify and modify unrealistic or unachievable outcomes.

6. Outcomes Should be Time-Limited

The time allotted for achievement of the outcome should be stated. Time frames may be very limited such as "within four hours," "on the first postop day," or "by the end of the first teaching session." These suggest a more specific time for evaluating the achievement of the outcome. Outcomes may also be stated to include broader perspectives such as "by the time of discharge" or "throughout hospitalization." However, it must be pointed out that when these broader time periods are utilized, the nurse periodically evaluates the client's progress rather than waiting until the time of discharge or until the end of a hospitalization.

Examples

Nursing Diagnosis: Impaired physical mobility related to recurrent leg pain

OUTCOME:	
Incorrect	**Correct**
Ambulates with assistance in room	Ambulates with assistance in room within 48 hours

Nursing Diagnosis: Constipation related to side effects of codeine

OUTCOME:

Incorrect	Correct
Moves bowels	Bowel movement within two days

7. Outcomes Should be Determined by the Client and the Nurse Together

During the initial assessment, the nurse begins involving the client in the planning of care. In the interview, the nurse learns about what the client perceives as the primary health problem. This leads to the formulation of nursing diagnoses. The client and nurse should validate the diagnoses and outcomes. In the context of discussion, they can exchange expectations and modify any unrealistic or unacceptable outcomes. The inclusion of the client as an active participant in the plan of care will help to facilitate the achievement of the outcomes.

Example. Carol McAloon is caring for Mark Soffer, a diabetic with recurrent foot problems. During the interview the client expresses concern about his ability to care for his feet properly. Carol says, ''By the time you leave the hospital, we will review the proper way to wash and dry your feet, the signs of an infection, and what to do if you find an infection. How does this sound?'' Mr. Soffer says, ''Great, that's what I want to know!''

During this conversation, the nurse has set outcomes and validated them with the client. By the time of discharge, the client will

☐ Demonstrate proper foot care

☐ Describe signs of infection

☐ State the course of action to follow if infection occurs

One of the consequences of failure to validate outcomes with a client may be the client's refusal to participate in the plan of care. This may occur if the client feels the outcomes are impossible to achieve or are in conflict with personal values.

Example. Reverend Johnson had a hernia repair four hours ago. The nurse in the ambulatory surgery unit notes that he is diaphoretic, pale, and lying in a rigid position. The nurse repeatedly offers an injectable pain medication which the client refuses.

Compare

The nurse's outcome for the client	*The client's goal for himself*
Asks for pain medication when needed	Get through this without having to take a shot

The nurse's outcome and the client's outcome are in conflict. In this situation strategies must be used to resolve the disagreement and to formulate an outcome that is acceptable to both of them. By exploring the client's reasons for refusal of the injection and offering acceptable pain management techniques, the nurse involves the client in choices about his care. Options might include oral analgesics, relaxation, or distraction techniques.

INDIVIDUAL RESPONSES AND OUTCOMES

Outcomes can be written to manage a variety of individual responses, including appearance and functioning of the body, specific symptoms, knowledge, skills, and emotions.

Appearance and Functioning of the Body

This category includes a number of observable manifestations. The following outcome written for a woman undergoing chemotherapy fits into this category: "Throughout chemotherapy, no evidence of ulcerations in oral cavity." This is a readily observable outcome that relates to the condition of her oral mucous membranes.

Other Examples:

NURSING DIAGNOSES	OUTCOMES
Constipation related to decreased peristalsis and change in diet	Within 48 hours, bowel sounds present, expels flatus/BM
Potential impaired gas exchange related to incisional pain	Lung sounds present and clear bilaterally each shift
Impaired corneal tissue integrity related to hazards associated with contact lenses	No evidence of corneal abrasion within the next three months

The outcomes illustrated above refer to the appearance and functioning of the client's body. It is important to note that a nursing diagnosis can be accompanied by more than one outcome. At times, several outcomes may be needed to define the prevention, modification, or resolution of a client response. In other situations, outcomes may change as the client progresses.

Specific Symptoms

Outcomes may be written to address the reduction or alleviation of symptoms that are interfering with the client's health status. Examples of symptoms include nausea, vomiting, diarrhea, constipation, burning sensation while urinating, frequent urination, pain, stiffness, weakness, and many others. The nurse identifies the symptoms during the assessment phase, develops appropriate nursing diagnostic statements during the diagnostic phase, writes outcomes to address them and determines interventions to alleviate them during the planning phase.

Examples:

NURSING DIAGNOSES	OUTCOME
Chronic pain related to inflammatory process	Takes pain medication when needed
Fear related to outcome of diagnostic studies	Verbalizes decreased fear within 48 hours

Knowledge

Outcomes may be formulated that involve the recall of information taught to the client. In order to determine whether the material has been mastered, outcomes should be developed that demonstrate comprehension and retention of certain information. Clients may be asked to list, describe, state, define, identify, or otherwise demonstrate knowledge acquisition and integration.

Example:

NURSING DIAGNOSIS	OUTCOME
Knowledge deficit (diabetic management)	By the end of the first teaching session: defines diabetes; explains relationship between diet, exercise, and activity

Psychomotor Skills

Psychomotor skills are often the subject of outcomes. Examples include the following:

☐ Injection of medications

☐ Transfer from bed to wheelchair

☐ Catheterization of self or others

☐ Counting pulse rate

☐ Performing CPR on mannequin

☐ Inserting intravenous catheters

☐ Testing urine or blood for glucose

The outcomes that are written for psychomotor skills identify what the client should be able to do as a result of the teaching plan.

Examples:

NURSING DIAGNOSES	OUTCOMES
Altered health maintenance related to lack of knowledge about foot care	By the end of the second teaching session, demonstrates proper technique for foot care
Altered parenting related to lack of knowledge of newborn care	By the time of discharge, feeds, bathes, and diapers newborn

Emotional Status

Outcomes may be written about the emotional status of the client. These outcomes frequently address how the client or family is responding to a crisis or stressful event. This may be an illness, family disruption, or a maturational crisis. After assessing the emotional response, the nurse develops an outcome that identifies the desired behavior that should result from nursing interventions.

Examples:

NURSING DIAGNOSES	OUTCOMES
Ineffective individual coping related to lack of support systems	Verbalizes planned coping strategies prior to discharge
Hopelessness related to perceived lack of alternatives	After third counseling session, verbalizes hope for the future

SUMMARY

Outcomes should be derived from the human response component of the nursing diagnostic statement. They should also be client-centered, clear, concise, observable, measurable, time-limited, realistic, and determined by the client and nurse together. Outcomes may refer to individual responses including appearance and functioning of the body, specific symptoms, knowledge, psychomotor skills, and emotional status. Consideration of these factors will enable the nurse to formulate outcomes that are individualized and easily evaluated.

Guidelines for Writing Outcomes

1. Outcomes should be related to the human response identified in the diagnostic statement
2. Outcomes should be client-centered
3. Outcomes should be clear and concise
4. Outcomes should describe behavior that is measurable and observable
5. Outcomes should be realistic
6. Outcomes should be time-limited
7. Outcomes should be determined by the client and the nurse together

5–2 TEST YOURSELF

IDENTIFICATION OF CORRECTLY AND INCORRECTLY WRITTEN OUTCOMES

The following is a list of nursing diagnoses and outcomes. Decide whether each outcome is correctly or incorrectly written. If incorrectly stated, identify the guideline violated from the list.

Nursing Diagnosis	Outcome	Correct/Inc Rule
1. Anticipatory grieving related to awareness of impending death	Dies with dignity	
2. Impaired physical mobility related to effects of left-sided weakness	By time of discharge transfers safely from bed to wheelchair	
3. Situational low self-esteem related to feelings of inadequacy 2° loss of job	Verbalizes positive feelings about self daily	
4. Altered health maintenance related to lack of knowledge about insulin injections	Injects self with insulin	
5. Potential for trauma related to decreased level of consciousness	Prevent accidents	
6. Hyperthermia related to effects of anesthesia	Temperature within normal limits 24 hours after surgery	

Nursing Diagnosis	Outcome	Correct/Inc Rule
7. Potential altered patterns of urinary elimination related to infection 2° catheterization	Client will be free of frequency/urgency in urination, cloudy/foul-smelling urine, dysuria, and temperature elevation	
8. Body image disturbance related to fear of rejection secondary to mastectomy	Verbalizes complete acceptance of loss of breast prior to discharge	
9. Fear related to unknown outcome of surgery	Before surgery, verbalizes fears regarding outcome of surgery	
10. Ineffective individual coping related to feelings of hopelessness	Client will receive support from staff	
11. Altered nutrition: more than body requirements related to imbalance between caloric intake and activity	Loses two lb per week until weight of 110 lb is achieved	
12. Sleep pattern disturbance related to auditory/visual hallucinations	Decrease in number of auditory/visual hallucinations	

5–2 TEST YOURSELF □ ANSWERS

NURSING DIAGNOSIS	OUTCOME	CORRECT/INC RULE
1. Anticipatory grieving related to awareness of impending death	Dies with dignity	/ 4
2. Impaired physical mobility related to effects of left-sided weakness	By time of discharge transfers safely from bed to wheelchair	/
3. Situational low self-esteem related to feelings of inadequacy 2° loss of job	Verbalizes positive feelings about self daily	/
4. Altered health maintenance related to lack of knowledge about insulin injections	Injects self with insulin	/ 4,6
5. Potential for trauma related to decreased level of consciousness	Prevent accidents	/ 2
6. Hyperthermia related to effects of anesthesia	Temperature within normal limits 24 hours after surgery	/
7. Potential altered patterns of urinary elimination related to infection 2° catheterization	Client will be free of frequency/urgency in urination, cloudy/foul-smelling urine, dysuria, and temperature elevation	/ 3,6
8. Body image disturbance related to fear of rejection secondary to mastectomy	Verbalizes complete acceptance of loss of breast prior to discharge	/ 5
9. Fear related to unknown outcome of surgery	Before surgery, verbalizes fears regarding outcome of surgery	/
10. Ineffective individual coping related to feelings of hopelessness	Client will receive support from staff	/ 2,4
11. Altered nutrition: more than body requirements related to imbalance between caloric intake and activity	Loses two lb per week until weight of 110 lb is achieved	/
12. Sleep pattern disturbance related to auditory/visual hallucinations	Decrease in number of auditory/visual hallucinations	/ 1,6

5–3 TEST YOURSELF

REVISION OF INCORRECTLY WRITTEN OUTCOMES

The outcomes that were incorrectly written in the previous exercise are listed below. Revise each outcome so that it is correctly stated.

Nursing Diagnosis	Outcome	Revised
1. Anticipatory grieving related to awareness of impending death	Dies with dignity	
2. Altered health maintenance related to lack of knowledge about insulin injections	Injects self with insulin	
3. Potential for trauma related to decreased level of consciousness	Prevent accidents	
4. Potential altered patterns of urinary elimination related to infection 2° catheterization	Client will be free of frequency/urgency in urination, cloudy/foul-smelling urine, dysuria, and temperature elevation	
5. Body image disturbance related to fear of rejection secondary to mastectomy	Verbalizes complete acceptance of loss of breast prior to discharge	
6. Ineffective individual coping related to feelings of hopelessness	Client will receive support from staff	
7. Sleep pattern disturbance related to auditory/visual hallucinations	Decrease in number of auditory/visual hallucinations	

5–3 TEST YOURSELF □ ANSWERS

NURSING DIAGNOSIS	OUTCOME	REVISED
1. Anticipatory grieving related to awareness of impending death	Dies with dignity	Prior to death, verbalizes acceptance of death
2. Altered health maintenance related to lack of knowledge about insulin injections	Injects self with insulin	Within 48 hours verbalizes need to learn health maintenance skills
3. Potential for trauma related to decreased level of consciousness	Prevent accidents	No injuries or accidents throughout hospitalization
4. Potential altered patterns of urinary elimination related to infection secondary to catheterization	Client will be free of frequency/urgency in urination, cloudy foul-smelling urine, dysuria, and temperature elevation	Voids at least 300 ml of clear urine four times daily within one week
5. Body image disturbance related to fear of rejection secondary to mastectomy	Verbalizes complete acceptance of loss of breast prior to discharge	Verbalizes feelings about loss of breast before discharge
6. Ineffective individual coping related to feelings of hopelessness	Client will receive support from staff	Identifies four available support systems prior to home visit
7. Sleep pattern disturbance related to auditory/visual hallucinations	Decrease in number of auditory/visual hallucinations	Within 24 hours, sleeps at least four hours uninterrupted q 24 hours

5–4 TEST YOURSELF

DEVELOPING CORRECTLY WRITTEN OUTCOMES FROM CASE STUDIES

Develop a correctly written outcome for each of the case studies presented below. Use the guidelines listed earlier in the chapter to correctly phrase the outcome.

Case Study #1

Cassie Tilton is an 88 year old woman transferred to your unit from a skilled nursing facility. Her history reveals that she had a "flu-like" syndrome for the past five days with persistent vomiting and diarrhea. Her vital signs are: B/P 108/56, pulse rate 112, respirations 28, and temperature 101.4°F. Her mucous membranes are dry and her skin turgor is decreased. She indicates that she feels weak, tired, and thirsty.

NURSING DIAGNOSIS: Fluid volume deficit related to vomiting and diarrhea

OUTCOME:

Case Study #2

Chip Ireland is a 35 year old businessman admitted to the outpatient surgicenter for a tonsillectomy. He indicates that he has had recurrent tonsillitis for the last three years. Postoperatively, he complains of being thirsty and requests a cold drink. You observe that he has difficulty swallowing and coughs up the water. He states "my throat is too sore; it feels like it is swollen." Upon examination, you note the presence of redness and edema in the operative area.

NURSING DIAGNOSIS Impaired swallowing related to edema and effects of surgery

OUTCOME:

Case Study #3

Dave Davis, a 54 year old self-employed mechanic, is admitted to your unit at 6:00 AM for an elective cholecystectomy. During your assessment, you observe that he is unusually apprehensive, moderately diaphoretic, restless, and pacing around the room. His vital signs are: B/P 156/88, pulse rate 108, and respirations 28. His voice trembles as he tells you that he has never had surgery before and states "My brother had a simple appendectomy when he was 18 and died on the table; nothing they did could save him."

NURSING DIAGNOSIS: Fear related to perceived threat of death

OUTCOME:

Case Study #4

Emily Fantin is an 86 year old woman who calls the office nurse and requests free samples of laxatives. She complains "I've spent so much money on laxatives at the drug store, I take them twice a day so that my bowels will move three times a day. My mother always told me to take laxatives to keep myself regular. By the way, do you have any sample enemas?" Upon further questioning you find out that Emily lives alone and does her own cooking. She eats mostly frozen dinners or prepared foods with few fruits and vegetables. In addition, she shops at a local convenience store with a limited supply of fresh produce. She relies on Metamucil daily, and Ex Lax and Milk of Magnesia approximately four times a week. She states that she gets very little exercise.

NURSING DIAGNOSIS: Perceived constipation related to long-standing family health beliefs

OUTCOME:

5–4 TEST YOURSELF □ ANSWERS

Case Study #1

Cassie Tilton is an 88 year old woman transferred to your unit from a skilled nursing facility. Her history reveals that she had a "flu-like" syndrome for the past five days with persistent vomiting and diarrhea. Her vital signs are: B/P 108/56, pulse rate 112, respirations 28, and temperature 101.4°F. Her mucous membranes are dry and her skin turgor is decreased. She indicates that she feels weak, tired, and thirsty.

NURSING DIAGNOSIS: Fluid volume deficit related to vomiting and diarrhea

OUTCOME: Within 48 hours, moist mucous membranes, vital signs within normal limits for client

Case Study #2

Chip Ireland is a 35 year old businessman admitted to the outpatient surgicenter for a tonsillectomy. He indicates that he has had recurrent tonsillitis for the last three years. Postoperatively, he complains of being thirsty and requests a cold drink. You observe that he has difficulty swallowing and coughs up the water. He states "my throat is too sore; it feels like it is swollen." Upon examination, you note the presence of redness and edema in the operative areas.

NURSING DIAGNOSIS: Impaired swallowing related to edema and effects of surgery.

OUTCOME: Before discharge from surgicenter, swallows at least 240 ml of fluid at a time

Case Study #3

Dave Davis, a 54 year old self-employed mechanic, is admitted to your unit at 6:00 AM for an elective cholecystectomy. During your assessment, you observe that he is unusually apprehensive, moderately diaphoretic, restless, and pacing around the room. His vital signs are: B/P 156/88, pulse 108, and respirations 28. His voice trembles as he tells you that he has never had surgery before and states "my brother had a simple appendectomy when he was 18 and died on the table, nothing they did could save him."

NURSING DIAGNOSIS: Fear related to perceived threat of death

OUTCOME: Verbalizes decreased fear prior to surgery

Case Study #4

Emily Fantin is an 86 year old woman who calls the office nurse and requests free samples of laxatives. She complains "I've spent so much money on laxatives at the drug store, I take them twice a day so that my bowels will move three times a day. My mother always told me to take laxatives to keep myself regular. By the way, do you have any sample enemas?''

NURSING DIAGNOSIS: Perceived constipation related to long-standing family health beliefs

OUTCOME: Within two months, verbalizes satisfaction with one bowel movement q one to two days

REFERENCES

Kalish R: The Psychology of Human Behavior, 5th ed. Monterey, CA: Brooks/Cole, 1983.
Maslow A: A theory of human motivation. Psychology Review 50:370, 1943.

BIBLIOGRAPHY

Christenson P: Goals and objectives. I Griffith J and Christensen P: Nursing Process, 2nd ed. St. Louis: CV Mosby, 1986.
Hanna DV and Wyman NB: Assessment + diagnosis = care planning: a tool for coordination. Nursing Management 18(11): 106–109, 1987.
Inzer F, and Aspinal MJ: Evaluating patient outcomes. Nursing Outlook Mar; 29: 178–181, 1981.
Kozier B, and Erb G: Fundamentals of Nursing Concepts and Procedures, 3rd ed. Menlo Park, CA: Addison-Wesley, 1987.
MacLeod and MacTavish M: Solving the nursing care plan dilemma: nursing diagnosis makes the difference. Journal of Nursing Staff Development 4(2): 70–73, 1988.
McElroy D, and Herbelin K: Writing a better patient care plan. Nursing 18(2): 50–51, 1988.
Nussbaum J: Care Planning for Nurses, 2nd ed. Thorofare, NJ: Charles B. Slack, 1981.
Orthopedic nursing practice: process and outcome criteria for selected diagnoses. Orthopedic Nursing 6(2): 11–16, 1987.
Popkess–Vater S: On a scale of one to ten . . . rating subjective outcomes. American Journal of Nursing 88(9): 1263–1264, 1988.

6

PLANNING—Nursing Interventions and Documentation

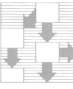

INTRODUCTION

STAGE 3—NURSING INTERVENTIONS
    Definition
    Development of Nursing Interventions
    Comparison of Nursing and Medical Interventions
    Characteristics of Interventions
    Provision of a Safe and Therapeutic Environment
    Teaching-Learning Opportunities
    Utilization of Appropriate Resources
    Guidelines for Writing Nursing Interventions

STAGE 4—DOCUMENTATION: THE NURSING CARE PLAN
    Definition
    Purposes
    Characteristics
    Components
    Types of Care Plans

SUMMARY

The stages of the planning phase of the nursing process are (1) setting priorities, (2) developing outcomes, (3) designing nursing interventions, and (4) documentation. The first two stages were addressed in the previous chapter. Once priorities have been established and outcomes developed, the next stages of planning begin.

Nursing interventions are developed in a number of ways, including hypothesizing and brainstorming. The third stage involves writing nursing interventions which describe how the nurse will assist the client to achieve the proposed outcomes. These interventions are based on (1) the information obtained during the assessment interview and (2) the nurse's subsequent interactions with the client and family. The desirable characteristics of nursing interventions include consistency, based on scientific principles, and individualized to the client. They should be implemented to assure a safe environment, to use teaching learning opportunities and to address the utilization of appropriate and available resources. The final phase—documentation—involves communicating the written plan of care to other members of the nursing staff. The nursing care plan is designed to share information about the client's significant health care needs, the outcomes identified by the nurse, and the planned interventions. Ideally, the care plan is written by a registered nurse following the first contact with the client, is readily available, and contains current information. The types of care plans in use include individually constructed, standardized, and computerized. As computer technology becomes more widespread in health care, nurses will have increased access to the power of the computer for developing care plans. This chapter will address these last two stages of the planning phase—developing nursing interventions and documenting the plan of care.

STAGE 3—NURSING INTERVENTIONS

Definition

Nursing interventions are specific strategies designed to assist the client in achieving outcomes. They are based on the related factor identified in the nursing diagnostic statement. Therefore, nursing interventions define the activities required to eliminate the factors contributing to the human response.

Example. "Potential for trauma related to hazardous home environment." The nursing interventions in this case would focus on reducing the environmental hazards in the client's home.

Development of Nursing Interventions

Once the nursing diagnoses and outcomes have been established, decisions are made on how to meet the outcomes and how to promote, maintain, or restore the client's health. Successful nursing interventions depend upon the nurse's ability to generate and choose alternatives that are most likely to be effective. Both hypothesizing and brainstorming are useful in the identification of possible alternatives.

Hypothesizing

The nurse hypothesizes when predicting that certain alternatives are appropriate to reach the desired outcome. Nursing interventions are proposed that (1) have been successful in the past in solving a particular problem and (2) are likely to be effective based on the client's knowledge, skills, or resources. This technique allows the nurse to apply scientific principles, develop creative approaches to problem-solving, and facilitate the delivery of individualized care.

Brainstorming

Brainstorming is a group technique utilized to generate ideas from more than one person. The purpose of this approach is to stimulate creative alternatives. An atmosphere of freedom and openness must be created for effective brainstorming to take place. Brainstorming can be done with the interdisciplinary team or among nursing staff. It may occur during a care planning session or interdisciplinary care conferences. After all possible alternatives are developed, each should be judged in terms of its feasibility and probability of success. The nurse chooses those that are most appropriate for the client.

Whether approaches are developed by hypothesizing or brainstorming, they are translated into nursing interventions and communicated in the written plan of care.

Comparison of Nursing and Medical Interventions

Medical or physician's orders usually focus on the activities involved in diagnosing and treating the client's medical condition. These orders are delegated to nurses and other health care personnel. Medical orders often include administration of medications, diagnostic tests, dietary requirements, and treatments.

Nursing interventions focus on the activities required to promote, maintain, or restore the client's health. They may be categorized as dependent, interdependent, or independent.

Dependent Interventions

Dependent interventions relate to the implementation of medical orders. They indicate the manner in which the medical order is to be carried out.

Example.   The physician writes an order to weigh a client three times weekly. The nurse defines how the order will be implemented. "Weigh Monday, Wednesday, and Friday. Use bedscale."

Example.   The physician writes an order for "colostomy care." The nursing interventions define colostomy care based on the individual needs of the client. These interventions could include
"Perform colostomy care every two days or when appliance is leaking."
"Use skin barrier and Bongort pouch size $1\frac{3}{4}$"."
"Review each step verbally with client and his wife."

Interdependent Interventions

Interdependent nursing interventions describe the activities that the nurse carries out in cooperation with other health team members. The interventions may involve collaboration with social workers, dieticians, therapists, technicians, and physicians.

Example.   Barrett Bleakley is a client who is in kidney failure. The medical order states "restrict fluids to 600 ml by mouth plus 720 ml 5% dextrose in .45 sodium chloride solution IV every 24 hours." To define how this will be achieved, the nurse and the dietician calculate the amount of fluid Barrett may receive each shift. The nursing interventions are as follows.

1.   Administer IV fluids at 30 ml/hr (total of 240 ml per shift) via IV pump.
2.   PO fluid intake:

    7:30 AM–3:30 PM—Total of 315 ml po
                     240 ml on dietary trays
                      75 ml for medications

3:30–11:30 PM—Total of 195 ml po
120 ml on dietary tray
75 ml for medications

11:30 PM–7:30 AM—Total of 100 ml po for medications

Independent Interventions

Independent nursing interventions are the activities that may be performed by the nurse without a direct physician's order. The type of activities that nurses may order independently are defined by nursing diagnoses. They are the responses that nurses are licensed to treat by virtue of their education and experience.

Example. Constance Lance is a confused 82 year old woman who fell and broke her hip. The nurse recognizes that she is at risk for developing a postoperative wound infection and writes the following nursing diagnosis, outcome, and interventions:

Nursing Diagnosis: Potential for infection related to debilitated state and confusion

Outcome: No evidence of infection throughout hospitalization

Interventions:
1. Use sterile technique when changing dressing.
2. Monitor incision for warmth, redness, swelling, or drainage.
3. Restrain hands if client is observed to be touching dressing.
4. Check temperature every four hours for the first 24 hours after surgery, then BID until discharge.

Characteristics of Interventions

Nursing interventions should have certain desirable characteristics. They should
1. Be consistent with the plan of care.
2. Be based on scientific principles.
3. Be individualized to the specific situation.
4. Be used to provide a safe and therapeutic environment.
5. Employ teaching-learning opportunities for the client.
6. Include utilization of appropriate resources (ANA, 1973).

1. Consistency

Nursing interventions should not be in conflict with the therapeutic approaches of other members of the health team. When nurses and other professionals are working at cross-purposes, confusion and frustration result. It is important that members of various disciplines communicate their goals and define approaches to achieve those goals. Any differences of opinion need to be resolved to promote consistency in care.

Example.   Kathy Smith works as an office nurse for a family practice physician. Eric Baker, a nine year old insulin-dependent diabetic, has been receiving insulin for three years. Up to this point, Eric's mother has been responsible for the insulin injections. Kathy believes that Eric, who is very bright, is ready to learn how to inject himself. When Kathy writes her interventions to begin teaching, the physician objects. "He's too young to learn how to give himself insulin. I don't want him to be taught that yet."

The physician and the nurse disagree in this situation. It is important that they resolve this conflict to promote a consistent approach to Eric's care.

2. Scientific Basis

The second characteristic of interventions is use of a scientific rationale that supports the nurse's decisions and forms the foundation for nursing action. This rationale is developed from the nurse's knowledge base, which includes natural and behavioral sciences and the humanities. Each nursing intervention should be supported by scientific principles. The following examples demonstrate nursing interventions and associated scientific principles.

Examples

NURSING INTERVENTION	SCIENTIFIC PRINCIPLE
1. Encourage client to identify hazards in his home	1. Elderly clients are at greater risk for injuries and falls
2. Teach client to rotate insulin injection sites	2. Repeated use of the same site may cause fibrosis, scarring, and decreased insulin absorption

3. Increase fluids to 2500 ml daily
    7–3   1300 ml
    3–11 800 ml
    11–7 400 ml
	3. Adequate fluid intake is necessary to maintain normal stool consistency and kidney function

Although scientific principles are usually not included in the written nursing intervention, the nurse must have a thorough understanding of the rationale for nursing actions. This allows modification of the nursing intervention, if necessary, without violating the principles upon which it is based.

Examples

NURSING INTERVENTION	RATIONALE
Turn q2h and massage bony prominences with lotion	Reduction of pressure and increased circulation decrease the potential for skin breakdown

While turning the client, the nurse notices a reddened area on the right heel and adds an order for a skin barrier. The rationale is the same.

Apply Duoderm to right heel	Reduction of pressure on the skin surface decreases the potential for skin breakdown

Occasionally the principles may be incorporated into the nursing intervention for clarification or explanation.

Example.   "Encourage client to feed self starting 1/15/90 to promote independence."

3. Individualization

One purpose of nursing interventions is to communicate how one client's care differs from that of another with a similar nursing or medical diagnosis. When developing interventions, the nurse chooses approaches that will address the client's specific physical and emotional needs. The following are guidelines that should be used in the development of individualized nursing interventions.

1. Focus on the related factor(s) of the nursing diagnosis.
2. Include the input of the client and family in choosing alternatives.
3. Consider client and family strengths and weaknesses.
4. Take into account the urgency and severity of the situation.

Focus on the Related Factor.   The nursing diagnostic statement provides a basis for establishing individualized nursing interventions. As explained previously, the nursing diagnosis has two parts—the human response and the related factor(s). The related factor(s) specifies the origin of the human response and provides direction for specific nursing interventions. The nurse's knowledge of the client and the problem directs the formulation of individualized nursing interventions.

Example.

Dona Vessels is a 17 year old hospitalized following a motorcycle accident. She is in skeletal traction for a fractured left leg.

Betsey Moehlich, an 84 year old, is a resident of a nursing home. She is thin, slightly dehydrated, and is confined to bed.

Both clients have the nursing diagnosis, "potential impaired skin integrity related to immobility.'' Note that although the nursing diagnosis is the same for both clients, the nursing orders are individualized.

Outcome: No evidence of skin breakdown while on bedrest.

NURSING INTERVENTIONS

Dona	Betsey
1. Apply foam mattress to bed	1. Apply air mattress to bed
2. Massage bony prominences with lotion q4h	2. Assist client to change position q2h (see turning schedule). Include prone position at least once per shift.
3. Encourage client to use trapeze to change position	3. Massage bony prominences with lotion q4h after turning.

Note that although the nursing diagnosis is the same for both clients, the nursing interventions are individualized.

Client Input.   After nursing diagnoses are established, outcomes are formulated with the client's input. The involvement of the client in outcome development increases the potential for individualization of nursing interventions. Likewise, after nursing interventions are formulated, they are reviewed with the client. This ensures that the planned interventions are understood by and are acceptable and applicable to the individual client. Frequently, clients will participate more actively in their care if their ideas have been solicited.

Example.   Ida Gold, an 85 year old woman, was recently discharged from the hospital after a total knee replacement. She is being cared for at home by a private duty nurse. She complains of being tired from having inadequate amounts of sleep. The private duty nurse explores the reasons for her fatigue and determines that Ida is having trouble sleeping because she is experiencing pain in her knee at night. Ida agrees to take a warm bath in the evening to increase her comfort level, followed by pain medication at bedtime.

> **NURSING DIAGNOSIS**
> Sleep pattern disturbance related to nocturnal knee pain

> **OUTCOME**
> Sleeps at least six hours a night without interruption.

Strengths and Weaknesses.   When developing individualized nursing interventions, the strengths and weaknesses of the client and the family must be considered. The client's assets should be identified and utilized in planning care. Strengths may include motivation, intelligence, a supportive family, education, and economic resources.

NURSING DIAGNOSIS

Knowledge deficit (diabetes management)

OUTCOME

Within one week: Verbalizes pathology and management of diabetes. Performs blood glucose monitoring accurately.

Example. Erin Mirabelli is a 22 year old newly diagnosed insulin-dependent diabetic. Erin is a highly motivated and self-disciplined young woman. She worked her way through college and graduated with a degree in biology. She is currently employed as a laboratory technician in industry. She maintains an active schedule, including aerobics and weight lifting.

The nurse practitioner decided to utilize Erin's strengths in planning her education on diabetic management. Erin was provided with self-learning packages on the fundamentals of pathology and management. She was also identified as a good candidate for blood glucose monitoring to determine her blood sugar and subsequent insulin needs.

The client's weaknesses or deficits should also be identified. The absence of motivation, intelligence, family support, economic resources, or education may act as a deterrent to health. Other deficits might include chronic illness, debilitation, depression, social withdrawal, or a language barrier.

In the following situation, the nurse considered the client's physical deficits when planning care.

NURSING DIAGNOSIS

Impaired physical mobility related to weakness

OUTCOME

Ambulates independently within two weeks

Example. Carmen Donatelli is a 76 year old man who had abdominal surgery last week. He was admitted to a rehabilitation facility to improve his strength prior to returning home. The physician's orders included "Ambulate TID." The nurse explained to Carmen that the usual procedure was to ambulate mid morning, mid afternoon, and after dinner. Carmen said, "I have trouble seeing at night. I don't want to walk in the hall after dinner." The nursing intervention was modified on the basis of Carmen's visual deficit to read: "Ambulate TID 9 AM, 1 PM, and 5 PM."

In this case, the nurse develops nursing interventions based on an assessment of Carmen's physical limitations.

These two examples demonstrate that individualized nursing interventions result from the nurse's consideration of the client's strengths and weaknesses when making decisions for care.

Severity and Urgency of Condition. At times, the severity or urgency of the client's problem may influence the nursing intervention. This occurs when the altered human response may result in harm to the client or to others.

Example. Michael York, an elderly client, has an adverse reaction to a sleeping medication. He becomes confused and violent when the nurse attempts to re-orient him. This situation requires immediate independent intervention. The nurse implements the following individualized nursing orders.

☐ Safely protect the client in bed with a jacket restraint.

☐ Assign a nursing assistant to stay until the client is re-oriented.

☐ Inform the physician of the change in the client's behavior.

☐ Medicate with tranquilizer prn.

> **NURSING DIAGNOSIS**
> Potential for violence (directed at others) related to adverse reaction to sleeping medication

> **OUTCOME**
> Does not injure self or others throughout hospitalization

4. Provision of a Safe and Therapeutic Environment

When planning interventions, the fourth characteristic to consider is the satisfaction of the client's physical and emotional needs. A *safe* environment is one in which the client's physiological needs are met and the client is protected from potential injury. A *therapeutic* environment utilizes effective interpersonal relationships to assist the client in resolving the altered human response.

Safe Environment. As described in Chapter 5, physiological needs—for air, food, rest, water—must be satisfied before higher level needs can be addressed. In a safe environment, these basic needs are provided for by nursing and medical interventions. Examples of nursing interventions that assist in the satisfaction of basic needs follow.

☐ Provide 2000 ml of clear fluids in 24 hours (food).

☐ Assess need for oxygen and provide via mask at 4 L/min (air).

☐ Encourage client to drink 60 ml prune juice each morning (elimination).

☐ Provide 30 minute rest intervals after meals (rest/sleep).

Those clients who are particularly at risk for injury include infants and children and those who are elderly, debilitated, or under anesthesia. There are numerous nursing actions designed to create a safe environment for these individuals. Common nursing interventions include the following.

FRAIL ELDERLY

☐ Restrain with Posey belt when necessary.

☐ Place bedside table within reach (for client on bedrest).

☐ Monitor client while smoking.

☐ Instruct client on potential hazards in the home.

☐ Assist client into tub, checking bath water temperature carefully.

CHILD

☐ Teach parents to child-proof the house.

☐ Teach parents to keep rail of crib up at all times.

☐ Teach parents to place safety net over top of crib.

☐ Teach parents not to leave dangerous objects within reach of crib.

ANESTHETIZED CLIENT

☐ Monitor vital signs every 15 minutes.

☐ Keep side rails up at all times.

☐ Observe for evidence of vomiting.

Therapeutic Environment. Nursing interventions are developed to identify strategies that are effective in the promotion, maintenance, or restoration of health. The interventions may consist of treatments, assessment, teaching, consultations, or any other types of actions likely to be helpful.

Examples

☐ Teach client about foods to avoid while taking anticoagulants.

☐ Assess for presence of incisional pain; medicate prn.

☐ Consult with social service regarding nursing home placement.

☐ Assist client with range of motion exercises for legs qid.

The caring environment is therapeutic for the client. The nurse demonstrates concern by the nonverbal components of behavior—tone of voice, touch, and eye contact. The nurse also conveys compassion by such actions as treating the client with respect and courtesy, by listening, and by being helpful.

Nursing interventions that help to demonstrate caring include the following.

☐ Notify client's son when client returns from recovery room.

☐ Assist client to identify support groups in the community.

☐ Encourage client to verbalize feelings about loss of spouse.

5. Teaching-Learning Opportunities

The teaching-learning process for the client includes the acquisition of new knowledge, attitudes, and skills and related changes in behavior. The nursing interventions involved in the teaching-learning process include the following.

☐ Assess client's learning needs.

☐ Determine client's readiness to learn.

☐ Identify the factors that influence client's ability to learn.

☐ Develop individualized outcomes that are realistic and attainable.

☐ Determine strategies to assist client and family to achieve desired outcomes.

☐ Present content in an understandable fashion using appropriate resources.

☐ Evaluate client's progress toward achievement of outcomes.

☐ Modify the plan as required.

Evaluation of the client's progress and modification of the plan will be addressed further in Chapter 9.

Assess Learning Needs.   During the assessment phase of the nursing process, the nurse should gather data to evaluate the client's individual learning needs. Clients should be encouraged to identify the needs they perceive as important. These needs may be evidenced by direct questions, such as "What happens when they do an ultrasound?" "Why can't I eat after midnight when I'm going for surgery tomorrow?" "How do I get dressed with this cast on?"

Learning needs may also be identified by observing the client's condition or behavior. For instance, the visiting nurse notes that the skin around Mr. Conover's colostomy stoma is red and excoriated. The nurse questions the client and determines that he has not been using a skin barrier because it is "too expensive." The school nurse observes that Maria Brown does not wash her hands before leaving the bathroom. These situations demonstrate indirect identification of client learning needs.

At times, clients may directly identify their learning needs by requesting information to promote, maintain, or restore their health.

Example.   Rorie Parrella is a 30 year old who had a biopsy for a benign breast mass. The nurse questions the client regarding her ability to do breast self-examination. The client indicates that she is not sure how to do it but would like to learn.

Here the nurse's intervention which consists of teaching self breast examination will assist the client to maintain her health by early detection of additional masses.

Identify Factors Influencing Ability to Learn.   The process of planning teaching interventions includes the recognition that there are a number of factors that affect the client's ability to learn, including pre-existing knowledge, level of education, age, motivation, perceived locus of control, state of health, and lifestyle.

Clients' current *level of knowledge*, including their misconceptions and misinformation, frequently affects their ability to learn. Some knowledge is prerequisite for additional learning. For example, clients who need to change a sterile dressing may encounter great difficulty if they do not know the basics of good hand-washing.

Level of education frequently defines clients' knowledge of health and disease. If the information presented is above that level, the client may be unable to learn. The reverse may also be true. If information is presented at a level significantly below the client's level of education, the client might feel insulted and therefore fail to learn the material.

Age also affects ability to learn. The very young child may have difficulty in grasping concepts unless they are presented in very concrete terms. Some elderly clients may have ingrained ideas or "myths" that affect their ability to accept new changes. Additionally, they may have physiological deficits that interfere with their ability to learn (e.g., vision or hearing problems).

Clients must also be *motivated* to learn. Generally, they will readily learn whatever is most important to them. This substantiates the need for an accurate assessment of the client's perceived needs. However, not all clients desire information. Some prefer to delegate the responsibility for promoting, maintaining, or restoring their health to family members or health care personnel. Others in a state of denial may refuse to acknowledge the need to learn about their illness. Therefore, it is very difficult for these clients to learn effectively.

The client's perceptions about *locus of control* will also affect readiness to learn. Locus of control is defined as the belief in one's ability to control reinforcements or results. If an individual perceives that results come from outside forces, such as luck, fate, or powerful others, this person is said to have an *external* control orientation. An individual with an *internal* control orientation perceives that the outcomes of one's own behavior are contingent upon one's own behavior and abilities (Bigbee, 1983). A client who has an internal control orientation will be more likely to be motivated to learn than individuals who believe that fate is in charge of their health status.

The client must be *physically and emotionally prepared* for the teaching–learning experience. The nurse should plan to use interventions directed toward relief of pain, fear, anxiety, or fatigue before attempting to involve the client in learning activities. The state of health of the client may affect ability to learn. The client with a critical illness, severe debilitation, or sensory-perception deficits may be unable to process or absorb information. This may also be the case for clients with terminal disease, since they may lack motivation or ability.

The client's *lifestyle* may affect ability to learn. This is particularly pertinent when considering low socioeconomic groups and people of certain cultures. The client's learning problem may be associated with deficits in the types of experiences that make learning a desirable outcome. The client may not be stimulated in his or her culture to learn content perceived to be unnecessary or unimportant. Certain personality types—e.g., dependent or irresponsible persons—may also have inherent motivational problems.

Develop Individualized Outcomes. The learning outcomes for each client involve knowledge, attitudes, and skills. For example, the nurse may be required to teach the client who needs an ostomy so that the client will be able to

- ☐ Describe how the surgery has altered the gastrointestinal tract (knowledge)
- ☐ Explain how the ostomy will affect the client's relationship with spouse (attitude)
- ☐ List types of equipment necessary to manage the ostomy (knowledge)
- ☐ Cleanse the stomal area and apply a pouch (skill)
- ☐ Irrigate the ostomy (skill)
- ☐ Express confidence in the ability to manage the ostomy (attitude)

Outcomes must be realistic. The involvement of the client in outcome decisions helps to assure that they will be realistic. Accurate assessment of the client's motivation and abilities is also critical.

Example. Steven Sturgeon is seen in a drug rehabilitation clinic. The nurse develops the following teaching goal: "identifies the effects of prolonged drug abuse at the end of the first teaching session." This outcome is not realistic for Steven, since he is still experiencing the effects of the drugs he is taking. A more realistic outcome might be "verbalizes a desire to stop taking drugs."

Example. For a newly diagnosed diabetic, the nurse may write this outcome: "correctly injects self with insulin prior to discharge." This goal may be unattainable for a variety of reasons—(1) the client may be discharged before the skill has been mastered, (2) the client may be unwilling or unable to achieve self-injection, or (3) the client may not require insulin therapy.

Determine Teaching Strategies. The teaching strategies utilized by the nurse should be individualized to the client's needs and the type of outcome desired. Knowledge outcomes frequently require the mastery of facts and concepts. These are most effectively taught by using written materials and audiovisual aids reinforced by discussion.

Skill outcomes are more likely to be achieved if the client is exposed to demonstration, discussion, practice, and reinforcement. Attitudes are more difficult to influence and to measure. However, discussion, role-modeling, and problem-solving experience assist the client in gaining insight into and accepting new attitudes.

The nurse may choose a variety of approaches, depending upon the client's needs, the goal of teaching, the environment, available resources, time, etc. Individual or group instruction may be utilized to accomplish learning outcomes.

Present Content. The nurse should identify the specific strategies and resources required to accomplish individual learning outcomes. Teaching methods previously described, when presented at the client's level of understanding, increase the possibility that new knowledge, skills, or attitudes will be acquired by the client. The pace of the program should be consistent with the client's ability to learn and should build on the client's previous knowledge. Learning is also facilitated when the nurse is a warm, accepting individual who encourages the active participation of the client. Retention is increased when (1) a number of the senses are involved in the learning process, (2) facts and skills are repeated, (3) the learner has the opportunity to apply the information, and (4) immediate feedback is provided.

Regardless of the strategy utilized in the teaching process, the interaction between the nurse and the client will affect the amount of learning that occurs. Supplemental teaching materials often enhance the client's ability to absorb content. Audiovisual aids, such as transparencies, films, filmstrips, slides, and audiotapes, may assist in the learning process. Models, posters, programmed instruction, and other printed materials appropriate to the reading level of the client may be utilized in specific instances. The nurse should be careful to review and evaluate these materials before using them. The materials selected should be appropriate, purposeful, and consistent with the goals of the teaching program. Additional resources should include sufficient time and personnel to assure that the client receives timely pertinent information.

6. Utilization of Appropriate Resources

The last characteristic of nursing interventions is the incorporation of appropriate resources. The nurse must consider whether the nursing intervention is realistic for the client situation. The intervention should be practical in terms of equipment, financial factors, and human resources.

Equipment. It is necessary to be aware of the types of equipment readily available within an agency and in the community. The nurse should utilize the assistive device that is most useful, at the least cost, and yet acceptable to the client.

For example, a client with potential impaired skin integrity related to decreased mobility may be placed on a foam, air, or water mattress. Availability, cost, and appropriateness will determine which device is selected.

Financial Factors. In addition to the selection of equipment, financial factors will influence the services available to the client. Clients with low income may be eligible for certain services, while other programs do not have income criteria. Social workers can often provide useful information about the financial aspects of available resources.

Human Resources. Human resources commonly utilized in the planning phase include health care personnel, family, and significant others. When formulating nursing interventions, the nurse must evaluate the need for and availability of these human resources. The nurse must also consider family resources when making plans that might involve them. Aspects to consider include their commitment to assist in the situation, financial resources, and degree of understanding of the client's needs.

In summary, nursing interventions should be realistic in the utilization of nursing staff, client, family, agency, and community resources.

Guidelines for Writing Nursing Interventions

Nursing interventions provide the health care team with a blueprint for reaching established outcomes and resolving the altered human response. A set of nursing interventions should be written to accomplish each outcome. To be effective, they must be written as clearly and concisely as possible. To avoid confusion or repetition of activities, they should describe who will implement them. When nursing interventions are dependent on previous activities, they should be numbered to designate sequence. All interventions should consist of

☐ Signature and date

☐ Precise action verb and modifiers

☐ Specification of "who, what, where, when, how, and how often"

☐ Individualized approaches for the client

1. Nursing Interventions Should be Dated and Signed

All interventions should be dated to identify the date of origin. The signature is included to reflect the nurse's personal and legal accountability. The signature allows coworkers (1) to give feedback on the effectiveness of the intervention, (2) to obtain clarification, and (3) to explore the rationale for the intervention (Carnevali, 1983).

2. Nursing Interventions Should Include Precise Action Verbs and List Specific Activities to Achieve the Desired Outcomes

All nursing interventions should clearly communicate the expected activities. Employing action verbs is useful in defining the specific actions. Verbs that are not precise create confusion for the caregiver. For example, if the intervention is "teach colostomy care," the nurse could (1) demonstrate the steps used in applying a colostomy pouch; (2) identify the equipment required in colostomy care; (3) provide printed instructions and discuss their content with the client; or (4) ask the client to perform a return demonstration. In this example, the verb "teach" is not precise. A more specific verb would give clearer directions to the nurse.

3. Nursing Interventions Should Define Who, What, Where, When, How, and How Often Identified Activities Will Take Place

Specifications of "who, what, where, when, how, and how often" are necessary to make the nursing order meaningful. In the example "irrigate wound vigorously," the nurse needs to know

☐ Which wound—perhaps the client has more than one.

☐ Who will irrigate—the nurse, client, or family?

☐ When to irrigate—prior to physical therapy? Once a day? Each time the dressing is changed?

☐ How to irrigate—vigorously by pouring the solution? Using a bulb syringe? With normal saline, peroxide, Betadine (povidone-iodine), or antibiotic solution?

Putting all of this together, the nursing interventions may read
"4/29—Irrigate lower abdominal incision at 8 AM, 2 PM, and 10 PM.
 Using a bulb syringe, irrigate vigorously with neomycin solution, followed by normal saline.
 Demonstrate wound irrigation technique to client and family members.
 Replace dressing with two gauze sponges and one 8 in × 8 in pad.
 Use paper tape (client's skin is very sensitive)."

The nurse should also include the duration of time, when indicated. For example, "OOB in chair for 30 minutes tid."

4. Nursing Interventions Should be Individualized to the Client

If routine procedures are spelled out in procedure manuals or protocols, the title of the procedure may be used in the nursing interventions to eliminate writing the entire procedure. Some examples of this might be "tracheostomy care" or "urinary catheter care." If modifications of the procedure need to be made, they are to be included in the nursing interventions. Using the example of "tracheostomy care," the nursing interventions may read
"Tracheostomy care at least once a shift and when there is a noticeable build-up of secretions.
Do not change trach strings. To be changed by MD only."

A modification of Hickman catheter care might read
"Perform Hickman catheter care three times weekly—Monday, Wednesday, and Friday.
Do not use Betadine—client is allergic."

6–1 TEST YOURSELF

IDENTIFICATION OF CORRECTLY AND INCORRECTLY WRITTEN INTERVENTIONS

The following is a list of interventions. Decide whether each intervention is written correctly or incorrectly. If written incorrectly, identify the guideline violated.

GUIDELINES

1. Nursing interventions should be dated and signed.

2. Nursing interventions should include precise action verbs and list specific activities to achieve the desired outcomes.

3. Nursing interventions should define where, when, who, how, and how often identified activities will take place.

4. Nursing interventions should be individualized to the client.

		CORRECT	INCORRECT	GUIDELINE
9/12 P. Dolds, RN	1. Make client comfortable.			
8/7 T. Call, RN	2. OOB in chair for $\frac{1}{2}$ hour BID.			
5/19 S. Snell, RN	3. Teach about diabetes management.			
8/29 B. Jackson, RN	4. No evidence of signs of infection.			
8/17 D. White, RN	5. Force fluids.			
3/2 C. Wilson, RN	6. Teach client to do 10 ankle pumps q1h while awake.			
	7. Hickman catheter care daily at 10 AM			
1/6 B. Walker, RN	8. Provide preferred fluids.			

6–1 TEST YOURSELF □ ANSWERS

		CORRECT	INCORRECT	GUIDELINE
9/12 P. Dolds, RN	1. Make client comfortable.		✔	2,4
8/7 T. Call, RN	2. OOB in chair for ½ hour BID.	✔		
5/19 S. Snell, RN	3. Teach about diabetes management.		✔	2
8/29 B. Jackson, RN	4. No evidence of signs of infection.		✔	This is an outcome
7/17 D. White, RN	5. Force fluids.		✔	3
3/2 C. Wilson, RN	6. Teach client to do ten ankle pumps q1h while awake.	✔		
	7. Hickman catheter care daily at 10 AM		✔	1
1/6 B. Walker, RN	8. Provide preferred fluids.		✔	4

6–2 TEST YOURSELF

REVISION OF INCORRECTLY WRITTEN NURSING INTERVENTIONS

The following interventions in Test Yourself 6–1 were incorrectly written. Revise each one so that it is correctly stated.

9/12
P. Dolds

1. Make client comfortable.

5/19
S. Snell, RN

3. Teach about diabetes management.

8/29
B. Jackson, RN

4. No evidence of signs of infection.

7/17
D. White, RN

5. Force fluids.

7. Hickman catheter care daily at 10 AM.

1/6
B. Walker, RN

8. Provide preferred fluids.

6–2 TEST YOURSELF □ ANSWERS

9/12 P. Dolds, RN	1. Make client comfortable.	9/12 P. Dolds, RN	Position on left side with two pillows.
5/19 S. Snell, RN	3. Teach about diabetes management.	5/19 S. Snell, RN	Teach correct foot care.
8/29 B. Jackson, RN	4. No evidence of signs of infection.	8/29 B. Jackson, RN	Maintain sterility of urinary drainage system.
7/17 D. White, RN	5. Force fluids.	7/17 D. White, RN	Administer 3000 cc/24 hours: 7–3 2000 cc 3–11 500 cc 11–7 500 cc
	7. Hickman catheter care daily at 10 AM	4/9 D. Como, RN	Hickman catheter care daily at 10 AM
1/6 B. Walker, RN	8. Provide preferred fluids.	1/6 B. Walker, RN	Provide preferred fluids. Client likes cola and juice.

6–3 TEST YOURSELF

DEVELOPMENT OF NURSING INTERVENTIONS

Develop correctly written nursing interventions for each nursing diagnosis and outcome presented in the following case studies. Use the guidelines listed in Test Yourself 6–1 to correctly phrase the interventions.

1. Cassie Tilton is an 88 year old woman transferred to your unit from a skilled nursing facility. Her history reveals a "flu-like" syndrome for the past five days with persistent vomiting and diarrhea. Her vital signs are: B/P 108/56, pulse rate 112, respirations 24, and temperature 101.4°F. Her mucous membranes are dry and skin turgor is decreased. She indicates that she feels weak, tired, and thirsty.

NURSING DIAGNOSIS: Fluid volume deficit related to vomiting and diarrhea

OUTCOMES: Within 48 hours: moist mucous membranes, vital signs within normal limits for client, intake greater than output

INTERVENTIONS:

2.   Chip Ireland is a 35 year old businessman admitted to the outpatient surgicenter for a tonsillectomy. He indicates that he has had recurrent tonsillitis for the past three years. Postoperatively he complains of being thirsty and requests a cold drink. You observe that he has difficulty swallowing and coughs up the water. He states "my throat is too sore; it feels like it is swollen." Upon examination, you note the presence of redness and edema in the operative area.

NURSING DIAGNOSIS: Impaired swallowing related to edema and effects of surgery

OUTCOME: By the time of discharge (from surgicenter) demonstrates ability to swallow at least 240 cc fluid

INTERVENTIONS:

3.   Dave Davis, a 54 year old self-employed mechanic, is admitted to your unit at 6:00 AM for removal of his gallbladder. During your assessment, you observe that he is unusually apprehensive, moderately diaphoretic, restless, and pacing around the room. His vital signs are: B/P 156/88, pulse rate 108, and respirations 28. His voice trembles as he tells you that he has never had surgery before and that his brother had a simple appendectomy at the age of 18. The brother died on the table; nothing they did could save him.

NURSING DIAGNOSIS: Fear related to perceived threat of death

OUTCOME: Verbalizes decreased fear prior to surgery

INTERVENTIONS:

4.   Emily Fantin is an 86 year old woman who calls the office nurse and requests free samples of laxatives. She complains "I've spent so much money on laxatives at the drug store; I take them twice a day so that my bowels will move two times a day. My mother always told me to take laxatives to keep myself regular. By the way, do you have any sample enemas?" Upon further questioning you find out that Emily lives alone and does her own cooking. She eats mostly frozen dinners or prepared foods with few fruits and vegetables. In addition, she shops at a local convenience store with a limited supply of fresh produce. She relies on Metamucil daily, and Ex Lax and Milk of Magnesia approximately four times a week. She states that she gets very little exercise.

NURSING DIAGNOSIS: Perceived constipation related to long-standing family health beliefs

OUTCOME: Within two months verbalizes satisfaction with one bowel movement every one to two days

INTERVENTIONS:

6–3 TEST YOURSELF □ ANSWERS

1.   Cassie Tilton is an 88 year old woman transferred to your unit from a skilled nursing facility. Her history reveals a "flu-like" syndrome for the past five days with persistent vomiting and diarrhea. Her vital signs are: B/P 108/56, pulse rate 112, respirations 24, and temperature 101.4°F. Her mucous membranes are dry and skin turgor is decreased. She indicates that she feels weak, tired, and thirsty.

NURSING DIAGNOSIS: Fluid volume deficit related to vomiting and diarrhea

OUTCOMES: Within 48 hours: moist mucous membranes, vital signs within normal limits for client, intake greater than output

INTERVENTIONS:
   1. Monitor and document vital signs and mental status every four hours for 24 hours.
   2. Assess and document frequency, color, and amount of emesis and diarrhea.
   3. Assess skin turgor, dryness, and mucous membranes every four hours for 24 hours, then every eight hours if vomiting and diarrhea have subsided.
   4. Monitor urine color and specific gravity every eight hours.
   5. Monitor intake and output every eight hours.
   6. Encourage p.o. fluid intake as tolerated. Provide 1500 cc per 24 hours: 7–3: 700 cc, 3–11: 600 cc, 11–7: 200 cc.
   7. Offer small amounts of fluids taken slowly.
   8. Instruct client to inform nursing staff if thirsty.
   9. Maintain IV fluids as ordered.
   10. Administer and evaluate the effectiveness of medications ordered to control vomiting and diarrhea.
   11. Monitor serum electrolyte value and report abnormalities.

2.   Chip Ireland is a 35 year old businessman admitted to the outpatient surgicenter for a tonsillectomy. He indicates that he has had recurrent tonsillitis for the past three years. Postoperatively he complains of being thirsty and requests a cold drink. You observe that he has difficult swallowing and coughs up the water. He states "my throat is too sore; it feels like it is swollen." Upon examination, you note the presence of redness and edema in the operative area.

NURSING DIAGNOSIS: Impaired swallowing related to edema and effects of surgery

OUTCOME: By the time of discharge (from surgicenter) demonstrates ability to swallow at least 240 cc fluid

INTERVENTIONS:
   1. Apply ice collar to neck per physician order.
   2. Administer and evaluate effectiveness of pain medication.
   3. Offer ice chips and gradually increase to sips of cold water and bland juice.
   4. Continue to assess edema every 15 minutes for one hour.
   5. Instruct client to notify nurse of breathing difficulty or increased swelling.

3. Dave Davis, a 54 year old self-employed mechanic, is admitted to your unit at 6:00 AM for removal of his gallbladder. During your assessment, you observe that he is unusually apprehensive, moderately diaphoretic, restless and pacing around the room. His vital signs are: B/P 156/88, pulse rate 108, and respirations 28. His voice trembles as he tells you that he has never had surgery before and that his brother had a simple appendectomy at the age of 18. The brother died on the table; nothing they did could save him.

NURSING DIAGNOSIS: Fear related to perceived threat of death

OUTCOME: Verbalizes decreased fear prior to surgery

INTERVENTIONS:
1. Encourage client to continue to verbalize fears and ask questions.
2. Acknowledge fear and provide realistic reassurance.
3. Explain and reinforce pre and postop routine.
4. Identify previously useful coping strategies and evaluate usefulness in dealing with fears.
5. Confer with surgeon and anesthesiologist regarding client's fears and need for preoperative visit.
6. Assess usefulness and client's openness to doing relaxation exercise preoperatively.

4. Emily Fantin is an 86 year old woman who calls the office nurse and requests free samples of laxatives. She complains "I've spent so much money on laxatives at the drug store; I take them twice a day so that my bowels will move two times a day. My mother always told me to take laxatives to keep myself regular. By the way, do you have any sample enemas?" Upon further questioning you find out that Emily lives alone and does her own cooking. She eats mostly frozen dinners or prepared foods with few fruits and vegetables. In addition, she shops at a local convenience store with a limited supply of fresh produce. She relies on Metamucil daily, and Ex Lax and Milk of Magnesia approximately four times a week. She states that she gets very little exercise.

NURSING DIAGNOSIS: Perceived constipation related to long-standing family health beliefs

OUTCOME: Within two months verbalizes satisfaction with one bowel movement every one to two days

INTERVENTIONS:
1. Discuss misconceptions regarding need for defecation two times a day.
2. Provide information regarding hazards of relying on laxatives.
3. Discuss with client benefits of increasing physical activity. Devise and supervise exercise plan. (specify): _____.
4. Assess daily fluid intake. Suggest at least 2000 cc per day.
5. Explore uses of hot water, coffee, tea, or lemon juice in early AM, and substituting natural bulk and fiber from fruits and vegetables of choice for laxatives.
6. Explore alternatives to shopping at the convenience store such as neighbors, delivery service, or Meals on Wheels.

STAGE 4—DOCUMENTATION: THE NURSING CARE PLAN

The fourth and final stage of the planning phase is recording the nursing diagnoses, outcomes, and interventions in an organized fashion. This is accomplished through documentation on the nursing care plan.

Definition

The nursing care plan is a method of communicating important information about the client. The format of the care plan assists the nurse in processing the information gathered during the assessment and diagnostic phases. The care plan acts as a receiving center when the nurse uses it to document the results of the planning phase. It facilitates communication by the sending of pertinent information. It also provides a mechanism for the evaluation of care provided. Development of pertinent care plans requires the nurse to have assessment, diagnostic, communication, and judgment skills.

Purposes

Nursing care plans are written in a variety of settings and are designed to promote quality care by facilitating (1) individualized care, (2) continuity of care, (3) communication, and (4) evaluation (Bower, 1982).

The care plan serves as a blueprint for directing nursing activities toward the fulfillment of the client's health needs. It provides a mechanism for the provision of consistent and coordinated care. The care plan is utilized as a communication tool among nurses and other members of the health care team. Furthermore, it provides a guideline for documentation on the nurse's notes. ''For instance, it lists what observations to make and how often, what nursing measures to take and how to implement them, and what to teach the patient and/or his family before he's discharged'' (Documentation, 1988). Finally, it guides the nurse in the evaluation of the effectiveness of care delivered.

Characteristics

Regardless of the setting in which they are written, nursing care plans have certain desirable characteristics. They are

1. Written by a registered nurse.
2. Initiated following the first contact with the client.
3. Readily available.
4. Current.

Written by a Registered Nurse

The American Nurses' Association, Joint Commission, and many nurse practice acts have addressed the development of nursing care plans. They have defined the role of the registered nurse as including responsibility for the initiation of the care plan. Based on educational preparation, the registered nurse is the most qualified person to complete this function. The client and other health care providers should be involved in the development of the plan. The client may contribute by defining and validating outcomes and nursing interventions.

Example. Frankie Cattner, a six year old boy, has been seen in the school nurse's office twice within the last month. Each visit was precipitated by an acute asthmatic attack. After questioning Frankie, the school nurse determines that each attack occurred shortly after he spent the day with a friend who has six cats. Frankie and the nurse agree to a mutual goal of the reduction or elimination of these attacks. They also agree to the following approach: Frankie will invite his friend to play at his house or in public parks.

The involvement of the client in this situation enhances the probability of successful resolution of his problem.

The nurse may also utilize the assistance of other health care providers in the development of the nursing care plan. These may include LPNs, aides, and members of other disciplines, such as social services or speech therapy.

Example. Glenn Weiser, a 57 year old man, is being followed up at home by the visiting nurse. He is aphasic as a result of a stroke. His sister manages his daily care and verbalizes her frustration over Glenn's inability to communicate his needs. The nurse presents the problem to a speech therapist, who recommends the use of a picture board. This enables the client to point to the things he needs and decreases the frustration of the client and his sister.

In addition to participating in the development of the plan, other health care providers may be utilized in its implementation. Specific nursing activities may be delegated to other nursing personnel, such as LPNs or nursing assistants. However, the responsibility and accountability for the initiation of the care plan rest with the registered nurse.

Initiation Following First Contact

The nursing care plan is most effective when it is initiated after the nurse's first contact with the client. Immediately after obtaining the data base, the nurse should begin to document actual or potential diagnoses, outcomes, and interventions. A partially developed plan will assist the nurse to focus on the client's needs. Additional interaction with the client may result in further development and refinement of the plan of care.

The nurse who obtains the data base has the most information about the client. Therefore, it is more likely that this nurse will be able to develop a comprehensive plan. Occasionally a comprehensive data base may not be collected because of time constraints, condition of the client, or the initiation of treatment modalities. In this situation the nurse may

1. Develop a preliminary plan based on the available information.
2. Gather the absent data during subsequent contacts with the client.
3. Refine the preliminary plan.

4. Delegate the responsibility for obtaining the absent data and refining the preliminary plan to another registered nurse.

The trend toward decreasing the length of stay for hospitalized clients emphasizes the importance of initiating the care plan on the first contact with the client. By identifying the client's needs at the time of admission, the nurse promotes efficient and coordinated care.

Readily Available

The nursing care plan should be readily available to all personnel involved in the care of the client. It may be located on the client's medical record, at the bedside, or in a centralized location. Ready access to the care plan facilitates its usefulness and its value as a communication tool.

Current

Since the nursing care plan is the blueprint for directing the client's care, it must contain current information. Therefore, it is essential that all components of the nursing care plan be updated frequently. Nursing diagnoses, outcomes, and interventions that are no longer valid are either eliminated or revised. The method of updating the care plan varies with the type of nursing care plan format utilized and the agency policy. This is addressed more fully in Chapter 9.

Example. Elaine Conner is a hospitalized client whose IV infusion infiltrated three days ago. The nurse made a diagnosis of "pain related to edema in right forearm." The nursing interventions include "warm soaks via heating pad for $\frac{1}{2}$ hour, tid at 10 AM, 4 PM and 10 PM." Today when a different nurse attempts to apply the soaks as ordered, Elaine informs her that they were discontinued yesterday.

As a result of an outdated care plan, the nurse's time was not utilized effectively. Furthermore, the client may lose confidence in the nurse's ability to deliver appropriate care.

Components

The nursing care plan may be structured in several ways, depending on the system in use in the agency. However, the components of the nursing care plan usually consist of

1. Nursing diagnoses
2. Outcomes
3. Nursing interventions

Each of these components has been previously described in detail.

The nursing care plan is frequently supplemented by the use of a Kardex. This form usually consists of a checklist of frequently ordered medical and nurs-

Vital Signs:	Nutrition:	Activity:	
TPR ____	Feed ____ Set-Up ____	Bedrest ____	BRP ____
BP ____	Diet:	Chair ____	OOB ____
Neuro ____	Fluids: (Force, Restrict)	Siderails	
Weight ____ Scale ____		Release ____ Restrain Order ____	

Bath:	Respiratory Therapy:	Physical Therapy	Cardiac Rehab. I II III IV
Complete ____	Mask ____ Humidifier ____	Referrals: (Pt. Ed., Hospice, Dietary)	
Partial ____	Cannula ____ Trach. ____		
Tub ____	Liters O$_2$ ____	Discharge Plans:	
Shower ____	Rx:	Home ____ Rehab. ____ Extended Care ____	

Elimination:	Fluid Balance:	Initials Signature Title
Last BM ____ Enema ____	I & O ____	
Commode ____	Heplock ____ Hyperali-mentation ____	
Stoma ____	IV ____	
Foley ____	Kelly Drip ____	
Change Date ____	Foley ____	
Care ____	N/G Tube ____	
C & A ____	Suction ____ Feed ____	
Insulin Coverage ____	Irrigation ____	

FIGURE 6–1. Kardex documentation form. (Courtesy of Mercer Medical Center, Trenton, NJ.)

ing functions (Figure 6–1). Diagnostic studies and treatments may be recorded on the Kardex in specific areas. The nursing implications associated with these modalities are defined in the nursing care plan.

Example. The doctor orders a myelogram utilizing Amipaque (metrizamide). The nurse places the order on the Kardex, assesses the client's knowledge of the procedure, and develops the care plan as follows.

NURSING DIAGNOSIS	OUTCOME	INTERVENTIONS
Knowledge deficit (myelogram)	Explains the usual pre and postmyelogram care	1. Review booklet on myelograms with client on evening of 6/11 2. Explain pre- and postmyelogram guidelines for fluid intake and position 3. Encourage client to verbalize feelings about the outcome of the myelogram

Types of Care Plans

There are several different types of care plans in use. Those that are most common include individually constructed, standardized, and computerized care plans.

Individually Constructed

Care plans written from scratch are documented on forms that are divided into columns with the usual headings of nursing diagnoses, outcomes, and interventions.

Advantages. The individually written plan enables the documentation of the nursing diagnoses, outcomes, and interventions that are most pertinent to a particular client. No extraneous or inapplicable information is included in the care plan.

Disadvantages. Development and documentation of this type of care plan is time consuming. In recognition of these difficulties, the Joint Commission has softened the requirements for individually constructed care plans. As this book is published there are indications that standardized plans of care will become more common. Other new forms of documenting care planning will emerge.

Standardized

Standardized care plans have been introduced into several types of agencies to facilitate the preparation and use of care plans. According to Mayers (1983), "a standard care plan is a specific protocol of care that is appropriate for patients who are experiencing the usual or predictable problems associated with a given diagnosis or disease process." Standardized care plans consist of actual, or potential nursing diagnoses, outcomes, and interventions that are printed in a care plan format. Individualization is possible through the use of blank spaces as illustrated on Table 6–1. Additional standardized care plans are found in the appendix. The nurse may cross off items that do not apply to the client or add additional nursing diagnoses, outcomes, and interventions. The care plans may be developed by the nursing staff of a particular agency or may be derived from the literature. Sources of published standardized care plans include articles or books. Table 6–1 is a standardized plan for the client with pain.

Standardized care plans may be used in one of two ways: (1) they may be placed in a centrally located area and referred to by nurses when developing handwritten individually constructed care plans, or (2) they may be placed directly on the Kardex, dated, and signed.

Advantages. The advantages of standardized care plans include the following.

1. They are usually developed by clinical experts who have carefully researched the literature. They are useful in educating nurses who are not familiar with a certain medical or nursing diagnosis.

TABLE 6–1. ACUTE PAIN

Pain related to effects of surgery, effects of ischemia, inflammatory process, effects of trauma, effects of invasive procedures, and prolonged immobility

Outcomes

Reports pain promptly when experiencing it

Verbalizes decreased pain within 30 minutes following initiation of comfort measures

Interventions

1. Help client identify pain relief measures that have been helpful in the past.
2. Explore with client feelings and attitudes related to use of pain medication and fear of addiction.
3. Instruct client/family:
    □ to report pain promptly
    □ to describe using 0–10 scale
    □ regarding prescribed regimen for pain relief
    □ to evaluate and report effectiveness of interventions
4. Assess for pain using verbal and nonverbal messages q_____ including location, quality, intensity, duration, precipitating/aggravating/relieving factors, and associated symptoms.
5. Explain source of pain/discomfort if known
6. Collaborate with physician to establish a pain control regimen:
    □ Medications
    □ Use of hot/cold application
    □ Patient controlled analgesia
    □ TENS
7. Provide therapeutic comfort measures based on appropriateness and client willingness/desire
    □ Position change (specify position of comfort) _____
      _____
    □ Back rub/massage
    □ Relaxation techniques and guided imagery
    □ Diversional activities (specify) _____
    □ Alteration in environment (specify) _____
8. Reassure and support client/family during episodes of pain.
9. Provide quiet environment and organize care to promote periods of uninterrupted rest.
10. Medicate prior to activities to promote participation.
11. Assess and document findings and effectiveness of interventions.

2.   They reduce the amount of time spent in writing nursing care plans. This increases the efficiency of nursing care planning.

3.   They provide information specific to a particular client and require less time to complete. Additionally, because they outline the expected nursing care, they enhance the quality of the delivery and documentation of care.

Disadvantages.   Using standardized care plans can be limiting because it is rare that all of the client's specific problems will be addressed by one standardized care plan. The nurse must individualize the standardized care plan to reflect the client's unique needs.

Computerized

The basic elements of care plan systems, nursing diagnoses, outcomes, and interventions are also present in computerized systems. The nursing care plan may be prepared at a terminal in the client's room or in a central location. Once data are validated and entered, a printed version may be generated daily, on each shift, or on demand (Figure 6–2). There are a number of mechanisms by which care plans are generated. Three commonly used systems are (1) standardized plans based on the medical diagnosis, (2) standardized plans based on the nursing diagnosis, and (3) individually constructed plans.

PATIENT CARE PLAN

GENERAL HOSPITAL	5/16/84 11:41 AM	PAGE 1

TRN-09   000187023 2555555   TRN
TESTPAT JACK   SEX: M
ADM: 5/15/84   SRV:URO   SMK: N
DOB: 10/06/21 62 COND: G   LEVEL: 1
HT: 5/11 F/I   WT: 180/000 P/O
10000 INTERNIST OTHER
ALG: PENICILLIN
DX: NEPHROLITHIASIS

KNOWLEDGE DEFICIT RELATED
TO SURGICAL EXPERIENCE

OUTCOME:	Describes type of surgery
OUTCOME:	States usual pre-op preparation
OUTCOME:	Identifies usual postop routine
OUTCOME:	Verbalizes feelings about impending surgery
INTERVENTION:	Assess knowledge of surgery and explore past surgical experience(s) at the time of admission
INTERVENTION:	Review surgical routine (preps, meds, dressing)
INTERVENTION:	Reinforce pre-operative teaching re: Sequence of events on day of surgery (pre-op stretcher to OR, RR return to room/ICU) Postop equipment (dsg., IV, tubes) Provisions for relief of pain and other symptoms (include need to request and frequency limitations) Turning, coughing and deep breathing Incentive spirometry if ordered Change in bowel/bladder functions Progressive diet changes Progressive self care

FIGURE 6–2. Computerized care plan. (Courtesy of HBO & Company, Atlanta, GA. All rights reserved.)

Medical Diagnoses.   In these systems, the computer provides the nurse with nursing diagnoses, outcomes, and nursing interventions commonly associated with the medical diagnoses. These are very similar to the printed standardized care plans discussed earlier. The nurse who is formulating the plan selects the appropriate items from the standardized data base. Additional diagnoses, outcomes, and interventions may be entered to reflect other concerns of the client.

Nursing Diagnoses.   Other computerized systems are more directly associated with the specific nursing diagnoses identified at the time of the detailed nursing assessment. The computer lists each diagnosis, and the nurse defines outcomes and nursing interventions by selecting from a menu of appropriate choices. The nurse may add other specific outcomes and interventions for an individual client, if appropriate. Some systems are constructed to allow clients to participate actively in the selection of outcomes and appropriate interventions. The nurse assists clients in choosing outcomes or interventions that they feel will best meet clients' needs. Selections are made from a menu that includes appropriate outcomes or nursing orders (Wesseling, 1980).

Individually Constructed.   In these systems, the nurse develops the care plan in a fashion similar to that used in a manual individualized plan. The nurse is not prompted to focus on specific diagnoses but uses a menu to select those diagnoses, outcomes, and interventions that apply to the individual client. Additional outcomes or interventions not identified in the menu may also be added when necessary.

Most computerized care planning systems facilitate frequent updating of the plan. The nurse identifies problems that have been resolved, and they are eliminated from the plan. Other options may include (1) revision of diagnoses, outcomes, and interventions to reflect the changing status of the client or (2) addition of new diagnoses, outcomes, and interventions. Printed care plans, which are a permanent part of the medical record, document the client's progress as reflected by the changing plan of care.

Computerized care plans increase the potential for accurate and thorough documentation of the delivery of care. The computer identifies specific nursing approaches listed on the plan and prompts the nurse to document the outcome of the intervention. This process also encourages frequent review of the plan as well as modification, when appropriate.

More sophisticated programs compare the client's data with a list of defining characteristics for specific nursing diagnoses. If the client's data match the defining characteristics, the program will display the nursing diagnosis. The nurse then has the option of choosing the displayed diagnosis or rejecting it and selecting another. If the displayed diagnosis is accepted, the system will present expected outcomes and interventions that would be applicable. The nurse chooses the appropriate outcomes and interventions or enters the individualized ones.

Advantages.   The advantages of computerized care plans include the following.

1.   Preparation of a computer-generated care plan from a standardized plan takes less time than handwriting an individualized care plan.

2.   The computerized care plan can be designed to determine the staffing needs of the unit.

3.   Care plans that are prepared on a printer are easy to read.

4.   Automated care planning consistently uses a systematic method to develop care plans, thereby decreasing the possibility of error.

5.   Utilizing computer-assisted care planning permits the identification of common nursing diagnoses for research and planning purposes.

Disadvantages.   Along with the many advantages, some disadvantages do exist and include the following.

1.   Adequate numbers of computers must be available to the nursing staff. If sufficient hardware is not available because of cost or space considerations, the care planning process will become more difficult.

2.   Errors that occur in computerized nursing care plans may be harder to detect. Nurses have a tendency to lend more credence to computer printouts than they would to handwritten records.

3.   The computer may develop a care plan that may be logically consistent but is not applicable to a client.

SUMMARY

The development of nursing interventions is the third stage of the planning phase of the nursing process. Nursing interventions define the activities that assist the client in achieving desired outcomes. Nursing interventions are consistent with the plan of care, based on scientific principles, and individualized to the specific client situation. They are also used to provide a safe and therapeutic environment. Additionally, nursing interventions include teaching-learning opportunities for the client and the utilization of appropriate resources.

Nursing interventions are developed through a scientific approach and include date, signature, precise action verbs, specific aspects of interventions, and modifications in standard therapy. The registered nurse is responsible and accountable for the development of nursing interventions.

The fourth stage of the planning phase consists of documentation of the plan on a nursing care plan. Care plans may be individualized, standardized, or computerized. Much time is wasted when care plans are not developed. Nurses who are unfamiliar with the client's care may spend time in reviewing the client's record and asking questions of other nursing personnel or of the client. This hit or miss approach leads to a great deal of wasted effort and inefficient care, which could be avoided by documentation of the plan. Care plans are necessary to provide a framework for the delivery of care and to ensure continuity.

REFERENCES

American Nurses' Association: Standards of Nursing Practice. St. Louis: American Nurses' Association, 1973.

Bigbee J: Locus of control and the obese adolescent: a pilot study. In Chinn O (ed): Advances in Nursing Theory Development. Rockville, MD: Aspen, 1983.

Bower F: The Process of Planning Nursing Care, 3rd ed. St. Louis: CV Mosby, 1982.

Carnevali D: Nursing Care Planning. Diagnosis and Management, 3rd ed. Philadelphia: JB Lippincott, 1983.

Documentation. Springhouse, PA: Springhouse Corporation, 1988.

Mayers M: A Systematic Approach to the Nursing Care Plan, 3rd ed. Norwalk, CT: Appleton-Century-Crofts, 1983.

Wesseling E: Automating the nursing history and care plan. In Zeilstorff R: Computers in Nursing. Rockville, MD: Aspen, 1980.

BIBLIOGRAPHY

Anthony M, Williams A, Hoagland B, and Cunningham D: Nursing interventions: independent or not. Nursing Management 1988 Dec; 18(12):14–15.

Fairless P: 9 ways a computer can make your work easier. Nursing 1986 Sep; 16(9):54–56.

Fraher J: Nursing diagnoses and care plans in critical care. Critical Care Nurse 1983 Nov–Dec; 3(6): 94–98.

Heater B, Becker A, and Olson R: Nursing interventions and patient outcomes: a meta analysis of studies. Nursing Research 1988 Sep–Oct; 37(5):303–307.

Hinson I, Silva N, and Clapp P: An automated Kardex and care plan. Nursing Management 1984 Jul; 15(7):35–36, 38–40, 42–43.

Marriner A: The Nursing Process: A Scientific Approach to Nursing Care, 3rd ed. St. Louis: CV Mosby, 1983.

McFarland G, and McFarlane E: Nursing Diagnosis and Interventions. St. Louis: CV Mosby, 1989.

Sandborn C, and Blount M: Standard plans: for care and discharge. American Journal of Nursing 1984 Nov; 84(11):1394–1396.

Walters S: Computerized care plans help nurses achieve quality patient care. Journal of Nursing Administration 1986; Nov; 16(11):33–39.

7 IMPLEMENTATION

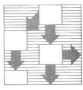

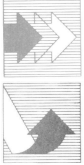

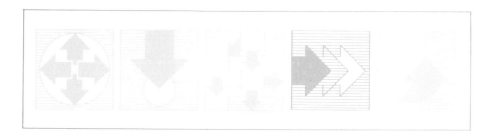

INTRODUCTION

Implementation is the initiation of the nursing care plan to achieve specific outcomes. The implementation phase begins after the care plan has been developed and focuses on the initiation of those nursing interventions that assist the client to accomplish desired outcomes. Specific nursing interventions are implemented to modify the factors contributing to the client's problem.

Nurses implement plans of care in a variety of health care environments. Regardless of the settings in which nurses practice, the nursing process is utilized to provide care to clients. The nurse utilizes three stages to complete the implementation phase—(1) preparation, (2) intervention, and (3) documentation.

STAGE 1—PREPARATION

The first stage of the implementation phase requires the nurse to prepare for the initiation of nursing interventions. This preparation involves a series of activities, including the following.

1. Reviewing the nursing interventions identified in the planning phase
2. Analyzing the nursing knowledge and skills required
3. Recognizing the potential complications associated with specific nursing activities
4. Determining and providing necessary resources
5. Preparing an environment conducive to the types of activities required

Reviewing Anticipated Nursing Interventions

Nursing interventions are designed to promote, maintain, or restore the client's health. When preparing to implement a nursing intervention, the nurse should review it to ensure that it remains current and includes certain desirable characteristics. These characteristics were identified in Chapter 6 and are summarized below.

Nursing interventions should

☐ Be consistent with the plan of care

☐ Be based on scientific principles

☐ Be individualized to the specific situation

☐ Be used to provide a safe and therapeutic environment

☐ Include teaching-learning opportunities for the client

☐ Consider utilization of appropriate resources

Nursing interventions that include these characteristics help to ensure that the client will receive quality nursing care.

Analyzing Knowledge and Skills Required

After reviewing the interventions in the plan of care, the nurse should identify the level of knowledge and types of skills required for implementation. This allows the nurse to determine the person who is best qualified to perform the required activities. It may be a member of the nursing department—clinical nurse specialist, registered nurse, licensed practical nurse, or nursing assistant.

Example. Missy Stevens is a 16 year old who will be having surgery later today. Her preop nursing interventions include "teach coughing and deep breathing 5/8 PM."

The nurse recognizes that this intervention requires knowledge of the relationship between adequate ventilation and effective removal of secretions and postoperative respiratory complications. The intervention also requires skills to explain the rationale, demonstrate the procedure, and encourage the client to practice coughing and deep breathing preoperatively. The nurse determines that the practical nurse who is caring for Missy is capable of initiating this intervention.

Personnel from other disciplines may also be involved in the implementation of nursing interventions. They may include the respiratory therapist, dietician, social worker, or speech therapist.

Example. Zack Cronin is an elderly client recently transferred to an extended care facility after a total hip replacement. He often verbalizes frustration over his inability to put on his socks and shoes. Nursing interventions for Mr.

Cronin include "teach client to put on socks and shoes using long-handled shoe horn."

The nurse recognizes that this intervention requires specific knowledge about total hip surgery, body mechanics, and the use of assistive devices. In this case, an occupational therapist will be requested to assist in teaching Mr. Cronin.

Recognizing Potential Complications

The initiation of certain nursing procedures may involve potential risks to the client. The nurse needs to be aware of the most common complications associated with the activities specified in the client's nursing interventions. This allows the nurse to initiate preventive approaches that decrease the risk to the client.

Example. Pat Ponticiello is a 35 year old woman who is three days post-op following an abdominal hysterectomy. Her catheter has been removed and nursing interventions include "ambulate to bathroom twice each shift; utilize nursing measures to encourage voiding—e.g., running water; check for bladder distention q4h (10 AM, 2 PM, 6PM, etc.); catheterize q8h prn."

In this case, both bladder distention and catheterization pose a risk for the client. Distention may result in an atonic bladder, while infection may be associated with catheter insertion. Based on this knowledge, the nurse palpates and percusses the abdomen carefully to identify the presence of distention. Should catheterization be necessary, the nurse utilizes meticulous sterile technique to avoid the introduction of organisms at the time of insertion.

Other less invasive procedures may also result in complications for the client.

Example. Sarah Johnson is a 56 year old woman with a medical diagnosis of cancer of the liver. One of Sarah's nursing diagnoses is "altered nutrition: less than body requirements related to decreased appetite secondary to chemotherapy." The physician orders 2500 ml of tube feedings daily. Associated nursing interventions include "monitor continuous tube feedings q2h (even hours); check tube placement q shift—8 AM, 4 PM, 12 AM, and prn."

In this case, the nurse is aware of the potential for aspiration in the client with a feeding tube. Based on this knowledge, the position of the tube is monitored to prevent or detect dislodgement and associated aspiration of feedings. The nurse also utilizes other techniques to avoid diarrhea. These include dilution of feedings to half-strength, use of continuous rather than intermittent feedings, and maintenance of constant flow rate with the assistance of a feeding pump.

The client may also be at risk for common complications associated with illness or treatment modalities. For example, this is typified by the pulmonary and embolic complications that may occur following surgery. Nursing interventions designed to prevent these problems include

"Encourage coughing and deep breathing q2h (even hours)."
"Incentive spirometer q2h"
"Turn and reposition q2h (even hours)."

"Apply antiembolism stockings upon return from postanesthesia care unit."

"Remind client to do at least ten ankle pumps per hour."

A common hazard in the elderly client is altered skin integrity associated with prolonged immobility. The nurse frequently initiates interventions to minimize the risk to these clients. They may include

"Turn q2h (odd hours) as specified on turning schedule."

"Massage bony prominences with lotion after turning."

"Bathe qod (even dates)—add Alpha Keri to water."

"Apply transparent dressing to reddened area on sacrum—change on the 7–3 shift q4d and prn."

The preventive approaches outlined above reflect a comprehensive nursing effort to protect the client in these circumstances. These may be necessary until the client is completely recovered, immobility is decreased, or the client is able to initiate such measures independently.

Providing Necessary Resources

When preparing to initiate nursing interventions, a number of concerns about resources should be addressed. These include time, personnel, and equipment.

Time

There are a variety of time considerations that affect the nurse's ability to implement the plan. First, the nurse must be careful to select the appropriate time for the initiation of specific interventions.

Example. Donna Kelsey is an 18 year old recovering from abdominal surgery, performed two days ago for a perforated appendix. Nursing interventions include "teach client to do dressing change on 1/3." The nurse enters Donna's room to begin teaching and finds her walking around the room, clutching her abdomen. Donna indicates that she has "gas pains."

In this case, the nurse recognizes that this is not the appropriate time to begin teaching. The client is obviously uncomfortable and will probably be unable to concentrate on or retain the information provided.

Example. James Boardman is a 56 year old who is receiving intravenous antibiotics for an infected wound. The medication is ordered every eight hours. When selecting administration times, the nurse chooses 6 AM, 2 PM, and 10 PM rather than 2 AM, 10 AM, and 6 PM.

In this case, the nurse's choice avoids disruption of the client's sleep at 2 AM. This allows Mr. Boardman to conserve the energy required for the healing process.

The nurse must also be sure to allow adequate time for completion of the nursing intervention. A thorough understanding of the actions necessary to implement the nursing intervention will allow the nurse to anticipate the time required. Careful organization will prevent the problems associated with hasty implementation.

Example. Kate Clinger is a community health nurse who is seeing a number of clients in a clinic. As she examines Jason Kovar, she discovers a serious skin irritation around his colostomy. Kate recognizes that the initiation of the measures required to manage the problem will involve a great deal of time. Therefore, she asks another nurse to see the waiting clients so that she can adequately treat Mr. Kovar's skin problem.

Personnel

The nurse should evaluate the availability of sufficient numbers of personnel required to implement the intervention.

Example. Henry Smithson is a 27 year old athlete who is recovering from chest surgery. He is six ft tall and weighs 255 lb. In preparing to ambulate this client for the first time, the nurse anticipates the need for assistance by at least one additional staff member. This will prevent injury to the client or the nurse during the ambulation process.

Equipment

Another consideration when preparing to implement nursing interventions is the identification and procurement of necessary supplies. Again, the nurse must have a thorough understanding of the identified nursing action. This allows the anticipation of required equipment.

Example. In preparing to assist with the insertion of a urethral catheter, the nurse recognizes that a variety of equipment is required. These supplies include a light, a drape, a catheter, a drainage bag, lubricant, cotton balls, and antiseptic solution.

The nurse's inability to anticipate the need for the equipment in this case may result in inefficient performance of the catheterization. Therefore, the nurse should determine and provide the supplies necessary to ensure that the intervention is accomplished in an efficient and timely fashion.

Preparing a Conducive Environment

Successful implementation of nursing interventions requires an environment in which the client feels comfortable and safe. Chapter 2 described a number of approaches designed to create a therapeutic environment in which clients and nurses can work toward resolving the factors that are contributing to the presence of unhealthful responses in the client.

Comfort

The creation of a comfortable environment involves consideration of both physical and psychosocial components. Physical concerns include the immediate environment (e.g., room and space), privacy, noise, odor, lighting, and temperature.

Example. Ed Kearney is a 78 year old man who had a cataract extraction three days ago. Following discharge from the hospital, he is being managed by his family at home with the assistance of a visiting nurse. Mr. Kearney requires a daily change of his eye patch and administration of medication. Before removing the dressing, the nurse ensures the client's comfort by pulling the shades and darkening the room to avoid the pain associated with exposure to light.

The nurse must also consider psychosocial concerns when preparing to implement nursing actions. These frequently require the use of interpersonal skills to provide an environment in which clients are comfortable in expressing their needs, fears, feeling, and concerns, and frustrations.

Example. Valerie Lezan is a 10 year old girl who fractured her leg. When Maria Burden, the nurse in the emergency department, begins to help Valerie remove her blouse, she says, "Please don't do that. I don't want you to look at my chest." Maria hands Valerie a gown and says, "I will stand outside your curtain while you change."

In this situation the nurse demonstrates respect for Valerie's need for privacy. Management of psychosocial concerns usually involves both verbal and nonverbal communication skills, including interviewing, counseling, listening, and demonstrating.

Safety

A number of factors must be considered when the nurse attempts to create a safe environment. These include the client's age, degree of mobility, sensory deficits, and level of consciousness or orientation.

Age. When considering age, certainly the very young and the elderly are at great risk of injury. However, any environment that is unfamiliar to the client may be hazardous.

The infant and the toddler may be unable to communicate sensations such as pain or burning. Additionally, young children tend to explore their environment and the objects in it. Therefore, the nurse, in preparing to initiate procedures, must ensure that special consideration is given to the child's safety.

Example. Kevin Chen is a four year old admitted to pediatrics with a diagnosis of insulin-dependent diabetes. Kevin requires intravenous therapy and frequent insulin injections.

In managing Kevin's care, the nurse is careful to ensure that his IV line is securely taped to reduce the possibility that he will put it out. The control clamp is also placed out of Kevin's reach to prevent him from inadvertently increasing the infusion rate. When preparing to administer injections, the nurse also checks the medication dosage carefully and secures assistance if necessary to prevent injury at the time of injection.

Developmental changes associated with aging also require the nurse to prepare a safe environment for the elderly client. Decreased muscle strength and reflex speed prevent the older individual from recovering lost balance. Aging may also be accompanied by decreased visual and hearing acuity.

Degree of Mobility. The client's degree of mobility may be affected by disease or trauma, external restrictions such as traction or casts, or the need to conserve energy or equilibrium.

Example. John Cambria is a 28 year old man admitted to the hospital for lumbar strain. His physician has ordered bedrest, with bathroom privileges for bowel movement only.

In anticipating the care of Mr. Cambria, the nurse is careful to place necessary supplies, such as water and the call bell, within his reach. This helps the client to avoid moving or reaching incorrectly, reducing the potential for further back strain. The nurse also instructs him to call for assistance when getting out of bed to avoid the potential for injury associated with a sudden drop in blood pressure after long periods of bedrest.

Sensory Deficits. The client who has decreased perception in sight, hearing, smell, taste, or touch may be at risk for injury. The nurse may be required to adapt the environment to protect the client's safety.

Example. Gladys Goldstein is a 26 year old quadriplegic who has developed an inflammation on her left thigh. She is seen in the outpatient clinic by a physician. Her medical orders include continuous warm soaks to her left thigh.

In this case, because Gladys has no feeling in her lower extremities, the nurse will attempt to ensure that the hazards of the treatment are reduced. This may be accomplished by instructing Gladys and her husband to check the temperature of the solutions and to inspect her skin frequently for evidence of burns.

Example. Sadie Bush is an 89 year old client who has been blind for ten years as a result of glaucoma. She is being admitted to a nursing home because she is no longer capable of caring for herself.

The nurse who admits Sadie may spend a great deal of time orienting her to this new environment and rearranging furniture to minimize the possibility that Sadie may be injured.

Clients with less serious visual deficits may be encouraged to wear corrective lenses. The nurse should also remind the client with a hearing deficit to wear a hearing aid if available. In addition, the nurse may touch the client to attract attention, approach from the client's good side, or be sure to be seen by the client before attempting to communicate or initiate other interventions.

Level of Consciousness/Orientation. Clients who have decreased levels of consciousness or who are disoriented often require special attention or interventions to promote safety. Clients may be lethargic, stuporous, confused, or disoriented. These responses require the nurse to adjust the environment to prevent injury.

Example. Tyrone Magee is a 54 year old man who is recovering from a cerebral concussion. He is frequently disoriented and is found wandering in the hall looking for his dog.

The nurse who is managing Mr. Magee's care reorients him and returns him to his room. In addition, she puts the bed in the lowest position, arranges the room so that he will not fall, and keeps a light on in his room at night.

The care of an unconscious client may require similar adaptations.

Example. Al Rogers, age 62, is comatose following a massive CVA (stroke). He is restless at times and has had many seizures in the last 24 hours.

In this situation, the nurse may initiate a number of measures to protect the client. They may include padding the side rails, frequent changes in position, special skin care, and passive range of motion exercises.

STAGE 2—INTERVENTION

The focus of the implementation phase is the initiation of nursing interventions designed to meet the client's physical or emotional needs. The nurse's approach may involve the initiation of independent, dependent, and interdependent actions. The approaches designed to meet the client's physical and emotional needs are numerous and varied, depending on individual, specific problems.

The implementation phase builds on the assessment, diagnosis, and planning phases of the nursing process. The initial detailed assessment was covered in Chapter 2. The assessment process utilized during the implementation phase is ongoing and involves the nurse's ability to collect and process data before, during, and after the initiation of nursing interventions. For example, before getting a postoperative client out of bed, the nurse observes that he is short of breath and slightly diaphoretic. Based on these findings, the nurse assesses the client's vital signs and chooses to defer his ambulation at that time.

The client's physical and emotional needs are identified in the assessment phase of the nursing process. A nursing diagnosis and outcomes are formulated, and individualized nursing interventions are written. During the implementation phase, the nurse initiates these interventions. The following subsections discuss the type of interventions used based on the North American Nursing Diagnosis Association Taxonomy. A definition is provided for each pattern along with a listing of the nursing diagnoses within the pattern. Some of the possible related factors for each pattern are also listed. The focus for nursing interventions associated with each pattern is described and illustrated with examples. Interventions are directed toward identifying usual patterns, detecting specific related factors, developing preventive or corrective approaches to alleviate the related factor, and providing client education. See Appendix I for a similar discussion utilizing functional health patterns.

Human Response Patterns

Exchanging.—human response pattern involving mutual giving and receiving

NURSING DIAGNOSES	POSSIBLE RELATED FACTORS
Altered nutrition: more than body requirements	Eating in response to stress or emotional trauma
Altered nutrition: less than body requirements	Nausea and vomiting
Altered nutrition: potential for more than body requirements	Family/cultural eating patterns
Potential for infection	Broken skin
Potential altered body temperature	Inappropriate clothing for environmental temperature
Hypothermia	Exposure to cold environment
Hyperthermia	Inability to regulate environmental temperature
Ineffective thermoregulation	Extremes of age
Dysreflexia	Bowel distention
Constipation	Ignoring urge to defecate
Perceived constipation	Cultural/family health beliefs
Colonic constipation	Lack of privacy
Diarrhea	Effects of medications
Bowel incontinence	Excessive use of laxatives
Altered patterns of urinary elimination	Pain/spasm in bladder or abdomen
Stress incontinence	Weak pelvic muscles
Reflex incontinence	Effects of neurological impairment
Urge incontinence	Ingestion of alcohol
Functional incontinence	Altered environment
Total incontinence	Inaccessible toileting facilities
Urinary retention	Fear of postoperative pain
Altered tissue perfusion (renal, cerebral, cardiopulmonary, gastrointestinal, peripheral)	Effects of vasospasm Decreased blood volume
Fluid volume excess	Effects of pregnancy
Fluid volume deficit (1)	Persistent fever
Fluid volume deficit (2)	Excessive use of alcohol
Potential fluid volume deficit	Excessive diaphoresis
Decreased cardiac output	Decreased myocardial contractility
Impaired gas exchange	Effects of inhalation of toxic fumes
Ineffective airway clearance	Viscous secretions
Ineffective breathing pattern	Fatigue

NURSING DIAGNOSES	POSSIBLE RELATED FACTORS
Potential for injury	Hazards associated with catheterization
Potential for suffocation	Vehicle engine running in closed garage
Potential for poisoning	Unsafe work environment
Potential for trauma	Riding in car without seat belt
Potential for aspiration	Reduced level of consciousness
Potential for disuse syndrome	Immobility
Altered protection	Inadequate nutrition
Impaired tissue integrity	Excessive use of contact lenses
Altered oral mucous membrane	Inadequate oral hygiene
Impaired skin integrity	Irritating wound drainage
Potential impaired skin integrity	Presacral edema

The list of nursing diagnoses and possible related factors for the exchanging pattern has been provided above. The implementation of nursing interventions for this pattern may be directed toward (1) identification of unhealthy patterns through assessment, (2) determination of the factors precipitating their potential or actual occurrence, (3) identification of available resources, (4) provision of specific education, and (5) implementation of corrective or preventive approaches.

Example. Patrick Jordan has returned home from the hospital to live with his wife. During the public health nurse's first visit several safety hazards are noted. The nurse instructs the elderly couple on how to correct the hazards with such interventions as taping down loose area rugs, installing a light at the top of the stairs, and installing grab bars in the bathroom.

Implementation:

Here, the nurse recognizes that the couple can reduce their potential for trauma by making some changes in their environment. The nurse's concrete suggestions help reduce the chances of the elderly couple experiencing falls.

Example. Constance Sohodski is a 40 year old woman who works as a computer operator. She tells the industrial nurse, "I'm so embarrassed. Since I've gained all this weight, every time I cough or sneeze I leak urine. If this gets worse I'm going to start getting wet spots on the back of my dresses. What should I do?"

The focus of interventions for this client with stress incontinence would include (1) advising client to see her urologist for an examination, (2) instructing her on the use of Kegel pelvic floor exercises, (3) encouraging her to urinate at frequent intervals to avoid a full bladder, and (4) suggesting the use of sanitary pads or adult diapers.

Example. Carla Ramirez is seen for the first time in a prenatal clinic. She is 17 years old and pregnant with her second child. When seen in the clinic she

---

NURSING DIAGNOSIS
Potential for trauma related to safety hazards

OUTCOME
No evidence of accident/injury within next 6 months

NURSING DIAGNOSIS
Stress incontinence related to obesity

OUTCOME
Identifies method to remain dry within 1 week

indicates that she had potato chips and soda for lunch. Carla states that she is unmarried, receives public assistance, and lives with her parents and nine siblings.

Implementation:

The nurse identifies that this client has specific nutritional needs associated with her pregnancy. Assessment also indicates a number of factors that will interfere with the client's ability to satisfy these needs. Therefore, the nurse will implement interventions designed to increase the potential for Carla to obtain the food, milk, and vitamin supplements required during pregnancy.

NURSING DIAGNOSIS
Altered nutrition: less than body requirements related to lack of financial resources

OUTCOME
Eats foods from each food group daily

Communicating.—human response pattern involving the sending of messages

NURSING DIAGNOSIS	POSSIBLE RELATED FACTORS
Impaired verbal communication	Language barrier
	Oral inflammation

The focus of nursing interventions is to identify related factors for the communication deficit and to design strategies to facilitate communication.

Example. David Long has had surgery on his larynx and is unable to speak. The nurse provides him with a pen and paper and a poster of common objects and words. When David is unable to write his messages because of fatigue, he uses the poster to communicate his needs.

Implementation:

In this example the nurse provides two methods for the client to use to specify his needs. The nurse also ensures that David's call bell is always within reach, since he is unable to verbally call for help.

NURSING DIAGNOSIS
Impaired verbal communication related to effects of surgery

OUTCOME
Communicates needs non-verbally within 24 hours

Relating.—human response pattern involving establishment of bonds

NURSING DIAGNOSES	POSSIBLE RELATED FACTORS
Impaired social interaction	Effects of chronic illness
Social isolation	Unacceptable social behaviors or values
Altered role performance	Change in financial status
Altered parenting	Lack of effective role model
Potential altered parenting	Lack of knowledge: child rearing
Sexual dysfunction	Lack of privacy
Altered family processes	Loss or gain of significant other
Parental role conflict	Change in marital status
Altered sexuality patterns	Obesity

The implementation of nursing interventions may be directed toward (1) assisting the client to clarify perceptions about roles, (2) identifying barriers to performance of one's role, (3) identifying resources to alleviate the related factors, and (4) providing specific education.

NURSING DIAGNOSIS
Altered parenting related to prolonged separation from son

Example.   Tony Angeli is a navy submarine officer who is frequently at sea for prolonged periods of time. Therefore, his interactions with his youngest son, age eight months, have been minimal. He verbalizes his frustration and feelings of parental failure in a conversation with the clinic nurse.

Implementation:
Here, the nurse's interventions focus on counseling to assist the father in achieving a more positive feeling about his parental skills.

OUTCOME
Verbalizes positive statements regarding parenting abilities within one week

NURSING DIAGNOSIS
Altered sexual patterns related to anticipated sexual inadequacy

Example.   Dona Ramsey is a 52 year old client who is seen in the doctor's office six weeks following a hysterectomy. She verbalizes her concern about resuming sexual relations with her husband, indicating that she believes "it just won't be the same."

Implementation:
In this example, the nurse utilizes a supportive approach, explains the normalcy of the client's response, and encourages open dialogue between the client and her husband. Her fears may be unfounded, and in fact, their relationship may improve as a result of this type of dialogue.

OUTCOME
Resumes usual sexual patterns within 3 months

Valuing.—human response pattern involving the assignment of relative worth

NURSING DIAGNOSIS	POSSIBLE RELATED FACTORS
Spiritual distress	Effects of loss of significant others
	Beliefs opposed by family, peers, or health care providers
	Disruption in usual religious activity

Nursing interventions will be focused on (1) identifying the specific value or belief pattern involved, (2) determining particular sources of conflict, when appropriate, (3) obtaining available resources to facilitate the practice of religious beliefs or the resolution of conflicts, and (4) providing information regarding health management to assist the client in making informed choices regarding continued health practices.

Example. Maria Bucellato is an 82 year old woman who is hospitalized after falling on the ice and fracturing her hip. She says to the nurse, "I just don't know what I am going to do. I go to Mass at my church every Sunday. It doesn't feel right to miss church."

Implementation:

The nurse's interventions for this client would include arranging for the priest to visit the client. Additionally, the nurse would investigate the possibility of utilizing the hospital's closed circuit television system for showing videotapes of Sunday Mass.

NURSING DIAGNOSIS
Spiritual distress related to disruption in usual religious patterns

OUTCOME
Within 2 days identifies method of practicing religious beliefs while hospitalized

Choosing.—human response pattern involving the selection of alternatives

NURSING DIAGNOSES	POSSIBLE RELATED FACTORS
Ineffective individual coping	Inadequate leisure activities
Impaired adjustment	Incomplete grieving
Defensive coping	Perceived personal inadequacy
Ineffective denial	Fear of death, disability
Ineffective family coping: disabling	Chronically unexpressed feelings of guilt, despair, anxiety, or hostility
Ineffective family coping: compromised	Isolation of family members from one another
Family coping: potential for growth	Effective management of crisis needs
Noncompliance	Previous unsuccessful experiences with advised regimen
Decisional conflict	Lack of experience with decision-making
Health seeking behavior	Increased awareness of risks associated with smoking

The implementation of nursing interventions may be directed toward (1) assisting the client to identify personal patterns of response to individual or family stress, (2) identifying the sources of stress for the client as an individual, (3) developing positive coping strategies to avoid distress, (4) providing education regarding identified variables and the use of relaxation, and (5) obtaining additional resources when required.

Example. Paul West is an elderly client hospitalized in an intensive care unit. He has been in the unit for one week and suddenly begins screaming that he can't take it anymore. He complains that all the noises are "driving me crazy, I never get any rest, and I'm tired of all this fussing and these newfangled machines."

NURSING DIAGNOSIS
Ineffective individual coping related to sensory overload secondary to prolonged ICU stay

OUTCOME
Verbalizes three strategies to cope with prolonged illness

Implementation:

This is a classic response to the sensory overload associated with critical care areas. In this situation, the nurse utilizes interpersonal skills to assist the client in identifying alternative coping strategies. The use of relaxation techniques may be particularly beneficial if accompanied by a reduction in environmental stimulation. Adjusting the times when care is provided might allow Paul to obtain longer rest periods.

Moving.—human response pattern involving activity

NURSING DIAGNOSES	POSSIBLE RELATED FACTORS
Impaired physical mobility	Decreased strength and endurance
Activity intolerance	Interrupted sleep
Fatigue	Excessive social or role demands
Potential activity intolerance	Generalized weakness
Sleep pattern disturbance	Effects of stress
Diversional activity deficit	Preoccupation with job
Impaired home maintenance management	Lack of motivation
Altered health maintenance	Decreased economic resources
Feeding self-care deficit	Joint stiffness
Impaired swallowing	Reddened, ulcerated mouth
Effective breastfeeding	Basic breastfeeding knowledge
Ineffective breastfeeding	Knowledge deficit
Bathing/hygiene self-care deficit	Pain associated with activity
Dressing/grooming self-care deficit	Lack of self-confidence
Toileting self-care deficit	Immobility secondary to traction
Altered growth and development	Effects of separation from significant others

The nursing interventions are directed toward (1) identifying usual patterns and related factors, (2) implementing preventive, supportive, or therapeutic approaches to increase the amount of rest the client receives, (3) providing specific education, and (4) providing adaptive devices to assist with self care.

NURSING DIAGNOSIS
Bathing/hygiene self care deficit related to joint stiffness

Example. Mabel Miller is a 92 year old with rheumatoid arthritis who has been a resident at a long-term care facility for several years. She is presently experiencing an acute flare-up of her arthritis that is interfering with her ability to wash herself.

OUTCOME
Bathes self with assistance when pain free

Implementation:

Nursing interventions are designed to provide pain relief through application of heat for stiffness and cold compresses for swollen joints. The nurse contacts Mabel's doctor to request appropriate medication to control the symptoms. In addition, the nurse provides adaptive devices including a long-handled toothbrush, comb, and mitten washcloth.

Example. Sandra Morales is a 37 year old woman admitted to the hospital with advanced multiple sclerosis. She is divorced and lives with her elderly mother, who is in poor health. With the progression of her disease, Sandra is now confined to a wheelchair and verbalizes concern about her ability to manage the upkeep of her apartment and care of her mother.

Implementation:

The nurse recognizes that an active diagnosis of impaired home maintenance management exists. At this point, the nurse will explore available resources to assist Sandra and her mother in this present living situation. In the future it may be necessary to discuss long-term arrangements in alternative settings.

> **NURSING DIAGNOSIS**
> Impaired home maintenance related to limited mobility secondary to confinement to a wheelchair

> **OUTCOME**
> Identifies resources to assist with home maintenance

Perceiving.—human response pattern involving the reception of information

NURSING DIAGNOSES	POSSIBLE RELATED FACTORS
Body image disturbance	Effects of loss of arm
Self-esteem disturbance	Perceived unsatisfactory personal relationships
Chronic self-esteem disturbance	Effects of psychological abuse
Situational low self-esteem	Weight gain associated with pregnancy
Personal identity disturbance	Ingestion of illicit drugs
Sensory perceptual alterations	
visual	Failure to use protective goggles
auditory	Excessive ear wax
kinesthetic	Sleep deprivation
gustatory	Inflammation of nasal mucosa
tactile	Effects of aging
olfactory	Foreign body in nasal passage
Unilateral neglect	Effects of neurological trauma
Hopelessness	Prolonged activity restriction
Powerlessness	Loss of financial independence

The focus of nursing interventions includes (1) assisting the client to define the perception of self, (2) identification of related factors, (3) referral to available resources, and (4) assisting the client to develop problem-solving skills to deal with the effects of change, loss, or threat.

Example. Laurie Bower is a 10 year old girl who visits the school nurse's office frequently with vague physical complaints. The nurse's approach has been to investigate each complaint and to reassure Laurie. During these conversations, the nurse learns that Laurie feels awkward because she is five inches taller than all of her friends, including the boys in her class. She has also begun to menstruate and is afraid that others will find out and make fun of her.

> **NURSING DIAGNOSIS**
> Body image disturbance related to effects of puberty

OUTCOME
Verbalizes one
positive statement
about self daily

Implementation:
The nurse recognizes that this client's self-image has been affected by rapid body changes associated with puberty. Nursing approaches will focus on continuing their trusting relationship and assisting Laurie to deal with rapid physical changes. In addition, the nurse will help Laurie practice behaviors that will help her deal with peer pressure.

Knowing.—human response pattern involving the meaning associated with information

NURSING DIAGNOSES	POSSIBLE RELATED FACTORS
Knowledge deficit	Lack of interest in learning
Altered thought processes	Limited attention span

The implementation of nursing interventions may be directed toward (1) identifying the barriers to education, (2) providing specific educatonal resources, (3) determining the source of the client's deficits in perception, and (4) obtaining additional resources when required.

NURSING DIAGNOSIS
Altered thought
processes related to
unfamiliar
environment

Example. Bill McCandless is a 75 year old man admitted to a long-term care facility. He states on admission, "Where did my mother go? Has she finished shopping? When am I going to school? If I am late the principal will cane me."

OUTCOME
Oriented to time,
place and person
within 48 hours

Implementation:
The nurse recognizes that some of Bill's confusion may be related to being placed in a new environment. The nurse provides familiar objects (if available), presents information to Bill in a slow concise manner, and uses the calendar and clock in his room to orient him to time.

NURSING DIAGNOSIS
Knowledge deficit
(hypertension
regimen)

Example. Bill Janis is a policeman who is being seen in the physician's office for persistent hypertension. The nurse's interactions with this client reveal a total lack of knowledge regarding the disease process, the need for frequent monitoring, and the relationship between stress and the occurrence of hypertension.

OUTCOME
Within one month
explains
hypertension and
verbalizes
importance of
following prescribed
regimen

Implementation:
The nurse's action in this situation is clearly defined—the development and implementation of a comprehensive teaching plan. Consideration must be given to incorporating some of the client's usual patterns along with the recommended changes to facilitate compliance.

Feeling.—human response pattern involving the subjective awareness of information

Nursing Diagnoses	Possible Related Factors
Pain	Effects of therapeutic regimen
Chronic pain	Muscle spasm
Dysfunctional grieving	Lack of support system
Anticipatory grieving	Effects of potential loss of significant other
Potential for violence: self-directed or directed at others	Withdrawal from cocaine
Post-trauma response	Effects of motorcycle accident
Rape-trauma syndrome	
Rape-trauma syndrome: compound reaction	
Rape-trauma syndrome: silent reaction	
Anxiety	Loss of possessions
Fear	Threat of death

The focus of nursing interventions includes (1) identifying unhealthful patterns, (2) referral to available resources, (3) assisting client to clarify responses to traumatic events, and (4) identifying positive strategies to cope with loss.

Example. Dudley Jay is sharing a room in a boarding home with Anthony Marchetti. Anthony has several annoying personal habits, including eating other residents' food. When Dudley finds Anthony eating his cookies, Dudley hits him with a book. For the rest of the month Dudley finds opportunities to curse at Anthony, pinching, slapping, and hitting him when no attendants are present.

> **NURSING DIAGNOSIS**
> Potential for violence: directed at others related to inadequate impulse control

Implementation:

In managing Dudley's potential for violence, the nurse moves Dudley to another room. The nurse enlists the cooperation of the other residents in reporting the episodes of violence. Further, the nurse sits down with Dudley and Anthony to encourage discussion of their feelings about each other.

> **OUTCOME**
> No incidence of violence to others during next week

Example. Chris Sopko is a 17 year old runaway seen in the community health clinic with symptoms of depression, withdrawal, and sleep disturbances. He tells the nurse that he was raped by a homosexual four months ago. He describes feelings of guilt and disgust and indicates that this was probably his punishment for running away. Additionally, he is fearful that he may have contracted AIDS through the experience.

> **NURSING DIAGNOSIS**
> Rape-trauma syndrome

Implementation:

The nurse's interventions in this case are directed toward providing psychological support to this traumatized client. The therapeutic relationship should be maintained, and the nurse should reassure the client, help him to resolve his guilt feelings, and assist him to develop a realistic plan for the future. Additional counseling, therapy, and testing for AIDS may be necessary.

STAGE 3—DOCUMENTATION

The implementation of nursing interventions must be followed by complete and accurate documentation of the events occurring in this stage of the nursing process. There are five types of systems of record-keeping utilized in the documentation of client care. They are (1) source-oriented records, (2) problem-oriented records, (3) focus charting, (4) charting by exception, and (5) computer-assisted records. Each of these systems will be explored in this section.

Source-Oriented Records

The source-oriented system, or narrative charting, is the traditional charting system; it continues to be utilized by a number of institutions and agencies. In this system, information is recorded chronologically within specific time periods. The medical record is divided into sections according to the source of the data. Each discipline records information on a separate section—e.g., nurses' notes, physician progress notes, physical therapy notes, respiratory therapy notes, and social service notes.

The frequency of documentation in a source-oriented system is dependent upon the client's condition. In an acute-care setting, notes may be documented as frequently as every few minutes for a critically ill client. More commonly, the nurse documents observations once each shift and includes assessment data, implementation of nursing and medical orders, and the client's response to nursing or medical interventions. In alternative settings, such as nursing homes, community health centers, or physicians' offices, findings may be documented less frequently—daily, weekly, monthly, or less often, as indicated by institutional policy or client contact.

A sample of a source-oriented note is shown in Figure 7–1. Source-oriented records include some type of nurse's notes and may utilize additional forms such as flowsheets, patient teaching forms, discharge summaries, and the like. Samples of these forms are found in Figures 7–2 to 7–6.

The advantage of a source-oriented system is easy access to the location of the forms and subsequent documentation of each discipline. The disadvantages of this system include

☐ fragmentation of the documentation of the client's care according to the provider

Text continued on page 199

G-013

HAMILTON HOSPITAL

NURSES NOTES

(Patient Identifying Data)

DATE	HOUR	OBSERVATIONS AND REMARKS	SIGNATURE
12/27/85	7^{30} AM	Client alert, oriented and responsive to verbal and tactile stimuli. No complaints of pain or discomfort at this time. I.V. infusing via #18 angio in left forearm. Hypoactive bowel sounds in R & L upper quadrants only. Breath sounds clear bilaterally. Coughing and deep breathing independently. Turns with minimal assistance —	
	8^{00} AM	Tolerated 450 cc clear liquids @ breakfast	
	8^{15} AM	Assisted with partial bath. I.V. dsgs. changed - no evidence of redness, swelling @ site. Anti-embolism stockings removed and reapplied. Abdominal dressing changed - no redness, swelling noted	
	8^{45} AM	C/o incisional pain - medicated c̄ Demerol 100 mg. I.M —	
	9^{15} AM	Sleeping @ intervals with no c/o pain.	
	11^{45} AM	Foley catheter drained 300 cc clear amber urine - removed per M.D. order — encouraged to force fluids p.o —	
	12^{noon}	Tolerated 500 cc clear liquids for lunch - expelling flatus @ this time	
	1^{50} pm	C/o incisional pain - medicated c̄ Demerol 100 mg. I.M —	
	2^{15} pm	Voided 450 cc amber urine - c/o burning on urination - encouraged to continue forcing fluids —	
	3^{00} pm	Sleeping @ present	Janet M. Cipek RN

FIGURE 7-1. Source note. (Courtesy of Hamilton Hospital, Trenton, NJ.)

**MEMORIAL HOSPITAL
OF BURLINGTON COUNTY**

PATIENT CARE RECORD

DATE		11-7	7-3	3-11			11-7	7-3	3-11
HYGIENE	Self Care				SAFETY	Side rails up			
	Bedside					Restraint			
	Shower/Tub					Vest			
	Bath w/assistance					Wrist			
	Partial Bath					Ankle			
	Complete Bed Bath					Other			
	*Special Skin Care to Pressure Points					Released Q 2 hr			
	Back Rub				TREATMENTS	Oxygen Therapy			
	Foot Care					Mask I _____			
	Peri Care					Cannula I _____			
	Mouth Care					Egg Crate Mattress			
	H. S. Care					Surgical Stockings			
ACTIVITY	Unassisted					Removed 1 x /shift			
	Ambulatory w/assistance					Isolation Type _____			
	1-2 x /shift				SPECIAL TREATMENTS				
	3 or more x's/shift								
	Bedpan/Urinal w/assistance								
	1-2 x's/shift								
	3 or more x's/shift								
	Commode or BR w/assistance								
	1-2 x's/shift								
	3 or more x's/shift								
	Chair/Transfer w/assistance								
	1-2 x's/shift								
	3 or more x's/shift								
	Dangle w/assistance								
	Bedrest								
	Turns Self								
	Turn/Position w/assistance								
	1-2 x's/shift								
	3 or more x's/shift								
	Range of Motion								
NUTRITION	NPO								
	Self Feed								
	Feed w/assistance								
	Complete Feed								
	*Tube Feeding								
	Nasogastric								
	Gastrostomy				**NURSES SIGNATURE AND STATUS & INITIALS**			
	Intermittent								
	Continuous				11-7				
	Enteral Pump					Initials		Initials	
	Adequate Intake				7-3				
	*Inadequate Intake					Initials		Initials	
	Fluid Restriction Amt. _____				3-11				
	Force Fluids Amt. _____				**NOTE:**	Initials		Initials	
BOWEL	Stool Number					Document unusual or abnormal findings on Patient's Progress Record.			
	No Stool								
	Incontinent # x's				CODES:				
BLADDER	Voiding Q S					* Further documentation required on Patient's Progress Record.			
	Incontinent # x's					Please initial in space as applicable.			
	Foley Catheter								
SLEEP	Slept Well								
	Awake at Intervals								
	Awake Most of Time								

070177 (3/85)

FIGURE 7–2. Patient care flowsheets. (Courtesy of Memorial Hospital of Burlington County, Mount Holly, NJ.)

G-013

HAMILTON HOSPITAL

NURSES NOTES

(Patient Identifying Data)

DATE/TIME	DIAGNOSIS	OBSERVATIONS AND REMARKS	SIGNATURE
12/27/85	Pain	Client c/o incisional pain twice this shift.	
3^{15} pm		Medicated c̄ Demerol 100 mg IM @ 8^{45} am and	
		1^{50} pm. Sleeping @ intervals after medication	
		Ice bag to incisional area	
	Elimination	Foley catheter patent for 300 cc clear amber	
	(urinary)	urine - removed @ 11^{45} am per M.D. order.	
		Voided 450 cc amber urine @ 2^{15} pm - c/o	
		burning when voiding - encouraged to force	
		fluids - prefers apple juice and ginger ale.	
	(bowel)	Hypoactive bowel sounds in R&L upper	
		quadrants - only - expelling flatus	
	Nutrition	I.V. infusing via #18 angio in Ⓛ forearm	
		Tolerating "clear" liquids by mouth -	
		1200 cc this shift	
	S.N.N	Coughing and deep breathing independently - Turns	
		with minimal assistance - breath sounds	
		clear bilaterally. Abdominal dsg. changed -	
		no evidence of redness, swelling noted	
			Janet M. York RN

FIGURE 7-3. Modified source-oriented note. (Courtesy of Hamilton Hospital, Trenton, NJ.)

HAMILTON HOSPITAL
TEACHING RECORD
HYPERTENSION

Following Instruction, the patient/family will be able to;	INFORMATION PROVIDED DATE SIGNATURE	INFORMATION REINFORCED DATE SIGNATURE -
1. Define Hypertension		
2. List the risk factors which predispose to the development of hypertension.		
3. Identify own risk factors and explain method of managing each. a. diet-		
b. heredity-		
C. kidney disease-		
e. smoking-		
f. stress-		
g. obesity-		
4. Describe the relationship between stress and hypertension		
5. Name positive methods of managing own stress		
6. State the effects of diet on hypertension.		
7. Select low sodium/low calorie foods from menu.		
8. Describe the effects of alcohol nicotine, and caffeine on blood vessels.		
9. States name of medication(s) SPECIFY - _____		
10. EXplaines action, dosage, schedule and major side effects of each.		
11. Identify symptoms to report to physician.		
12. Identify post discharge resources. a. American Heart Association-		
b. Sharing and Caring -		
c. Stay-Well Programs-		
d. Other-		

COMMENTS: _____

_____

G152B
9/12/85

FIGURE 7-4.

CARDINAL CUSHING GENERAL HOSPITAL
235 NORTH PEARL STREET
BROCKTON, MA 02401
(508) 588-4000

PATIENT DISCHARGE CARE PLAN
NURSING DISCHARGE INFORMATION SHEET

Part I
NURSING UNIT _____ EXTENSION # _____

Discharge Date: _____ Time: _____ Destination: _____

Mode of transportation: Car _____ Ambulance _____ Other _____ Accompanied by: _____

Describe Physical Status at Discharge: _____

_____

Activities of Daily Living/Self Care Ability: (I) Independent   (D) Dependent   (A) Needs Assistance

Feeding _____ Bathing/Hygiene _____ Toileting _____ Dressing/Grooming _____

Special Devices: No _____ Yes _____ Specify type: _____

Special Instructions	Patient/Family Understanding/Response
Activity:	
Treatments:	
Therapies:	
Diet:	
Medications:	
Other:	

Follow-up Appointments: _____

_____

Disposition of Personal Belongings: (Circle One) Patient/Other, Specify _____

Nurse's Signature/Title _____ Patient Signature: _____

POST HOSPITAL PATIENT CARE PLAN—Part II

Discharged To: Home _____   Other _____

	Discharge Planner	Date
At Home Services Not indicated ____		
Agency/Facility	Phone	Service
	Date	Requested
Contact Person	Referred	
Agency	Phone	Service
	Date	Requested
Contact Person	Referred	

I HEREBY ACKNOWLEDGE RECEIPT AND UNDERSTANDING OF THE DISCHARGE PLAN–PART II AS INDICATED ABOVE.

#600-151 rev. 5/88

SIGNATURE OF PATIENT   PATIENT COPY - WHITE   MEDICAL RECORD COPY - YELLOW   DATE

FIGURE 7–5. Patient discharge care plan. (Courtesy of Cardinal Cushing General Hospital, Brockton, MA.)

P A T I E N T   C A R E   P R O F I L E

GENERAL HOSPITAL 5/16/84 11:45AM PAGE 1 SHIFT:1

ACTIVITIES OF DAILY LIVING
Vital Signs RT
OOB W/Assist pk
Bath W/Assist pk
Fluids Force
Transport by W/C pk
All Regular
Cranberry Juice at Bedside
NPO After Midnight
PRC: Hard of Hearing

ACTIVE ORDERS
CBC W DIFF 05/16 07:30A
SMA 18 BIOCHEM PRO 05/16 07:30A
PYELOGRAM INTRAVEN 05/16 AM
1: MAY HAVE LIQUIDS ON THE DAY OF EXAM UNLESS UPPER G.I.SERIES,GALL BLADDER SERIES OR SONOGRAM IS ORDERED

TREATMENTS
1: ANESTHESIA TO SEE PT.
2: SHAVE AND PREP-MID NIPPLE TO MID BACK AND FROM MID AXILLA TO HIP ON RIGHT SIDE
3: PRE OP ON CALL. DATE:5/17
4: STRAIN ALL URINE. D/E/N: pk
5: INTAKE & OUTPUT q SHIFT. D/E/N: pk

TRN-09 U00187023 2555555 TRN
TESTPAT JACK SEX: M
ADM: 5/15/84 SRV: URO SMK: N
DOB: 10/06/21 62 COND: G LEVEL: 1
HT: 5/11 F/I WT: 180/000 P/O
10000 INTERNIST OTHER
ALG: PENICILLIN
DX: NEPHROLITHIASIS

OUTCOME: Describes type of surgery
OUTCOME: States usual pre-op preparation
OUTCOME: Identifies usual post-op routine
OUTCOME: Verbalizes feelings about impending surgery
INTERVENTIONS:
1: Assess knowledge of surgery and explore past surgical experience(s) at the time of admission
2: Review surgical routine (preps, meds, dressing)
3: Reinforce pre-operative teaching re: Sequence of events on day of surgery (pre-op stretcher to O.R., R.R. return to room/ICU)
Post-op equipment (dsg., I.V., tubes)
Provisions for relief of pain and other symptoms (include need to request and frequency limitations)
Turning, coughing and deep breathing
Incentive spirometry if ordered
Change in bowel/bladder functions
Progressive diet changes
Progressive self care

DATE:	NURSING NOTES	SIGNATURE
8am	Clear yellow urine. No evidence of stones or (R) flank pain. Pt. prepared for IVP this am. Dr. Jones visited	Pat Kelly, RN
10³⁰ am	Returned from X-ray. Demerol 100 mg. IM IHD for (Rt) flank pain	Sally Smith, RN
11³⁰ am	Pain subsided. Pt. verbalized understanding of information in pre-op booklet and able to give return demonstration of TCDB.	Pat Kelly, RN
1³⁰ pm	Urine remains clear. No evidence of stones or (R) flank pain	Pat Kelly, RN

INT	SIGNATURE	INT	SIGNATURE	INT	SIGNATURE
pk	Pat Kelly, RN	SS	Sally Smith, RN		

FIGURE 7–6. Computer generated shift worksheet. (Courtesy of HBO & Company, Atlanta, GA. All rights reserved.)

☐ no clear definition of the client's problem or interdisciplinary approaches to management

☐ lack of integrated documentation of the client's responses to intervention

☐ inconsistent documentation of teaching when accomplished by many disciplines—e.g., nursing, nutrition, respiratory therapy

☐ greater difficulty in auditing the record when evaluating the quality of care delivered (Sorensen and Luckmann, 1979)

☐ narrative notes are not organized into topics, making it difficult to retrieve data about a particular problem

Problem-Oriented Records

The problem-oriented system of documentation parallels the nursing process. Each involves data collection, identification of client responses (nursing diagnoses), development and implementation of the plan of care, and evaluation of outcome achievement. In this system, information focuses on the client's problems (diagnoses) and is integrated and recorded by all disciplines, utilizing a consistent format. This facilitates multidisciplinary recording utilizing the same data base and progress notes. Therefore, data are more accessible and focus on the client's individual needs. The advantages of a problem-oriented system are as follows.

☐ Quality care is facilitated, since the entire health care team focuses on the same identified problems.

☐ All disciplines involved in the care of the client have rapid access to data reflecting the plan of care.

☐ The collaboration of all health team members is encouraged, since multidisciplinary findings are readily available.

☐ Learning is increased because each discipline identifies and observes what others have done.

☐ Evaluation of the quality of care is easily performed and deficiencies more clearly identified.

☐ Research is facilitated, since records tend to be more accurate and complete.

The disadvantages of a problem-oriented system may include the following.

☐ The education of a variety of disciplines in the utilization of the system may be lengthy and costly.

☐ Members of some disciplines may resist the utilization of an integrated system.

☐ If care is fragmented and nonindividualized, documentation will not resolve these problems.

☐ It is sometimes difficult to determine what information belongs in each component of the SOAPIE note.

☐ Some nurses find the use of the problem list to record nursing diagnoses to be redundant with the nursing care plan.

There are four major components of a problem-oriented system: (1) the data base, (2) the problem list, (3) a plan, and (4) the progress notes.

Data Base

The standard data base in a problem-oriented system includes the client's profile, history, and physical and diagnostic studies (e.g., laboratory and radiology reports). The information acquired becomes the source from which the client's needs and problems are identified. The methods for acquiring an accurate and complete data base have been discussed in detail in Chapter 2.

Problem List

The problem list is a cumulative listing of actual or potential client problems that may require intervention to improve the client's health or well-being. Problems may be identified independently by specific health care providers or collaboratively in client care conferences. The problem list is usually on the front of the chart and serves as the index or table of contents to the medical record. It includes the diagnoses of nursing, medicine, and other disciplines. Each problem on the list is designated by number (Table 7–1). This number reflects the sequence in which the problems have been identified, rather than their priority or intensity.

Although the number remains fixed, the status of each problem is dynamic. It may be active, in the process of resolution, or inactive. Signs or symptoms

TABLE 7–1. PROBLEM LIST

No.	Problem	Date Entered	Date Resolved
1	Cholecystitis	1963	1963
2	Pneumonia	1972	1972
3	Fractured left hip	2/2/90	
4	Pain	2/2/90	
5	Impaired physical mobility	2/2/90	
6	Potential for trauma	2/2/90	

may appear as components of the problem list to indicate the need for further investigation. If the client's condition improves and the sign or symptom subsides, it is eliminated from the problem list. If it persists, a diagnostic label is formulated, and it becomes an active component of the problem list. When a problem is resolved, the date is entered; however, the number assigned to the problem is not used to identify subsequent problems. In Table 7–1, problems 1 and 2 have been resolved, while 3, 4, 5 and 6 are active.

Plan

After identifying a problem, the health care provider must develop a plan of care for the client. Initial plans usually include diagnostic, therapeutic, and educational components. The diagnostic component includes the acquisition of additional data required to confirm the diagnosis (whether medical, nursing, or other). This may consist of medical orders for laboratory or radiology studies, such as urinalysis or chest x-ray. It may also include nursing intervention of gather additional data from the client—e.g., from available support systems or the client's feelings—or observation of specific skills or limitations.

Treatment might include intravenous therapy, frequent position change, and range of motion exercises. Education involves providing the client or family with the information and skills required to manage the client's illness or limitations. Table 7–2 reflects a sample plan for problem 6 on the problem list in Table 7–1. Note that outcomes are defined and specific orders necessary to achieve them are included.

TABLE 7–2. CARE PLAN FOR A PROBLEM FROM TABLE 7–1

Problem 6	Outcome	Interventions
Potential for trauma related to decreased vision and possible home hazard	No evidence of further trauma after discharge from hospital	☐ Consultation with ophthalmologist to evaluate visual acuity (diagnostic) ☐ Assist client to identify potential environmental hazards in the home (treatment) ☐ Instruct client and son on basic safety measures designed to prevent injury (education)

Progress Notes

The final component of the problem-oriented system is the progress notes. These are designed to document the client's response to the plan. Integrated progress notes include narrative entries from all disciplines. Evaluation of the information documented in these notes assists in measuring the client's progress toward outcome attainment. This also allows the evaluator to modify the plan accordingly. The frequency of the recording of progress notes may vary depending upon the setting or specific institutional policies. They may be done hourly, once each shift, daily, monthly, or only when significant changes occur.

The format for progress notes in this system is specific and structured. Originally the acronym SOAP was used when problem-oriented records were first developed. The letters represent Subjective data, Objective data, Assessment, and Plan. Subjective data include the client's feelings, symptoms, and concerns— e.g., fears about the outcome of diagnostic studies. Frequently the client's words or a summary of the conversation is documented in the subjective data. Objective data include the findings of various members of the health care team—e.g., lung sounds, blood pressure, or radiology reports. Nurses use this part of the note to include data from observations, assessment, and interviews with the family or other health care team members (Burke and Murphy, 1988). These data consist of the defining characteristics of the nursing diagnosis. Assessment includes the nurse's interpretation of the subjective and objective data. Some nurses include the nursing diagnosis in this section of the note. The plan consists of the steps that will be taken to assist the client with the resolution of the problem.

SOAPIE or SOAPIER are common variations of the original SOAP format. The I stands for the interventions performed to alleviate problems. The E is used to evaluate the effectiveness of the interventions in achieving the outcome. The R or Revision documents any changes in the nursing interventions based on the evaluation of the client's response.

Table 7–3 is a sample of progress notes utilizing the SOAPIE format. Note that the problem continues to be identified by number.

It is not necessary to include each component of the format in every set of progress notes. For example, there may be no subjective data if the client is unable to communicate. Therefore, no entries would be included in the S area.

TABLE 7–3. SOAPIE PROGRESS NOTES

DATE/TIME	PROBLEM	NOTES
8:30 AM	6	S—"I'm going to have to watch myself when I go home. I don't want to hurt myself again."
		O—Tense, wringing hands, expressed concern about hurting self.
		A—Aware of the relationship between hazards in the home and occurrence of injuries. Motivated to avoid harm to self.
		P—Encouraged to reorganize and correct hazards in home environment.
		I—Discussed home environment with client to identify hazards.
		E—Identified loose rug at top of stairs as hazardous. Plans to request home hazard survey by visiting nurse prior to discharge.

Focus Charting

Focus charting is a method of organizing information on the nurse's notes that was developed in Minneapolis. It includes three components:

1. The use of a focus to label the nurse's note
2. Organization of the nurse's note into the categories of data, action, and response
3. Flowsheets for documenting data.

Focus notes are used:

"to expand on the data recorded on a flowsheet to record an unusual or unexpected event.

to document patient response to medical or nursing care or teaching

to document the discharge plan

to describe the status of the patient at the time of transfer from one nursing unit to another or at the time of discharge to fully describe the psychosocial or emotional needs of the patient" (Lampe, 1988)

Focus Column

The phrases placed in the Focus column may include signs or symptoms, client concerns or behavior, short phrases from a nursing diagnosis, acute changes in the client's condition or significant events. The focus does not necessarily have to describe an actual problem. The focus of the note may be directed toward identifying potential problems or strengthening the client's health status.

Examples of Foci

Signs or symptoms	Dizziness
	Irregular pulse
	Vomiting
Client concerns or behavior	Withdrawn
	Anxiety about discharge
	Home care needs
Phrases from nursing diagnosis	Impaired mobility
	Potential for aspiration
	Ineffective breastfeeding
Acute changes in condition	Seizure
	Cardiac arrest
Significant event	Return from surgery
	Fall
	Blood transfusion

Nurse's Notes

The nurse's notes are organized into three categories:

Data—subjective or objective data that are related to the focus of the note

Action—nursing interventions that have been implemented

DATE/TIME	FOCUS	NOTES
6/19 8:00 AM	Constipation (phrase from nursing diagnosis)	D: Client states she has not had a B.M. for three days. A: MD informed of client's constipation. Laxative administered as ordered.
8:30 AM 12:00 PM	Fever (sign or symptom)	D: Temperature 102. A: Tylenol administered. Client encouraged to increase intake of fluids to 2000 cc until 9:00 PM. Advised to stay in bed and call for help if she wants to get out of bed since fever may make her dizzy.
1:00 PM	Fever	R: Temperature now 101.2°F Client following instructions to increase fluid intake. Has consumed 400 cc so far. J. Long RN ————
4:00 PM	Concern about discharge (client concern or behavior)	D: Client states, ''I was planning to go home tomorrow. How can I go home if I have this fever?'' A: Encouraged to talk about her feelings. Explained need to be sure fever has disappeared before she is ready to go home. R: Client states, ''I guess you are right. I'd be even more disappointed if I went home and had to come back to the hospital.''
8:15 PM	Fall (Significant event)	D: Roommate put on light and said client was lying on floor. Upon entering room client was found lying on floor in feces. Stated the laxative worked. Denies pain in legs, hips, head. A: Assisted to bed. House physician notified and examined client. Instructed client to remain in bed and use call light when wishing to get out of bed. R: Client verbalized understanding of instructions. J. Reynolds RN ————

Words in parentheses by each Focus are added for illustration and would not appear in an actual note.

FIGURE 7-7. Example of Focus note.

Response—evaluation of the effectiveness of the interventions in addressing the focus

Not every note will contain each category of information. For example, additional time may be needed before the nurse is able to evaluate the effectiveness of the interventions. Figure 7–7 shows an example of a Focus note.

ADVANTAGES

☐ The format of focus charting organizes information into two distinct columns.

☐ Use of key words in the focus column makes it easy to locate content on a specific aspect of patient care.

☐ The Data, Action, Response (DAR) format provides a complete concise description of each focus of care.

☐ Including subjective and objective data in the same section eliminates the need to distinguish between these types of data.

DISADVANTAGES

Some of the data that are described in the note may be redundant with the data recorded on the flowsheets.

Charting by Exception

Charting by Exception (CBE) is a documentation system that was developed in Milwaukee. Staff nurses developed CBE in an effort to streamline charting and reduce the amount of time spent on documentation.

Nursing/Physician Order Flowsheets are used to document assessment findings and nursing interventions for a 24 hour period (see Fig. 7–8). The column labeled

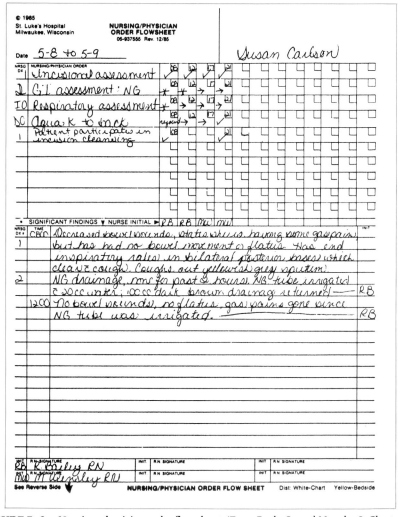

FIGURE 7–8. Nursing physician order flowsheet. (From Burke L, and Murphy J: Charting by Exception. New York: John Wiley & Sons, 1988. Reprinted with permission of John Wiley & Sons.)

nursing diagnoses is used to refer to a nursing diagnosis by number, a physician order (D.O.), or an incidental order (I.O.). An incidental order is a nursing intervention that does not require the formulation of nursing diagnosis or is an interdependent nursing intevention specific to a protocol or use of medical equipment.

The time that the nurse completes the intervention is indicated in the upper right hand corner of each square. Symbols used in each block include:

    ✔ A checkmark to indicate that there were no significant findings (Normal findings identified in Fig. 7–9).

    * An asterisk to refer the nurse to the "See Significant Findings" section of the flowsheet.

    → An arrow to indicate that significant findings remain unchanged from the previous assessment.

GUIDELINES FOR USE OF THE NURSING/PHYSICIAN ORDER FLOW SHEET

1. Indicate the Nursing Diagnosis which relates to the nursing order in the far left hand column of the category boxes. If the order is a physician order, indicate "D.O." ("Doctor Order") instead of the nursing diagnosis number.

2. Indicate the nursing or physician order. If the nursing order includes an assessment to be completed, use the following protocol:

    a. "NEUROLOGICAL ASSESSMENT" will include orientation, pupils, movement, sensation, quality of speech/swallowing & memory.

    b. "CARDIOVASCULAR ASSESSMENT" will include apical pulse, neck veins, CRT, peripheral pulses, edema, & calf tenderness.

    c. "RESPIRATORY ASSESSMENT" will include respiratory characteristics, breath sounds, cough, sputum, color of nailbeds/mucous membranes, & CRT.

    d. "GASTROINTESTINAL ASSESSMENT" will include abdominal appearance, bowel sounds, palpation, diet tolerance & stools.

    e. "URINARY ASSESSMENT" will include voiding patterns, bladder distention, & urine characteristics.

    f. "INTEGUMENTARY ASSESSMENT" will include skin color, skin temperature, skin integrity & condition of mucous membranes.

    g. "MUSCULOSKELETAL ASSESSMENT" will include joint swelling, tenderness, limitations in ROM, muscle strength & condition of surrounding tissue.

    h. "NEUROVASCULAR ASSESSMENT" will include color, temperature, movement, CRT, peripheral pulses, edema & patient description of sensation to affected extremity.

    i. "SURGICAL DRESSING/INCISIONAL ASSESSMENT" will include condition of surgical dressing and/or color, temperature, tenderness of surrounding tissue, condition of sutures/staples/steri-strips, approximation of wound edges, & presence of any drainage.

    j. "PAIN ASSESSMENT" will include patient description, location, duration, intensity, radiation, precipitating factors, & alleviating factors.

OR

Specify exactly which parts of assessment should be completed.

3. Top of sheet should be dated. Time should be indicated in the small box in upper right hand corner of each category box.

4. Upon carrying out an order that has no significant findings, a "✔" in the appropriate category box is sufficient to indicate it was done. If the order includes an assessment, the following parameters will be considered a negative assessment and constitute the use of a "✔":

    a. "NEUROLOGICAL ASSESSMENT" - Alert & oriented to person, place, & time. Behavior appropriate to situation. Pupils equal & reactive to light. Active ROM of all extremities with symmetry of strength. No paresthesia. Verbalization clear & understandable. Swallowing without coughing and choking on liquids & solids. Memory intact.

    b. "CARDIOVASCULAR ASSESSMENT" - Regular apical pulse. S1 & S2 audible. Neck veins flat at 45 degrees. CRT < 3 sec. Peripheral pulses palpable. No edema. No calf tenderness.

    c. "RESPIRATORY ASSESSMENT" - Respirations 10-20/min. at rest. Respirations quiet & regular. Breath sounds vesicular through both lung fields, bronchial over major airways, with no adventitious sounds. Sputum clear. Nailbeds & mucous membranes pink. CRT < 3 sec.

    d. "GASTROINTESTINAL ASSESSMENT" - Abdomen soft. Bowel sounds active (5-34/min.). No pain with palpation. Tolerates prescribed diet without nausea & vomiting. Having BMs within own normal pattern & consistency.

    e. "URINARY ASSESSMENT" - Able to empty bladder without dysuria. Bladder not distended after voiding. Urine clear & yellow to amber.

    f. "INTEGUMENTARY ASSESSMENT" - Skin color within patient's norm. Skin warm and intact. Mucous membranes moist.

    g. "MUSCULOSKELETAL ASSESSMENT" - Absence of joint swelling & tenderness. Normal ROM of all joints. No muscle weakness. Surrounding tissues show no evidence of inflammation, nodules, nail changes, ulcerations, or rashes.

    h. "NEUROVASCULAR ASSESSMENT" - Affected extremity is pink, warm, & movable within patient's average ROM. CRT < 3 sec. Peripheral pulses palpable. No edema. Sensation intact without numbness or paresthesia.

    i. "SURGICAL DRESSING/INCISIONAL ASSESSMENT" - Dressing dry & intact. No evidence of redness, increased temperature, or tenderness in surrounding tissue. Sutures/staples/steri-strips intact. Wound edges well-approximated. No drainage present.

    j. "PAIN ASSESSMENT" - If medication alone relieves pain & expected outcome is met, documentation on the Medication Profile is sufficient. No specific problem need be identified in the Nurses' Notes or Flow Sheet.

5. Upon carrying out an order that has significant findings, an asterisk is entered in the appropriate box. An asterisk " * " in the category box indicates to "See Significant Findings Section".

6. If status remains unchanged from previous asterisk entry, current entry may be indicated with an " → "

7. If an order no longer needs to be carried out, the next unused category box in that row should indicate "order D/Ced", and a line should be drawn through the remaining boxes. Any unused rows can be left blank.

8. Each Flow Sheet is used for 24 hours.

FIGURE 7-9. Guidelines for the nursing physician order flowsheet. (From Burke L, and Murphy J: Charting by Exception. New York: John Wiley & Sons, 1988. Reprinted with permission of John Wiley & Sons.)

Nurse's Notes are written in the SOAP or SOAPIER format to document the initial care plan and its revision as well as completion of orders that cannot be documented with checkmarks such as psychosocial assessments.

Forms kept at the bedside include the Nursing/Physician Order Flowsheet, the Patient Teaching Record, the Graphic Record, and the Patient Discharge Note.

ADVANTAGES

☐ Trends and changes in the client's status are easily detected through the specially designed flow sheets.

☐ Normal physical findings are concisely documented.

☐ Printed guidelines are available on the back of forms to increase the consistency of their use.

☐ Data are recorded immediately on bedside forms and are always available for review.

DISADVANTAGES

☐ It is uncertain if the legality of CBE will stand up in court. Few if any suits involving CBE charting systems have reached the courts since its introduction.

☐ Implementation of CBE requires a major change in an agency's documentation system affecting large numbers of forms.

Computer-Assisted Records

The expansion of computerized information systems in health care agencies has resulted in the development of a variety of documentation methods. Some systems generate a shift worksheet similar to the one shown in Figure 7–6. The six sections define the independent and dependent nursing activities for each client on a given shift. The worksheet reflects the nursing care plan and includes those client outcomes and nursing interventions that are appropriate for each shift. The nurse initials the actions that have been implemented. The nurses' notes are handwritten in a format similar to a source-oriented documentation system. Physicians' orders and nursing interventions may be handwritten on the worksheet after they are entered into the system. Discontinued orders may be deleted from the system at any time. After removing the orders from the computer, the nurse draws a line through the order on the worksheet. This process ensures that orders are current and that documentation reflects the actual care delivered (Hinson et al, 1984).

Other computerized systems utilize a problem-oriented type of documentation. The data base is initiated at the bedside, and a problem list is generated. The computer identifies unusual or abnormal findings and prioritizes those areas requiring additional attention. Each problem is addressed in the initial plan in order of priority. The nurse selects diagnoses, sets client outcomes, and chooses nursing interventions. (If standardized care plans are available in the system, this process may be expedited.)

Progress notes may be documented by using several approaches. One commonly used format involves choosing specific interventions to document. "The computer presents any appropriate descriptions associated with the order for elaboration" (McNeill, 1980). These may be simple statements (such as "completed" or "not completed") or more detailed descriptions of care. The system then sorts the information provided into subjective and objective data and follows the SOAPIE format. Another approach builds the progress notes by selection of data from displays. This allows documentation of current data and the addition of new findings. The nurse chooses from structured screens. These screens contain significant symptoms and physical findings that serve as a guideline for additional assessment and nursing management. The progress notes of all disciplines are documented in an integrated fashion.

A number of additional screens may be used to document nursing interventions, such as administration of medications. The nurse initials those medications given to the client either on the screen or on a worksheet generated by the program.

SUMMARY

Implementation is the phase of the nursing process that involves the initiation of the nursing care plan. The goal of implementation is the achievement of outcomes. The implementation phase is divided into three stages—preparation, interventions, and documentation. Preparation includes reviewing anticipated nursing actions, analyzing the nursing knowledge and skills required, and recognizing the potential complications associated with specific nursing orders. Preparation also involves determining and providing necessary resources, preparing an environment conducive to the types of inteventions required, and identifying the ethical and legal concerns associated with potential interventions.

The client's physical and emotional needs may be divided into nine human response patterns. (While each has an infinite variety of interventions associated with it, assessment, planning, and teaching are common approaches.)

Documentation, the last stage, may utilize a variety of charting formats. The traditional ones include source-oriented and problem-oriented. Focus charting, charting by exception, and computer-assisted records are increasingly being used to replace the more traditional and cumbersome charting formats of the past.

7–1 TEST YOURSELF

DOCUMENTATION OF IMPLEMENTATION

Charles Stewart is a 67 year old man who was admitted to the hospital two days ago with a diagnosis of stomach cancer. The following is a segment of his care plan.

NURSING DIAGNOSIS	OUTCOME	INTERVENTION
Altered nutrition: less than body requirements related to decreased oral intake	Loses no more than 5 pounds throughout hospitalization	1. Provide small frequent meals at 8 AM, 1 PM, 4 PM, 6 PM.
		2. Supplemental feeding: Ensure 90 ml at 11 AM and 9 PM.
		3. Assess likes/dislikes.
		4. Encourage food from home if permitted.
		5. Obtain dietary consult (date: 7/5).
		6. Monitor food intake.
		7. Weigh daily at 8 AM.

While you are caring for Mr. Stewart, he shares the following information with you. "I don't like strawberry Ensure, although the other flavors are all right. What I'd really like would be some of my wife's lasagna." When Mr. Stewart's trays were observed after each meal, you noted that he consumed all of his breakfast, two thirds of his lunch, and 45 ml of Ensure at 11 AM. His weight at 8 AM was 148 lb, which constitutes a loss of three pounds since admission. Therefore you suggest to Mr. Stewart's physician that a consultation with a dietician be obtained. She agrees, and the dietician visits at 1:30 PM. When Mrs. Stewart visits at 2:00 she agrees to bring in some lasagna for her husband.

Based on the information provided above, document the implementation of this segment of the plan of care using source-oriented, SOAPIE, or Focus charting.

7–1 TEST YOURSELF □ ANSWERS

Source-Oriented Note

DATE	TIME	NURSES' NOTES
7/5/91	8 AM	Discussed dietary preferences with client—indicates that he wants "my wife's lasagna or bread pudding." Weight 148 lb this AM. Consumed entire breakfast.
	10:00 AM	Dr. Klein visited—discussed weight loss—dietary consult order requested and received.
	11:00 AM	Consumed ½ Ensure feeding. Client indicates that "I don't like strawberry Ensure although the other flavors are all right."
	1 PM	Consumed ⅔ of lunch.
	1:30 PM	Visited by dietician—will make changes in diet and discontinue strawberry Ensure.
	2:00 PM	Wife visited—agreed to bring in lasagna.

Janet York-Blasser, RN

SOAPIE Note

DATE	TIME	
7/5/91	8 AM	S: "I don't like strawberry Ensure. I'd like some of my wife's lasagna." O: Weight 148 lb. Consumed all of his breakfast.
	11 AM	Drank 45 ml of Ensure.
	12 PM	Ate ⅔ of his lunch. A: Significant weight loss of three pounds since admission probably related to decreased caloric consumption.
	12:30 PM	P: Request order for dietary consult. I: Received order for dietary consult. Notified dietary department. E: Visited by dietician E: Visited by wife, who agreed to bring in lasagna.

Janet York-Blasser, RN

DATE	TIME	FOCUS	NURSES' NOTES
7/5/91	12:00 PM	Altered nutrition	*Data:* Dislikes strawberry Ensure, wishes to have wife's lasagna. Ate all of breakfast and $\frac{2}{3}$ of lunch, plus 45 ml of Ensure. Has lost three pounds since admission.
			Action: Requested a dietary consult
			Response: Order obtained for dietary consult.
	1:30 PM		Visited by dietician.
	2:00 PM		Wife agreed to bring in lasagna.
			Janet York-Blasser, RN

REFERENCES

Burke L, and Murphy J: Charting by Exception. New York: John Wiley & Sons, 1988.

Hinson I, Silva N, and Clapp P: An automated Kardex and care plan. Nursing Management 1984 Jul; 15(7):35–43.

Lampe S: Focus charting. Minneapolis: Creative Nursing Management. 1988.

McNeill D: Developing the complete computer-based information system. In Zielstorff R. Computers in Nursing, Rockville, MD: Aspen, 1982.

Sorensen K, and Luckmann J: Basic Nursing: A Psychophysiological Approach. Philadelphia: W.B. Saunders, 1979.

BIBLIOGRAPHY

Atwood J, Mitchelle P, and Yarnall S: The POR: A system for communication, Nursing Clinics of North America, 1974 June; 229–234.

Barry C, and Gibbons, L. Information systems technology: Barriers and challenges to implementation. Journal of Nursing Administration, 1990 February; 40–42.

Cline A: Streamlined documentation through exceptional charting. Nursing Management, 1989 February; 62–64.

Collins H: Legal risks of computer charting. RN, 1990 May; 81–86.

Iyer P, and Camp N: Nursing Documentation: A Nursing Process Approach. St. Louis: Mosby Yearbook, 1991.

Iyer P: Preventing falls in the elderly. Southern California Nursing Review, 1988 October; 14–16.

Kozier B, and Erb G: Fundamentals of Nursing Concepts and Procedures, Third edition. Menlo Park, CA. Addison Wesley, 1987.

Lampe S: Focus charting: streamlining documentation. Nursing Management. 1985 July; 16(7):43–46.

Lampe S, and Hitchcock A: Documenting nursing diagnosis using focus charting. In Mclane A (ed): Classification of Nursing Diagnosis: Proceedings of the Seventh Conference. St. Louis: CV Mosby, 1987, pp 337–387.

Masson V: Nursing the charts. Nursing Outlook. 1990: 38(4) 196.

McPhee A: Teaching students how to chart. Nurse Educator, 1988; July/August; 33–36.

Murphy J, and Burke L: Charting by exception, Nursing 90, May 1990, 65–67.

Niland M, and Bentz A: Problem oriented approach to planning nursing care. Nursing Clinics of North America, June 1974, 235–245.

Svanda C: Key words show what's important. RN, 1986 Dec.; 49(12): 32–33.

Wake M: Nursing care delivery systems. Journal of Nursing Administration, 1990 May; 47–51.

8

IMPLEMENTATION— Nursing Care Delivery Systems

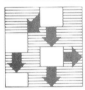

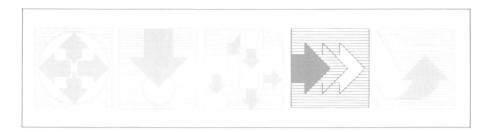

INTRODUCTION

Regardless of the type of setting in which nurses practice, one of four major models is utilized for implementing nursing care. These four approaches are (1) functional nursing, (2) team nursing, (3) primary nursing, and (4) case management. Their differences lie primarily in the systems used to organize and carry out the types of activities necessary to satisfy client needs. Nursing care may be accomplished by using individual models in their pure form or by adapting one or more methods. This chapter will explore each of the four models in terms of their definitions, advantages, and disadvantages.

FUNCTIONAL NURSING

Definition

In the functional approach to nursing care delivery, nursing responsibilities are divided by task and performed by varying levels of nursing personnel. All caregivers are involved in the client's care, but each individual is assigned to complete selected functions, such as monitoring vital signs, administering medications, or giving treatments. The individual functions are assigned to various levels of personnel based on the complexity of the task, including the knowledge, skills, and experience required to complete them.

For example, on an individual nursing unit on any given day, one RN may be in charge of unit management while another administers medications, and a third completes patient teaching. The LPN may be assigned to measure vital signs or bathe clients, while the nursing assistant makes beds or delivers meal trays.

In an office setting, the LPNs may take patient histories, record vital signs, and perform simple treatments. The RN similarly accomplishes physical assessment, administers medications, completes complex treatments, and provides education to the client.

Advantages

1. The emphasis in this model is on the efficient delivery of required care. Since the system allows the use of less skilled personnel to complete many tasks, it may also be more economical. Individual staff members become more skilled and efficient when assigned to the same tasks on a regular basis. This may also more effectively utilize the individual nurse's skills and experience. Some nurses are particularly skilled at initiating intravenous therapy or administering medications and tend to be more motivated and efficient when completing those tasks than when performing treatments or teaching clients.

2. The volume of supplies and equipment required may also be decreased because fewer numbers of personnel utilize them. Consistency of task assignment may also decrease maintenance costs of equipment, since staff members become more proficient in the use of the types of equipment required to complete their specific function.

3. This method also tends to facilitate the organization of work, since assignments are clearly defined. Therefore, the overlapping of responsibilities and the associated confusion are minimized.

Disadvantages

1. The primary concern with the functional model is the fragmentation of care to which it gives rise. Assigning a variety of personnel to specific tasks frequently becomes inefficient and impersonal. The client's care is often divided into segments, each of which must be managed by a different individual. One nurse administers medications, a second provides teaching, and a third monitors vital signs. This tends to make the client feel insecure and frustrated.

2. Continuity of care is difficult, if not impossible, since no single staff member has a complete picture of the client's needs and responses to nursing or medical interventions. This allows unnoticed gaps to occur in client care.

3. From the nurse's perspective, this type of care delivery may become monotonous. Administration of medications for weeks at a time may decrease the nurse's motivation and limit continued personal development because of reduced exposure to a variety of experiences.

4. Job satisfaction may also be diminished in a functional approach because the individual nurse's role in the client's recovery may not be clearly defined or perceived as valuable by the client, other staff members, or supervisory personnel.

5. Communication and decision-making may be compromised, since caregivers are focusing on individual aspects of the client's care. Frequently, the nurse manager is the only staff member who receives complete information on the client. The responsibility and accountability for decision-making is focused on the manager rather than on individual staff members who actually implement the plan of care.

TEAM NURSING

Definition

Team nursing is a system of nursing care delivery in which a group of professional and nonprofessional personnel work together to deliver nursing care to a number of clients. It was designed after World War II (1) to provide improved client care utilizing available staff and (2) to alleviate the problems associated with the functional method (Tappen, 1983). Team nursing is frequently utilized in nursing homes, hospitals, and community health settings. Comprehensive client care is provided by the staff member under the direction of a registered nurse who is the team leader. Other team members may include RNs, LPNs, and nursing assistants. However, the size and composition of a team are often dependent upon the setting.

The team leader is the key person in this model. Leaders must have particular knowledge and skills not only in client care procedures and techniques but also in management and decision-making strategies. The team leader has the authority and responsibility for assigning the care of a group of clients to team members. These assignments are based on client needs and the knowledge, skills, and experiences of team members.

The success of the team approach is dependent upon effective communication. This method relies on the use of written client care assignments, timely development and revision of nursing care plans, frequent participation in client care conferences, and frequent reports and feedback among team members.

Advantages

1. Although nursing care in a team approach is divided among several staff members, it is less fragmented than in the functional method. This is a result of the extensive communication and coordination built into the system. Continuity of care is facilitated, particularly in systems where teams are constant. Therefore, team nursing is more satisfying to clients, since they are able to identify and communicate more effectively with the personnel responsible for delivering care.

2. From the nurse's perspective, the team model is more satisfying because the skills of each team member are frequently identified, recognized, and utilized. This provides the opportunity for nurses to identify their role in the client's progress along the illness-wellness continuum. The participation of team members in client care conferences improves the quality of decision-making and facilitates the development of individual team members. The cooperation and communication inherent in the system increase the potential for the delivery of quality nursing care.

Disadvantages

1. The team nursing model can very easily become a duplication of the functional method. For example, if team members are responsible for individual

functions, such as administering medications, monitoring vital signs, or giving baths, it is difficult to differentiate this system from functional team nursing.

2. Team nursing may be less efficient than a functional system. The communication and coordination required for the success of the system are compromised if the team leader does not have skills in organization, leadership, communication, motivation, and nursing care delivery. This method can also be ineffective if staff members sre not client-centered, skilled in nursing practice, and able to communicate clearly.

3. The number of personnel caring for clients is not substantially reduced in a team approach. This may not be cost-effective and may dilute the quality of care provided, particularly in settings in which a large volume of non-nursing personnel provide direct care.

4. The dilution of individual responsibility and accountability may also decrease the quality of care provided.

5. Team nursing may also promote a task-oriented approach to client care.

PRIMARY NURSING

Definition

Primary nursing is a system of care delivery in which the registered nurse is responsible and accountable for directing the care of a client or group of clients. The primary nurse develops the plan of care and ensures that the plan is implemented around the clock. In the absence of the primary nurse, the care of the client is delegated to an associate nurse, who follows the plan of care as developed by the primary nurse.

Primary nursing may be utilized in a variety of settings, including hospitals and public health agencies. Primary nursing systems emphasize (1) the nurse's responsibility and accountability for management of care, (2) decentralized decision-making with authority held by the primary nurse, (3) the importance of accurate and complete assessment, diagnosis, and planning, (4) the client's involvement in validation and goal-setting, (5) the need for communication between primary nurses and other nurses, members of the health care team, and clients and their families, and (6) preparation for discharge through client and family teaching, identification of available resources, and referral to other systems when required.

In some settings, primary nurses select their own clients. More frequently, the unit is divided into districts or modules, with one primary nurse assigned to each area. This nurse provides direct care to a caseload, which usually does not exceed six clients. The head nurse functions as the coordinator of the unit and is a resource person for the primary nurses. The primary nurse plans and provides the care, administers medications and treatments, interacts with the physician and other health professionals, and reports on the client's status. Other levels of staff, including LPNs and nursing assistants, aid the primary nurse in the provision of care. Client care conferences, which involve primary and associate nurses as well as other members of the health team, are frequently utilized to discuss specific client problems and to develop strategies for resolving them.

The professional nurse functioning in a primary care setting must have (1) a thorough knowledge of the nursing process, (2) refined communication skills, (3) the ability to perform nursing procedures identified in nursing orders, (4) well-developed problem-solving techniques, and (5) a commitment to client-centered care.

Advantages

1.   The primary nursing method of delivery promotes consistent, total client care by virtue of the quality and frequency of interactions between the client and the nurse. Each primary nurse is responsible for coordinating all aspects of care, including physical and emotional care, teaching, and the medical regimen.

2.   This method promotes increased autonomy and responsibility in individual nursing practice. The nurse may be more satisfied because involvement in direct care is increased, and therefore the nurse's role in the client's recovery is more clearly defined. Additionally, the nurse is more accountable, since care responsibilities focus on the total care of a small number of clients rather than the partial care of many.

3.   Primary nursing also provides the opportunity for professional growth. The nurse's involvement in all aspects of the client's care, particularly the decision-making component, facilitates the acquisition of new knowledge and skills. Nurses frequently feel that they are more effective in a primary system because they have a more global view of the needs of the client and family.

4.   Clients are also generally more satisfied because of the increased frequency of interaction with one specific nurse who is particularly knowledgeable about them. This allows the client to identify clearly the primary nurse and creates an atmosphere of trust and open communication.

5.   Other health care providers, such as physicians, therapists, and dieticians, also appreciate the ability to interact with an individual nurse who is informed about the client.

Disadvantages

1.   Primary nursing requires competent practitioners who can function independently when implementing the nursing process. Not all nurses are comfortable in accepting the responsibility associated with this system.

2.   In some instances, primary nursing may be less economical than functional or team nursing, since this model may require a larger percentage of registered nurses. However, the abilities of the registered nurse can be spread through the use of a "nurse extender," a person working as an assistant to an experienced primary nurse. The RN delegates responsibilities to the nurse extender while the RN remains accountable for care planning.

CASE MANAGEMENT

Definition

Case management is the second generation of primary nursing. It evolved from the emphasis on decreasing length of stay and the focus on achieving timely client outcomes. Case management is the organization of care to achieve specific client outcomes within a timeframe that is consistent with the length of stay designated by the client's DRG. The goals of case management include:

1. to facilitate the achievement of expected and/or standardized patient outcomes
2. to facilitate early discharge or discharge within an appropriate length of stay
3. to promote appropriate and/or reduced utilization of resources
4. to promote collaborative practice, coordination of care, and continuity of care
5. to promote professional development and satisfaction of hospital-based registered nurses
6. to direct the contributions of all care providers toward the achievement of patient outcomes (Bower, 1988 A).

Case managers are nurses with expertise in a particular clinical area. They work with other similarly educated nurses in a group practice. The members of the group work in a variety of hospital units. "For example, nursing group practice members for patients with vascular disorders would include specifically identified nurses in the ambulatory care area, the general inpatient unit, the operating room, the intensive care unit, and the rehabilitation unit. Each of these nurses would be the primary nurse for the patients while they receive care in the various settings. One of the group practice members would be identified as an individual patient's case manager and would assume responsibility for the outcomes of the patient's care for the episode of illness" (Bower, 1988 B). The group practice works with other health care professionals to facilitate care which achieves the expected clinical outcomes within a reasonable timeframe.

Two types of tools are used by nurses in case management: (1) A *case management plan* is a comprehensive plan of care that outlines the client's diagnoses, expected outcomes, and interventions. The plan is developed collaboratively by nurses and physicians and includes both medical and nursing interventions. (2) The *critical path* or *patient outcome timeline* is a one-page summary of the case management plan. It identifies predictable, important events which must occur at set times to achieve an appropriate length of stay (ANA, 1988). For example, the client who has had abdominal surgery should be assisted out of bed and to a chair the day after surgery, and should be walking in the hall by the fourth day. The critical path plan also presents the key interventions needed to achieve the outcomes and is used each shift to monitor the client's progress.

Advantages

1.   There is enhanced collaboration between nurses and other health care professionals, clients, and their families.

2.   Nurses experience increased morale and job satisfaction, facilitating recruitment and retention efforts.

3.   Achievement of client outcomes within a fiscally responsible timeframe is enhanced.

4.   Resources of the hospital are utilized more efficiently.

5.   Clients are well informed and actively participate in their progress.

6.   Case management promotes the establishment of standards of care for specific case types.

7.   Part-time and agency nurses have a clearer indication of what needs to be done during the shift to move the client toward the outcomes.

8.   Timely discharge of patients is facilitated.

9.   Staff nurses have increased knowledge about the financial impact of the client's length of stay.

Disadvantages

1.   The model requires a great deal of planning and cooperation to establish the system.

2.   It may be difficult to obtain the cooperation of physicians in defining how to manage certain case types and to collaborate with nurses on a professional level.

Table 8–1 summarizes the differences between functional, team, and primary nursing, and case management. The following example depicts how the delivery systems might affect the care of a hypothetical client.

Example.   Paul Kumar, age 56, was admitted to the hospital for major abdominal surgery. His postoperative course was uncomplicated. Depending on the type of nursing care delivery system in place, his first day after surgery may have fit one of these descriptions.

Functional Nursing

At change of shift report the head nurse assigned everyone to a task for the day. Paul's day began when the nursing assistant woke him and all of the clients by taking their temperatures. The licensed practical nurse came by a few minutes later to take Paul's blood pressure. An hour later the medication nurse delivered his medications on the way down the hall with the drug cart. A registered nurse assisted him in washing since the nurse was assigned to do baths. A registered nurse doing the treatments for the day came in after lunch to change his dressing. Paul wanted to complain to someone that he waited until 11:00 AM for his morning bath so he shared his dissatisfaction with the head nurse. No one revised his plan of care to reflect his preference for an early bath. Change of shift report

TABLE 8–1.   COMPARISON OF NURSING CARE DELIVERY SYSTEMS

FACTOR: ASSIGNMENTS
Functional:
Head nurse assigns to staff members tasks that fall within their job descriptions.
Team:
Team leader assigns individual clients to nurses, usually based on the location of the client's room and the nursing care needs involved.
Primary:
Head nurse assigns individual clients to nurses, matching the client's needs to the nurse's skills.
Case Management:
The nurse case manager is assigned to the client based on the client's needs, the case manager's skills, and any prior relationship with the client.

FACTOR: RESPONSIBILITY FOR PLANNING CARE
Functional:
No one person is responsible for planning unless this is assigned as a functional task to a specific RN for a given period.
Team:
The team leader is responsible for planning the nursing care for the assigned group of clients.
Primary:
The primary nurse is responsible for planning the nursing care of all primary clients, from the time they are admitted to a nursing unit until they are discharged from that unit. The physician is usually not involved in the care planning discussion. The care plan and outcomes are reviewed with the client and family. The primary nurse evaluates the achievement of outcomes.
Case Management:
The case manager and physician review and revise a critical path plan within 24 hours of admission. The critical path and outcomes are reviewed with the client and family. The case manager and physician evaluate the client's progress and, if necessary, analyze reasons for the client not achieving the outcomes as planned.

FACTOR: RESPONSIBILITY FOR PROVIDING CARE
Functional:
Nursing care is delivered in a fragmented manner—many staff members interact with the client as the various tasks are carried out.
Team:
Typically, one nurse provides nursing care while another administers medications.
Primary:
The primary nurse delivers or oversees the delivery of all nursing care to the primary clients.
Case Management:
The case manager delivers or oversees the delivery of care to the client throughout the hospitalization.

FACTOR: DOCUMENTATION OF PLAN OF CARE
Functional:
Nursing care regimens are rarely documented; therefore individual approaches are inconsistent.
Team:
Because nursing case load is too large, documented nursing care plans are encouraged but can not always be demanded.

TABLE 8–1. COMPARISON OF NURSING CARE DELIVERY SYSTEMS
(*Continued*)

Primary:
Documented nursing care plans are facilitated by a smaller case load of each nurse and by consistency of assignment.
Case Management:
The case manager is involved in the development and revision of the plan of care.

FACTOR: REPORTING AT THE END OF THE SHIFT
Functional:
A "charge" nurse reports on clients to another charge nurse; most of the information shared is based on reports of other workers.
Team:
The team leader gives report on the group of clients to the oncoming team; most of the information is based on reports of other workers.
Primary:
The primary nurse gives a report on each assigned client to an oncoming nurse who will care for the client; the nurse who reports has interacted directly with all the clients whose reports are given.
Case Management:
Report is given by the primary nurse with a focus on comparison of the client's progress with the expected outcomes identified on the critical path.

FACTOR: DECISION-MAKING
Functional:
Decisions are made on a basis of separate tasks performed by individual staff members for each client on the unit.
Team:
The team leader makes final decisions about nursing care for the clients in the group on the basis of feedback from team members.
Primary:
Each primary nurse makes final decisions about the nursing care for the assigned clients. The primary nurse's power base rests within the nursing group and comes from peers and nurse managers.
Case Management:
Each case manager utilizes the group practice members to review the client's progress toward achieving the outcomes and any changes needed in the plan of care. The case manager's power base is the same as that of the primary nurse. In addition, the case manager's power base is strengthened by institutional and multidisciplinary support. The case manager, in collaboration with the physician, is directly involved in ensuring appropriate length of stay and utilization of resources.

FACTOR: COORDINATION AND OUTCOMES OF NURSING CARE:
Functional:
No one nursing staff member is held accountable for the coordination and outcomes of nursing care; the head nurse often answers to everyone for the entire staff.
Team:
The team leader, who plans care but often does not give it, is accountable for the care of each client in the assigned group, and for the coordination and outcomes of nursing care.

(*Table continued on following page*)

TABLE 8–1. COMPARISON OF NURSING CARE DELIVERY SYSTEMS
(*Continued*)

Primary:
The primary nurse is accountable for the coordination and outcomes of nursing care.

Case Management:
The case manager is accountable for the coordination and outcomes of care for an entire episode of illness, or from the time of the client's admission to the health care system until the time that the client no longer requires care.

FACTOR: ACCOUNTABILITY FOR FOLLOW-UP ON CLIENT'S CLINICAL PROBLEMS:

Functional:
Physicians, administrators, and other interdepartmental personnel can rarely pinpoint responsibility for follow-up on problems. "Passing the buck" is prevalent.

Team:
The team leader is responsible for follow-up on client problems, which are often reported by other staff. There is a moderate amount of "passing the buck" because of change in staff assignments from day to day.

Primary:
The primary nurse is responsible for follow-up on clinical problems of assigned clients. There is minimal, if any, "passing of the buck" because of consistency of staff assignments to the same clients.

Case Management:
The case manager is responsible for follow-up on problems of assigned clients throughout hospitalization, after discharge, and on subsequent admissions. There is no "passing the buck" since the case manager is held accountable for outcomes.

FACTOR: COMMUNICATION BETWEEN NURSES AND CLIENTS

Functional:
Client, family, and significant others find it difficult to identify a nursing staff member with whom to relate on a continuing basis.

Team:
Client, family, and significant others may be confused as to the identity of the nursing staff member to whom questions and problems may be directed.

Primary:
Client, family, and significant others can clearly identify the nurse and can share ideas, feelings, and problems freely with this person.

Case Management:
Client, family, and significant others can clearly identify the case manager and can share ideas, feelings, and problems.

FACTOR: COMMUNICATION BETWEEN NURSES AND STAFF OF OTHER DEPARTMENTS

Functional:
Physicians, administrators, and interdepartmental staff address questions and problems to nurses or to the head nurse on the unit, but often satisfactory answers are delayed or not available.

Team:
As in functional nursing, physicians, administrators, and interdepartmental staff address questions and problems, except to a team leader rather than a head nurse.

TABLE 8–1. COMPARISON OF NURSING CARE DELIVERY SYSTEMS
(*Continued*)

Primary:
All communications are directed to the primary nurse for each client.
Case Management:
The case manager is part of a group practice which includes key physicians and other members of the health care team. The group reviews its caseload and provides support to each other. Case managers are easily identifiable.

FACTOR: COST EFFECTIVENESS

Functional:
Nursing care is of poor quality owing to fragmentation. This results in many complaints from clients. Nursing staff are easily frustrated and turnover rate is usually high, thus increasing the cost of orientation and of staff development. The output from professional nurses is low since they are not required to perform the full job—the total nursing process—for which they are being paid.
Team:
Nursing care is of only moderate quality, since expertise in judgment and communication cannot be delegated from the care planners (team leaders) to the caregivers (team members). Turnover of nursing staff is moderate. The output from professional nurses is low also. The combination of a mix of registered nurses, licensed practical nurses, and nurses' aides increases cost effectiveness.
Primary:
The product is of high quality, since the person most prepared and best equipped to perform does so on a continuing basis for the same clients. Turnover is minimized and job satisfaction is high. Primary nursing units that rely heavily on a high number of registered nurses are more costly than team nursing units.
Case Management:
The product is of high quality since the care is coordinated and outcomes of care are closely monitored. Turnover is minimized and job satisfaction is high. Case management is likely to be cost effective, because the case manager is responsible for meeting client care outcomes within an appropriate length of stay and the use of resources.

was given by the head nurse based on all the information provided by the staff nurses.

Team Nursing

The shift began when the head nurse placed the nurses on a team. The team leader, a registered nurse, assigned an RN to take care of Paul. The registered nurse took Paul's vital signs, assisted him with his bath, and changed his dressing. Meanwhile, the team leader spent the day giving medications. When Paul complained to the team leader that he had to wait until 11:00 for his morning bath, the team leader explained that an emergency had caused a delay in the work schedule of his assigned nurse. The team leader made a few additions to Paul's care plan based on the RN's feedback and shared these during the change of shift report.

Primary Nursing

At change of shift report the head nurse reviewed the assignment. Paul's primary nurse had admitted him on the morning of his surgery and was assigned to provide his care. The primary nurse took his vital signs, helped him wash, provided his medications, and changed his dressing. Paul realized that this bath was delayed until 11:00 because he had been told by his primary nurse that it would be more comfortable for him to bathe after pain medication had taken effect. The primary nurse made a few additions to Paul's care plan and discussed these during change of shift report. Paul's nurse gave report directly to the nurse on the evening shift who was going to be taking care of Paul.

Case Management

Paul's case manager was a registered nurse who was part of the abdominal surgical group practice. After change of shift report, the case manager took Paul's vital signs and administered his medications. Paul's bath and dressing change were performed by his case manager. During the morning the case manager and the surgeon reviewed the critical path and saw no need to make revisions in it. Paul did not complain about his bath being done at 11:00, since he knew his first priority was to be kept comfortable with pain medication. His critical path indicated that he was to get out of bed with assistance in the afternoon. When the case manager gave report to the nurses on the next shift, Paul's response to ambulating to the chair was discussed.

SUMMARY

Functional, team, primary nursing, and case management are four methods of delivering nursing care. The differences among the systems are dependent upon the mechanisms utilized by nurses to organize and deliver care. Each method has advantages that influence the efficiency and effectiveness of the system. In the 1990's functional nursing is the least common method of delivering nursing care. Case management is projected to be the most commonly used method of nursing care delivery by 1992 (Wake, 1990).

REFERENCES

American Nurses' Association: Nursing Case Management. Kansas City, MO: American Nurses' Association, 1988.

Bower K: Managed Care: Controlling Costs, Guaranteeing Outcomes. Definition 1–3, Summer, 1988.

Bower K: Case Management: Meeting the Challenge. Definition 3–1, Winter, 1988.

Tappen R: Nursing Leadership: Concept and Practice. Philadelphia: FA Davis, 1983.

Wake M: Nursing care delivery systems. Journal of Nursing Administration 1990 May; 20(5):47–51.

BIBLIOGRAPHY

Altman J, and Thielbar S: Educational efforts to support primary nursing. Journal of Nursing Staff Development 1985 Fall; 1:119–123.

Blinkarn H, D'Amico M, and Virtue E: Primary nursing and job satisfaction. Nursing Management 1988 Apr; 19(4):41–42.

Chavigny K, and Lewis A: Team or primary nursing care? Nursing Outlook 1984 Nov-Dec; 32(6):322–327.

Culpepper R, Richiel M, Sinclair V, et al: The effect of primary nursing on nursing quality assurance. Journal of Nursing Administration 1986 Nov; 16(11):24–31.

Donnelly L: A new look at (of all things) team nursing care. Nursing Management 1986 Sep; 17(9):59.

Glandon G, Colbert K, and Thomasma M: Nursing delivery models and RN mix: cost implications. Nursing Management 1989 May; 20(5):31–33.

Loveridge C, Cummings S, and O'Malley J: Developing case management in a primary nursing system. Journal of Nursing Administration 1988 Oct; 18(10):36–39.

Manthey M: Myths that threaten. Nursing Management 1988 Jun; 19(6):54–55.

Manthey M: Primary practice partners (a nurse extender system). Nursing Management 1988 Mar; 19(3):58–59.

Mutchner L: How well are we practicing primary nursing? Journal of Nursing Administration 1986 Sep; 16(9):8–13.

Turnock C: Clinical update: task allocation. Nursing Times 1987 Nov 4–10; 83(44): Nursing Practice: 71.

Zander K: Nursing care management. Journal of Nursing Administration 1988 May; 18(5):23–30.

Zander K: Second generation primary nursing: a new agenda. Journal of Nursing Administration 1985 Mar; 15(3):18–24.

Zander K, Blaney C, Hayes J, et al: Nursing Group Practice: The "Cadillac" in Continuity. Definition 1–3, Spring 1988.

9

EVALUATION

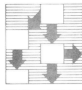

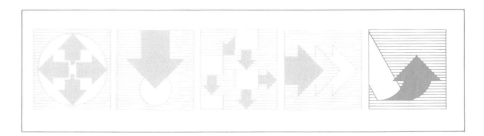

OVERVIEW

The process of evaluation is both ongoing and formal. Although evaluation is identified as the last phase in the nursing process, it is an *integral* part of each phase. Evaluation occurs whenever the nurse interacts with the client:

> As the nurse *assesses* the client, the data collected are being sorted, analyzed, and appraised for their significance. Evaluation is used in the *diagnostic* phase as the nurse reviews the defining characteristics and identifies the most appropriate diagnoses for a particular client. *Planning* includes setting priorities and making judgments about realistic outcomes that form the basis for evaluating the effectiveness of nursing interventions. Throughout *implementation* the nurse observes the client's behavior and revises the interventions based on the client's responses.

Evaluation can be conducted at the end point of the nursing process when it compares the client's health status with the outcomes defined by the plan of care. As a result of this activity the nurse determines if the care plan is appropriate, realistic, current, or in need of revision. If the client has not achieved the outcomes the nurse engages in problem-solving to determine how to revise the care plan.

The evaluation process consists of four steps:

1. Gathering data about the client's health status
2. Comparing the gathered data with the outcomes
3. Making a judgment about the client's progress toward achieving the outcomes
4. Revising the plan of care.

GATHERING DATA

Data is gathered for the purpose of evaluation through the same types of techniques used during assessment. These may include client interview, direct observation, physical examination or review of the medical record.

Client Interview

The client interview may be utilized while providing care to elicit information about the client's concerns, physical or emotional status, and knowledge of condition.

Direct Observation

Direct observation involves careful and thorough assessment of the cues related to a client's appearance and behavior.

Physical Examination

Physical examination involves use of the techniques of inspection, palpation, percussion, and auscultation to obtain data regarding the status of the client.

Review of Documents

Review of the client's medical record is useful in gathering data about the client's health status. Laboratory results and notations made by other health care professionals are analyzed to gain a complete picture of the client's progress. The nurse also looks at the progress notes and flowsheets to note data charted by nurses and other health care professionals.

COMPARISON OF DATA WITH OUTCOMES

After gathering data the nurse compares the client's current health status with the outcomes identified on the care plan.

Example. Nursing diagnosis: Altered skin integrity related to prolonged immobility. Outcome: Throughout hospitalization, no evidence of skin breakdown over bony prominences.

To evaluate this outcome the nurse would carefully inspect the client's skin, paying particular attention to the sacrum, elbows, hips, and heels. The inspection would occur as an ongoing part of care while the client is being bathed or positioned.

MAKING JUDGMENTS ABOUT PROGRESS

Add Other Outcomes

In the situation in whi
associated with the diagno
nursing diagnoses describe
to set outcomes at increasi
hydrated client with a nur
creased oral intake might h
24 hours." As the client's
read "consumes 2000 ml e

Example. William H
weight and physically inact
able to achieve the outcom
swimming twice a week an
times a week. Then, the nt
10 pounds in one month.

NURSING DIAGNOSIS

Health seeking behavior
(exercising and weight
loss)

In this example the
outcome to engage in reg
developed.

Example. Linda Va
diabetic. After two sessio
herself with insulin. The
involved learning to test

NURSING DIAGNOSIS

Knowledge deficit (insulin
injection technique,
blood glucose
monitoring)

After gathering data about the client's health status and comparing the data with the outcome, the nurse makes a judgment about the client's achievement of the outcome. There are two possible responses that are summarized in Figure 9–1:

1. The outcome was achieved and
2. The outcome was not achieved.

The numbers in the following paragraphs correspond to the numbers on Figure 9–1.

The Outcome was Achieved

1. The nursing diagnosis was resolved

If the outcome has been achieved, the nursing diagnosis identifies a human response which has been resolved and is no longer current.

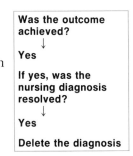

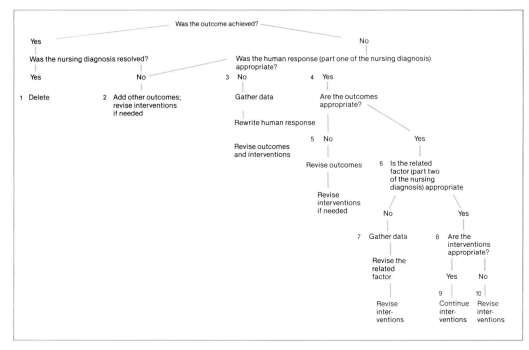

FIGURE 9–1. Flowsheet for evaluation.

fi
p
it
"
it
u

—

I

—

I

j
i
ς

i
i
i
l

Was the nursing diagnosis resolved?
↓
No

**Add other outcomes
Revise interventions
Reassess to
determine if the
human response was
appropriate**

DATE / INITIALS
9–10   KS
**NURSING
DIAGNOSIS   OUTCOME**

Ineffective   Within two
breastfeeding   days
related to   demonstrat
feelings of   ability to
inadequacy   breastfeed

FIGURE 9–2. Two meth

NEW OUTCOME

Within one day is able to
demonstrate correct
technique for blood
glucose monitoring

Revise the Interventions

When the nursing diagnosis is not resolved and the outcomes have been revised, the nurse should review the interventions specified in the plan of care and determine why they were not effective in assisting the client. Careful analysis of the approaches used may indicate alternative strategies that will assist the client in achieving the outcome.

Example.   Christine Parker was discharged from the hospital after having a colostomy. During the first home visit the nurse found that Christine was having trouble changing the ostomy pouch which collects feces. Christine said that since she dropped out of school in the fourth grade she could not read the pamphlet given to her by the nurse in the hospital. Recognizing that a different approach was needed to teach Christine, the visiting nurse used Christine's videocassette recorder and TV to show her a tape on colostomy care.

When the visiting nurse returned the following week Christine was able to independently change her pouch.

NURSING DIAGNOSIS	OUTCOME	ORIGINAL INTERVENTION	CUE
Knowledge deficit (colostomy care)	By the time of second visit is able to change pouch independently	1. Reinforce information in "Colostomy Care" pamphlet	Having difficulty changing pouch
		REVISED INTERVENTIONS	
		1. Show tape on colostomy care 2. Observe client's ability to change pouch after viewing tape	

Reassess to Determine if the Human Response was Appropriate

As was stated in Chapter 4, outcomes are developed from the first part of the nursing diagnosis, the human response. The interventions are derived from the related factor identified in the second part of the nursing diagnosis. This process is summarized below.

NURSING DIAGNOSIS		
Human response	related to	Related factor
↓		↓
Outcomes		Interventions

The evaluation process involves reviewing the nursing diagnosis when outcomes are not achieved.

The Outcome was Not Achieved

3. *The human response is not appropriate*

When the outcomes are not achieved the nurse first reviews the human response to determine if it accurately describes the client's status.

This process is done by comparing the defining characteristics associated with the diagnosis with the client's symptoms. If the diagnosis is not pertinent to the client's problems, assessment skills are used to gather more data. This may lead to the revision of the human response, outcome, and interventions.

> **Was the human response (part one of the nursing diagnosis) appropriate?**
> ↓
> **No**
>
> **Gather data**
> **Rewrite human response**
> **Revise outcomes and interventions**

Example.   Peter Greene, age 72, was admitted to the hospital a week ago with uncontrolled diabetes. He was very restless, changed position in bed frequently, and indicated anticipation of his wife's visit because she knew how to make him feel better. Although he was capable of washing himself, he told the nurse, Michelle Henley, that he wanted to wait until his wife came in.

Michelle put this data together and concluded that Mr. Greene's restlessness was caused by anxiety. However, when his wife arrived at 2:00, he continued to be restless. Wondering if something other than anxiety was at the root of Mr. Greene's symptoms, the nurse began asking him questions and assessing his physical status. When Michelle discovered that Mr. Greene had a distended bladder, he stated, "Things haven't been working right since that tube came out of my bladder last night." Michelle realized *urinary retention* was a more specific diagnosis for Mr. Greene and contacted his doctor.

ORIGINAL CARE PLAN		
NURSING DIAGNOSIS	OUTCOME	CUE
Anxiety related to unknown etiology	Verbalizes decrease in anxiety at the time of wife's visit	Restlessness Feelings of helplessness

REVISED CARE PLAN		
NURSING DIAGNOSIS	OUTCOME	CUE
Urinary retention related to effects of diminished sensory impulses	Empties bladder by voiding or by catheterization within one hour	Distended bladder Difficulty voiding

In this example the nurse originally put some cues together and developed a plausible diagnosis which did not accurately describe the symptoms the client was experiencing. Further assessment resulted in additional data and revision of the nursing diagnosis and plan of care.

Example. Carla Woerner is a 19 year old nursing student who has completed the first semester of her program. She visited the student health nurse stating she was upset about her grades. "I feel overwhelmed by all of this studying I have to do. I feel so helpless. I always got good grades in high school. Why can't I get A's in nursing school?" The nurse encouraged Carla to talk about her feelings and referred her to the academic advisor for information on study skills. Additionally, Carla was given an appointment to revisit the nurse in three weeks.

When Carla came in for her second visit she looked tired and disheveled. She had not bathed or changed clothes in a week. "It is no use," she told the nurse. "I'll never learn all of this stuff. My parents will be angry at me for wasting their money. I must confess I've thought about ending it all." When the nurse asked Carla about her desire to "end it all," Carla said, "My roommate has some sleeping pills. I've been wondering if it hurts to die." The nurse recognized that Carla was at high risk for suicide and arranged for her to be seen by the staff psychiatrist within half an hour.

ORIGINAL CARE PLAN		
NURSING DIAGNOSIS	OUTCOME	INTERVENTIONS
Situational low self-esteem related to perceived academic overload	Within three weeks makes positive statements about self	1. Refer to academic advisor for study skills review 2. Encourage to verbalize feelings 3. Set up revisit in three weeks

REVISED CARE PLAN		
NURSING DIAGNOSIS	OUTCOME	INTERVENTION
Potential for injury: self-directed related to feelings of failure	Does not harm self	1. Obtain immediate psychiatric attention.

In this situation the nurse identified that Carla did not achieve the outcome of verbalizing more positive feelings about herself. Additional assessment data revealed that Carla had a plan for committing suicide and was in immediate danger. The nursing diagnosis was revised along with the outcomes and interventions.

4.   The human response is appropriate

When the nurse reviews the human response and finds that it is appropriate to the client's status, the nurse then examines the outcomes to determine their applicability. The process of evaluating the outcomes includes asking the following questions:

1.   Is the outcome realistic?
2.   Was the outcome formulated with the client's strengths in mind?
3.   Is the timeframe appropriate?

> Was the human response appropriate?
> ↓
> Yes
>
> Are the outcomes appropriate?
> ↓
> No

5.   The outcome is not appropriate

If the outcome was not achieved because it was not appropriate, revision of the outcome and interventions would occur.

> Revise outcomes
> Revise interventions if needed

Example.   Linda Dote was admitted to the hospital after an argument in which her husband fractured her ribs and ruptured her spleen. On the second day after admission the nurse helped Linda set an outcome of being able to work out a plan to permanently move out of her home. During discussions Linda continued to say, "Part of me wants to leave him and part of me is afraid to try to make it on my own. I've never lived alone. I'm afraid I would be lonely." On the fourth day of her hospitalization, Linda's husband showed up with a dozen red roses and promises of never hitting her again. Although the nurse explained to her that this is a predictable phase in the cycle of violence, Linda was unwilling to listen. "Don't you see? He promised he wouldn't hurt me. I think he really means it this time." Recognizing that Linda was now uninterested in moving out, the nurse gave her written information on the local shelter for battered women. The nurse said, "Linda, you may need this information some day. You will be protected at the shelter and will have a chance to think while your husband cools off." Linda replied, "I am sure I will never need this phone number but I will keep it—just in case."

NURSING DIAGNOSIS	OUTCOME	INTERVENTIONS
Decisional conflict (separation from husband) related to fear of loneliness	By the time of discharge identifies a plan for alternative living arrangements	1. Assist client to identify alternative living arrangements 2. Encourage client to verbalize feelings
	REVISED OUTCOME	REVISED INTERVENTIONS
	By the time of discharge is able to describe how to contact shelter	3. Provide client with phone number of shelter 4. Assist client to identify advantages of temporarily utilizing shelter

The nurse in this example determined that Linda was not ready to achieve the outcome of planning a move into her own apartment. Since the nursing diagnosis was appropriate, the nurse revised the outcome and interventions to reflect a different strategy for assisting Linda.

Are the outcomes
appropriate?
↓
Yes

Is the related factor
(part two of the
nursing diagnosis)
appropriate?
↓
No

Gather data
Revise the related
factor
Revise interventions
if needed

6. *The outcome is appropriate*

The related factor in the nursing diagnosis is reviewed when an outcome is not achieved after the human response and outcome are evaluated to be applicable to the client. The nurse determines if the related factor is accurate in describing the etiology of the human response. Assessment data are used to determine if the related factor is descriptive and current.

7. *The related factor is not appropriate*

More data are gathered and revision of the related factor and interventions occurs when the nurse determines that the related factor is not appropriate.

   Example.   During Janie Howard's monthly visit to the outpatient department her blood pressure was found to be elevated. The clinic nurse concluded that Janie needed a review of the causes and treatment of high blood pressure and gave her pamphlets to read. Janie's blood pressure was still elevated during her visit the following month. While being questioned by the nurse, Janie said, "Oh, I know I need to take my pills. I just can't afford to keep refilling my prescription. Instead of taking one pill every day, I've been taking one every other day to make them last longer." At this point the nurse realized that financial concerns were the real reason for Janie's noncompliance. Janie was given a list of discount drugstores in the area and a new prescription for a medication which would be just as effective yet less expensive.

ORIGINAL CARE PLAN		
NURSING DIAGNOSIS	OUTCOME	INTERVENTIONS
Noncompliance (medication) related to lack of knowledge of hypertension	Takes prescribed medication daily	Educate on cause and treatment of hypertension
REVISED CARE PLAN		
NURSING DIAGNOSIS	OUTCOME	INTERVENTIONS
Noncompliance (medication) related to decreased financial resources	Takes prescribed medication daily	1. Contact physician for change in prescription 2. Provide client with discount drug store list

8. *The related factor is appropriate*

If the related factor is applicable to the client's status, the nurse reviews the interventions specified in the plan of care. The nurse sould consider the following questions:

   1.   Are the interventions individualized for the client?
   2.   Are the interventions realistic given the available resources?

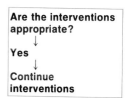

Are the interventions appropriate?
↓
Yes
↓
Continue interventions

Evaluation of the achievement of outcomes carries the nurse through the nursing process to the revision of the plan of care. The nurse may choose to continue the interventions after determining that they are appropriate. The nursing diagnosis may be one that is describing a human response which is difficult to alleviate through nursing intervention.

Example. Floyd Kendrick was hospitalized due to widespread bone cancer. He has been receiving pain medication every three hours around the clock. When asked about his pain, Floyd states, "The medicine keeps it under control."

NURSING DIAGNOSIS	OUTCOME	INTERVENTION	CUE
Pain related to effects of terminal illness	Throughout hospitalization states he feels comfortable	1. Medicate for pain every three hours 2. Evaluate level of pain every three hours	"The medicine keeps the pain under control"

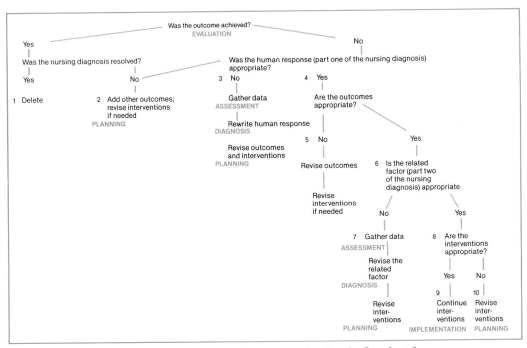

FIGURE 9–3. Diagram of how steps of the nursing process related to the flowsheet for evaluation.

In this situation the nurse recognizes that pain management will be a continuing concern. The nurse will continue to implement the care plan as stated since the interventions are realistic for the staff and individualized for the client. Figure 9–3 identifies how each step in the nursing process is linked to evaluation of outcomes.

QUALITY ASSURANCE

Up to this point the concept of evaluation has been discussed from the perspective of the individual nurse who evaluates the client's achievement of outcomes. The concept of *quality assurance* is defined as a planned and systematic evaluation of the care given to groups of clients.

History

The concern for quality assurance is not new. Beginning in the 1600s attention was paid to the rates of illness and death as indicators of quality of care delivered in institutions. In 1916, Dr. Codman was one of the first to call upon hospital officials to evaluate the quality of care delivered in their institutions. He said:

> "I am called eccentric for saying in public: that hospitals, if they wish to be sure of improvement, must find out what their results are. Must analyze their results to find their strong and weak points. Must compare their results with those of other hospitals. Must care for what cases they can care for well, and avoid attempting to care for the cases which they are not qualified to care for well. Must assign the cases to members of the staff (for treatment) for better reasons than seniority, the calendar, or temporary convenience. Must welcome publicity not only for their successes but for their errors, so that the public may give help when it is needed. Must promote members of the staff on a basis which gives due consideration to what they can accomplish for their patients. Such opinions will not be eccentric a few years hence." (Greeley Associates, 1984).

Although considered revolutionary in his day, Dr. Codman's points are valid and accepted today. Shortly after World War I, the demand for critical evaluation of health care began to escalate. The pressures by consumers for some type of systematic evaluation culminated in the passage of legislation. In 1972, Congress mandated professional review of health care services, singling out the care delivered to Medicare (people over 65 years of age), Medicaid (low-income populations), and Maternal-Child Health programs. Long-term care facilities which provide care to Medicare, Medicaid, and private pay residents are among the most heavily regulated of all health care facilities.

In the 1970s Professional Standards Review Organizations (PSROs) were created. In the 1980s the title of these organizations became Professional Review

Organizations (PROs), and their structure has been somewhat altered. The mission of the PROs includes the following:

1. To ensure that all health care reimbursed from federal funds is necessary
2. To ensure that care meets professional standards
3. To require that care be provided economically in an appropriate setting.

Joint Commission

The organization most actively involved in evaluating quality of care is the Joint Commission for Accreditation of Healthcare Organizations (JCAHO). It is responsible for evaluating hospitals, nursing homes, home care agencies, and a variety of other agencies. JCAHO has used a number of strategies for evaluating the quality of health care provided by facilities seeking accreditation. JCAHO reviews the *structure* of the facility, including whether it has appropriate equipment, buildings, policies, and procedures. Also evaluated is the facility's *process* of care to determine if it delivers health care appropriately. Following Dr. Codman's advice, JCAHO has put more emphasis on the evaluation of the facility's *outcomes* of care to ensure that the facility is obtaining good results with its resources.

The JCAHO ten-step quality assurance model is summarized in Figure 9–4. The model is applicable for hospitals, long-term care facilities, home health care agencies, and other agencies seeking to use a systematic method for monitoring quality of care. The remainder of the chapter explains the ten-step model and demonstrates the critical role of nursing in evaluating the delivery of quality care.

1. Assign responsibility

2. Delineate scope of care

3. Identify important aspects of care

4. Identify indicators related to these aspects of care

5. Establish thresholds for evaluation related to the indicator

6. Collect and organize data

7. Evaluate care when thresholds are reached

8. Take actions to improve care

9. Assess the effectiveness of the actions and document improvement

10. Communicate relevant information to the organizational quality assurance program

FIGURE 9–4. Joint Commission's Ten Step Monitoring and Evaluation Process.

The Ten-Step Model

Step 1—Assign Responsibility

The nurse holding the highest administrative position within a health care facility is ultimately accountable for quality assurance. This nurse may delegate responsibility for specific activities related to monitoring and evaluating care.

Step 2—Delineate Scope of Care

The nursing department or, in larger facilities, each clinical area develops a description of their clinical activities. This statement includes:

> "types of patients served
> conditions and diagnoses treated
> treatments or activities performed
> types of practitioners providing care
> sites where care is provided, and
> times when it is provided" (Fromberg, 1988).

Step 3—Identify Important Aspects of Care

Monitoring and evaluation activities are based on the most important activities of the nursing department. Highest priority is given to those aspects of care which are high volume, high risk, or problem prone.

> *High volume* aspects of care occur frequently or affect large numbers of clients.
>
> *High risk* aspects of care include those which place clients at risk for serious consequences or deprive them of substantial benefit if the care is not provided correctly.
>
> *Problem prone* aspects of care are those that have tended in the past to produce problems for staff or patients (Fromberg, 1988).

Table 9–1 provides examples of high volume, high risk, and problem prone aspects of care for various types of nursing settings.

TABLE 9–1. EXAMPLES OF HIGH VOLUME, HIGH RISK, AND PROBLEM PRONE ASPECTS OF CARE

Type of Aspect of Care	Service	Aspect of Care
High volume	Critical care	Cardiac monitoring
High volume	Postpartum	Providing comfort measures
High volume	Nursing home	Maintaining skin integrity
High risk	Postanesthesia care unit	Maintaining an open airway
High risk	Pediatrics	Administering medications
High risk	Home care	Detecting complications
Problem prone	Surgical unit	Managing the confused elderly postop client
Problem prone	Outpatient clinic	Follow-up on clients who miss appointments
Problem prone	Emergency department	Communicating with a client with a language barrier

Step 4—Identify Indicators

Indicators are the measurable components of the aspects of care. They are identified by the nurses who work within a particular setting and are based on nursing literature. Indicators may evaluate the structure, process, or outcome of care. As was mentioned earlier in the chapter, the *structure* of nursing care includes the resources such as the number of nurses, the mix of registered nurses and other support personnel, or the type of equipment that is available.

Examples of Structural Indicators

Turnover rate
Availability of emergency equipment on each nursing unit

Processes of nursing care focus on the delivery of nursing care. Nursing interventions that are considered processes of care include performing procedures, managing complications, and documentation.

Examples of Process Indicators

Accurate assessment of clients
Management of the client during a seizure
Proper completion of documentation forms

Outcomes of care are the complications and positive results of nursing interventions. Outcome indicators are the prime focus of the quality assurance monitoring and are illustrated in Table 9–2.

TABLE 9–2. EXAMPLES OF CLINICAL INDICATORS

HOSPITALWIDE
Development or worsening of pressure ulcers
Development of pneumonia in patients treated in special care units
Commission of important medication errors resulting in death or major morbidity

OBSTETRICAL CARE
A maternal length of stay more than five days after a vaginal delivery or more than
    seven days after a cesarean section
A maternal death up to and including 42 days postpartum
A successful or failed vaginal birth after cesarean section

ANESTHESIA CARE
Respiratory arrest within a specified time following anesthesia care
Development of injury to the brain or spinal cord within a specified time following
    anesthesia care
Dental injury during anesthesia care

(Modified from the Agenda for Change. Chicago: Joint Commission for Accreditation of Healthcare Organizations, June 1988, p 3.)

Examples of Outcome Indicators

Wound infections
Medication reactions
Client satisfaction with nursing care
Client understanding of teaching provided

Step 5—Establish Thresholds for Evaluation

When nurses identify the indicators they will be monitoring they establish thresholds for evaluation. Thresholds are the numerical values which, when reached, trigger an investigation into the causes of a problem. They are determined before data collection begins.

Example

INDICATOR	THRESHOLD
The client who has had ambulatory surgery is free of nausea and vomiting 24 hours after surgery	95%

In this example phone calls are made to clients who have had surgery the previous day. If 95 percent of them deny nausea or vomiting, no further investigation is required. When less than 95 percent deny these symptoms, the threshold has been reached and further evaluation is initiated.

Thresholds for evaluation are determined by the nurses who will be doing the monitoring in conjunction with the nurses whose performance will be monitored. Some indicators require 100 percent thresholds. These include serious events or outcomes in which it would not be appropriate to accumulate a series of such occurrences before doing further investigation.

Example. The threshold for failure to administer the correct blood to a client is 100 percent. Any incidents of incorrect blood transfusion would be immediately investigated.

Thresholds of 100 percent are also set for critical performance issues in which anything less than 100 percent would be unacceptable.

Example. The threshold for the correct application of a chest restraint would be 100 percent since improperly applied restraints can compromise the client's ability to breathe.

In other situations it is not realistic to set a threshold of 100 percent, particularly when there are some factors beyond the nurse's control.

Example.　The threshold for client satisfaction with nursing care might be 95 percent based on the premise that some clients will be dissatisfied regardless of all efforts made to please them.

Step 6—Collect and Organize Data

Data are collected from a variety of sources including reports, medical records, committee minutes, and questionnaires. Interviews, observation, or review of written materials are methods of data collection.

Step 7—Evaluate Care

When the cumulative data reach the threshold for evaluation, an intensive review of the data occurs. The data are evaluated to see if any patterns or trends exist.

Examples.　When reviewing falls on a geriatric unit it was determined that more falls occur on the night shift than on any other shift.

A new nursing employee was found to be consistently filling out the intake and output record incorrectly in comparison to the procedure for its use.

Step 8—Take Action to Solve Problems

The identification of trends or patterns helps to focus the problem-solving activities. Corrective action may involve providing more education, making changes in the health care facility's policies, procedures, equipment, or staffing, or changing an individual's performance through counseling or increasing supervision. When monitoring does not reveal a problem or an opportunity to improve care the monitoring continues to be performed. In this case the nurses examine the indicators, data collection methods, and thresholds to determine their usefulness and to make changes as needed.

Step 9—Assess Actions and Document Improvement

One of the most frequently overlooked steps includes the evaluation of the effectiveness of the corrective action. If the corrective action has not solved the problem, further analysis of the data occurs with planning and implementation of new corrective actions. Once again, evaluation of the impact of problem solving follows.

Step 10—Communicate Information to the QA Program

Quality assurance information is reported by nursing to the facility wide QA department. Reporting serves to inform others of the efforts to improve care and helps to prevent duplication of efforts. Reporting is accomplished through written summaries, such as the one shown in Figure 9–5.

DIVISION: Critical Care   **DATE:** 9/15/90

INDICATOR: Assessment of Chest Pain

OBJECTIVE OF MONITORING: To evaluate the documentation of assessment of chest pain

RESULTS OF MONITORING:

A random sample of 20 charts of emergency department clients was reviewed over a one-month period of time.

1. 100 percent of the charts contained a description of the location of chest pain and associated symptoms. (The threshold was 100%).
2. 90 percent had monitor rhythm strips attached to the chart (90% threshold).
3. 85 percent of the charts had documentation of radiation and quality of chest pain (90% threshold).
4. 70 percent of the charts contained vital signs including temperature (90% threshold).
5. 50 percent of the charts contained a description of past medical history (100% threshold).
6. 30 percent of the charts included a description of breath sounds (95% threshold).

DID MONITORING REVEAL A PROBLEM: Yes x No

PLAN FOR CORRECTIVE ACTION:

Who or What is Expected to Change?

Staff nurses are expected to improve documentation of radiation and quality of chest pain, vital signs, onset of chest pain, past medical history, and respiratory assessment.

Who is Responsible for Implementing Action?

Head nurse and clinical specialist.

What Action Was Taken?

1. Results of QA monitoring were shared with the staff at the July 8, 1990 staff meeting.
2. Documentation inservices were conducted in August 1990.
3. A new flowsheet was developed that is specific for cardiac clients.
4. The new emergency department sheet, which is being revised, will include such items as past medical history.
5. A videotape on breath sounds was placed in the emergency department library for review by the staff.

When Will Indicator Be Re-evaluated?

December 1990

FIGURE 9–5. Sample quality assurance report.

Example of the Ten-Step Process

1. Nancy Foot, the Vice President for Nursing of a 350-bed hospital, instructed the directors of each nursing division to formalize the nursing quality assurance program.

2. Bob Hiss, Director of the Medical Surgical Nursing Division, assisted the oncology unit to write its scope of care statement. The oncology unit determined that it cared for clients with cancer in various stages of their illness.

3. One of the oncology unit's high volume aspects of care was maintaining skin integrity.

4. The unit identified pressure sores as an outcome indicator and developed a number of questions to monitor this indicator.

5. The threshold for evaluation was set at 80 percent.

6. Monitoring was accomplished through observation of the client's skin and review of the medical record.

7. The nurses determined that four out of a sample of ten clients developed a pressure sore, or 60 percent did *not* develop a pressure sore. Since the threshold for evaluation (80%) was reached, the nurses did an intensive review.

8. The oncology nurses determined that the clients with the most skin breakdown were emaciated and had inadequate nutritional intake. As a result of their analysis, Bob Hiss made arrangements to utilize special beds as a preventive measure. In addition, the data was discussed with the physicians and dietitians. Thereafter, the dietitians began assessing each oncology client on admission to identify those with inadequate nutritional status.

9. Three months later the oncology nurses repeated the monitoring activity and determined that only one client out of a sample of 10 had developed a pressure sore.

10. These results were reported through Bob Hiss and Nancy Foot to the hospitalwide Quality Assurance Committee and the Board of Directors.

SUMMARY

Evaluation is an ongoing process used to judge each component of the nursing process. The term is used most commonly to describe decisions made about the client's achievement of outcomes. The plan of care is modified based on this analysis. Evaluation of the quality of care given to groups of clients has become increasingly more sophisticated. The trend in quality assurance is to evaluate the outcomes of care by comparing results against national standards.

REFERENCES

Fromberg R: The Joint Commission Guide to Quality Assurance. Chicago: Joint Commission for Accreditation of Healthcare Organizations, 1988, pp 50–57.
Greeley Associates: Continuous Monitoring and Data Based Quality Assurance. Salem, WI: Greeley Associates, 1984.

BIBLIOGRAPHY

Coyne C, and Killien M: A system for unit-based monitors of quality of nursing care. Journal of Nursing Administration 1987 Jan; 17(1):26–32.

Crockett D, and Sutcliffe S: Staff participation in nursing quality assurance. Nursing Management 1986 Oct; 17(10):41–42.

Osinski E: Developing patient outcomes as a quality measure of nursing care. Nursing Management 1987 Oct; 18(10):28–29.

Patterson C: Standards of patient care: the Joint Commission focus on nursing quality assurance. Nursing Clinics of North America 1988 Sep; 23(3):625–638.

10

LEGAL AND ETHICAL ISSUES AND THE NURSING PROCESS

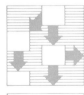

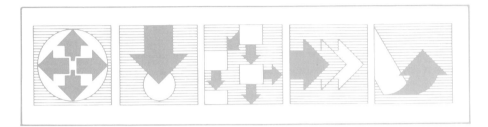

INTRODUCTION

Legal and ethical issues pervade all aspects of the nursing process. The information presented in this chapter addresses four basic principles of law. Ethical content will include definitions of morals and ethics, sources of ethics, ethical theories, examples of ethical dilemmas, and the steps in ethical decision-making.

PRINCIPLES OF LAW

There are four basic concepts which guide the legal system:

The Legal System is Constantly Evolving

Changes occur in the legal system in response to societal issues. As new technologies and health care issues raise legal questions, the courts attempt to come up with solutions. For example, the act of becoming a surrogate mother raises questions about the identity of the parents, the obligations of the surrogate mother, and the response to a request of a surrogate mother for custody of the child. As issues such as this one appear to be resolved, others arise to take their place. The legal issues being raised in the first half of the 1990s will be different from the ones affecting health care in the second half of the decade. As cases are resolved in court, the decisions being made subsequently influence the resolution of future cases and impact on nursing practice.

Each Individual has Rights and Responsibilities

This principle dictates that each person in the health care environment has rights to be protected and obligations to fulfill. The client's rights are considered when planning and delivering nursing care. Additionally, the nurse has rights and responsibilities as an employee and a professional.

Client's Rights

In the 1990s the concept of client rights has come under increased scrutiny. Clients as health care consumers have become aware of their rights as a result of two recent developments in health care:

1. The federal government's attempts to decrease the cost of health care to reduce the federal deficit have weakened the commitment to high quality health care for all. The Diagnostic Related Groupings System (DRG) with its emphasis on early discharge has created concerns about financial issues becoming more important than the client's need for health care.

2. Competition among a variety of health care providers has created an image of health care as being callous and commercial. This is in contrast to a more traditional view of health care as professional, caring, and concerned with quality of care (Rosenfield, 1988).

Consumer and health care groups have fought to protect the consumer by mandating certain rights. The Bill of Rights for Mental Health Patients is a federal law that guarantees client rights in nursing homes and home health agencies, and various state laws describe the rights of mentally or developmentally disabled persons, residents of health facilities, and for clients in general (Rosenfield, 1988).

The American Hospital Association has published a voluntary bill of rights for all hospitalized clients in both private and public facilities (see Fig. 10–1). The Bill of Rights describes the type of care the client can expect to receive while hospitalized. The nurse is responsible to be a client advocate in helping to ensure that all of the rights listed are respected. A few of these rights will be discussed below.

Right to Considerate and Respectful Care. As part of the therapeutic relationship the nurse determines how the client wishes to be addressed. Nurses should refrain from using such disparaging forms of address such as "Gramps," "Pops," "Grandma." Research has shown that hospitalized clients equate quality of care with how often they are called by name (Satisfaction Data, 1989).

Right to Refuse Treatment to the Extent Permitted by Law and to be Informed of the Consequences. When the nurse ignores a client's refusal of treatment, the nurse may be held liable for assault or battery. Battery is the intentional touching of another without consent and assault is the suggestion or threat of battery (Cazales, 1978). If the client refuses a treatment and the nurse says it will be performed anyway, *assault* has occurred. If the nurse actually performs the procedure, *battery* results.

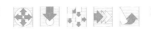

A PATIENT'S BILL OF RIGHTS

The American Hospital Association presents a Patient's Bill of Rights with the expectation that observance of these rights will contribute to more effective patient care and greater satisfaction for the patient, his physician, and the hospital organization. Further, the Association presents these rights in the expectation that they will be supported by the hospital on behalf of its patients, as an integral part of the healing process. It is recognized that a personal relationship between the physician and the patient is essential for the provision of proper medical care. The traditional physician-patient relationship takes on a new dimension when care is rendered within an organizational structure. Legal precedent has established that the institution itself also has a responsibility to the patient. It is in recognition of these factors that these rights are affirmed.

1.   The patient has the right to considerate and respectful care.

2.   The patient has the right to obtain from his physician complete current information concerning his diagnosis, treatment, and prognosis in terms the patient can be reasonably expected to understand. When it is not medically advisable to give such information to the patient, the information should be made available to an appropriate person in his behalf. He has the right to know, by name, the physician responsible for coordinating his care.

3.   The patient has the right to receive from his physician information necessary to give informed consent prior to the start of any procedure and/or treatment. Except in emergencies, such information for informed consent should include but not necessarily be limited to the specific procedure and/or treatment, the medically significant risks involved, and the probable duration of incapacitation. Where medically significant alternatives for care or treatment exist, or when the patient requests information concerning medical alternatives, the patient has the right to such information. The patient also has the right to know the name of the person responsible for the procedures and/or treatment.

4.   The patient has the right to refuse treatment to the extent permitted by law and to be informed of the medical consequences of his action.

5.   The patient has the right to every consideration of his privacy concerning his own medical care program. Case discussion, consultation, examination, and treatment are confidential and should be conducted discreetly. Those not directly involved in his care must have the permission of the patient to be present.

6.   The patient has the right to expect that all communications and records pertaining to his care should be treated as confidential.

7.   The patient has the right to expect that within its capacity a hospital must make reasonable response to the request of a patient for services. The hospital must provide evaluation, service, and/or referral as indicated by the urgency of the case. When medically permissible a patient may be transferred to another facility only after he has received complete information and explanation concerning the needs for and alternatives to such a transfer. The institution to which the patient is to be transferred must first have accepted the patient for transfer.

8.   The patient has the right to obtain information as to any relationship of his hospital to other health care and educational institutions insofar as his care is concerned. The patient has the right to obtain information as to the existence of any professional relationships among individuals, by name, who are treating him.

9.   The patient has the right to be advised if the hospital proposes to engage in or perform human experimentation affecting his care or treatment. The patient has the right to refuse to participate in such research projects.

10.   The patient has the right to expect reasonable continuity of care. He has the right to know in advance what appointment times and physicians are available and where. The patient has the right to expect that the hospital will provide a mechanism whereby he is informed by his physician or a delegate of the physician of the patient's continuing health care requirements following discharge.

11.   The patient has the right to examine and receive an explanation of his bill regardless of source of payment.

12.   The patient has the right to know what hospital rules and regulations apply to his conduct as a patient.

No catalogue of rights can guarantee for the patient the kind of treatment he has a right to expect. A hospital has many functions to perform, including the prevention and treatment of disease, the education of both health professionals and patients, and the conduct of clinical research. All these activities must be conducted with an overriding concern for the patient and, above all, the recognition of his dignity as a human being. Success in achieving this recognition assures success in the defense of the rights of the patient.

FIGURE 10–1. A patient's bill of rights. (Reprinted with permission of the American Hospital Association. Copyright 1972.)

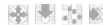

When a client refuses to consent to a treatment, the nurse should stop and notify the nursing supervisor. The supervisor and the doctor, depending upon the circumstances, may try to convince the client to accept the treatment. In rare instances the doctor may seek a court order to overrule the client's decision. For instance, this is sometimes done when a Jehovah's Witness with minor children refuses to accept a blood transfusion. The courts have held that it is in the state's best interests to protect the children from a parent's decision to risk death.

A mentally competent adult has the right to refuse care even in life-threatening situations.

Example. During an attempt to resuscitate a woman in the intensive care unit the client opened her eyes. She said to the nurse, "Let me go. Leave me alone." The physician, who was standing by her side, verified that the client wanted no further treatment. The resuscitation effort ended and the client was allowed to die.

Right to Expect that all Communications and Records Pertaining to Care Will be Kept Confidential. The ethical aspects of this issue will be discussed later in this chapter. Nurses are prohibited from sharing information about a client with anyone other than health care professionals directly responsible for the client's care. This principle applies to families who are seeking detailed information. It is best to ask the client's permission before giving information to friends and family.

Example. A nurse was on duty one night when a client's son asked about his mother's condition. The nurse answered his questions and the client protested to the hospital that her health was her own business. The nurse was officially reprimanded and a copy was placed in her personnel record (Baer, 1985).

The nurse should be sure to determine the procedure to follow if a family member wants to see the client's record. Most facilities require the client to give written permission and expect the nurse to notify the physician of the request.

Nurses should not discuss the client's condition in public areas. The elevator is one such place in which a casual comment could be overheard by a family member or friend. Additionally nurses should not talk about their clients outside of the hospital or agency.

Example. "A maternity nurse told her teenage daughter that a 17 year old classmate had given birth and planned to give her baby up for adoption. The nurse didn't realize that the teenage mother had been out of school for months to conceal her pregnancy. The teenage mother returned to school to find out that everyone knew of her pregnancy. Tracing the information to the nurse's daughter, she filed a complaint with the hospital. The nurse was fired" (Baer, 1985).

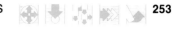

Nurse's Rights

Under this principle of law the nurse has rights and responsibilities as an employee and professional. For example, required testing for AIDS as a condition of employment violates a nurse's privacy and confidentiality and may lead to charges of discrimination. The nurse has a right to a safe working environment according to the Occupational Safety and Health Administration (OSHA) laws. The regulations permit a nurse to refuse to work in proven unsafe conditions. The employer is obligated to provide the nurse with safety equipment (Creighton, 1986 B). The nurse has a responsibility to use the equipment. For example, the nurse is expected to wear gloves when handling blood and body fluids. If the nurse does not utilize gloves when drawing blood and contracts hepatitis, the nurse would not be entitled to compensation from the employer.

Working with inadequate staffing is a controversial issue that affects the nurse's rights and responsibilities. "Prevention of litigation is a simple matter of providing a standard of nursing care equivalent to that which should be available to patients under ordinary circumstances. Extraordinary circumstances do not minimize the obligation to provide safe, professional care. Thus, the fact that there is a nursing shortage and hospital units must be staffed by tired or inexperienced nurses is not a defense. The institution's first legal responsibility is to the provision of safe and adequate care. Should staffing shortages make provision of safe and adequate care questionable, the hospital has an obligation not to offer care" (Fenner, 1988).

Accrediting agencies, such as JCAHO, reinforce the agency's legal obligation to provide appropriate numbers of nurses. "There are sufficient qualified nursing staff members to meet the nursing care needs of patients throughout the hospital" (JCAHO, 1990). When a patient is injured, staffing issues may be a factor in an ensuing lawsuit.

Example. In Leavitt v. St. Tammany Parish Hospital a woman put on her call light and waited at least 15 minutes. When no one responded, she got out of bed and fell. The court decided in her favor, saying that the hospital owed a duty to respond promptly to the client's call for assistance and that it breached its duty by having less than adequate staff available (Cushing, 1988 B).

The nurse has a responsibility to provide care when no other or too few staff are available to provide for the client's safety. No nurse can walk off a unit in these circumstances without being charged with abandoning the clients. "Abandonment is a gross departure from good and accepted nursing practice" (Cushing, 1988 A). However, in times of short staffing, nurses are frequently involved in more subtle challenges to their rights and responsibilities. A nurse may be asked to work two shifts in a row, to float to an unfamiliar area, or to accept assignments which would be legally unsafe. In these circumstances the nurse should:

1. Evaluate the reasons for challenging an assignment—is it unreasonable, unsafe, or a non-nursing responsibility, such as one normally performed by physicians?

Murphy and Connell (1987) studied 100 records of Arizona nurses who had violated the state's nurse practice act and discovered that 60 percent of the nurses had been disciplined for substance abuse and 40 percent for incompetence.

Nurses have also been disciplined or lost their licenses for failure to file tax returns and pay taxes, allowing the daughter of a nurse to pose as a nurse (Creighton, 1986 A), and failing to comply with regulations for nurse midwives. Advanced nursing practice was the basis of a Missouri case on the role of nurse practitioners. An Idaho nurse named Jolene Tuma provided a client with information on alternative cancer therapies and retained her license after the Idaho board sought to remove it for unprofessional conduct. The Idaho court ruled that the nurse practice act was sufficiently vague on what constituted unprofessional conduct (Cushing, 1986).

A Colorado nurse lost her license after being charged with seventeen allegations of failure to administer medication, treatment, and feedings to patients; fourteen allegations of making false or incorrect entries in patients' records regarding the administration of medication, treatment, and feedings; numerous allegations of sleeping on duty; three allegations of removing patients' call bells during the night; two allegations of leaving open the door of the medicine storage room; several allegations of patient abuse, including the forced feeding of one patient and hitting the stumps of two amputees against their bed rails; four allegations of failure to check on patients who were reportedly experiencing difficulties; one allegation of failure to recognize that a patient was not dead and could be resuscitated; numerous allegations of failure to make rounds; and charges of permitting unlicensed nurse's aides to administer medication. When the nurse appealed the revocation of her license, the Colorado Supreme Court upheld the decision (Tammelleo, 1986).

A Nurse's Actions are Judged on the Basis of What a Similarly Educated Reasonable and Prudent Person Would Have Done in a Similar Situation

This fourth principle refers to the concepts that are applied in nursing malpractice cases. In a society that has increasingly turned to the courts for resolution of disputes, standards are needed to judge nursing performance. The number of lawsuits being filed against nurses is increasing, although physicians are sued with greater frequency. According to the American Nurses Association, 6.2 nurses per 10,000 are sued each year. This is in contrast to 1,800 physicians per 10,000 (How Likely is a Lawsuit, 1990). Despite the relatively small number of nurses who are sued each year, nurses need to continue to be concerned with the legal aspects of nursing practice. Lawsuits against nurses are on the increase for a number of reasons:

1. The consumer has become better educated on what to expect from the health care system and nursing care.
2. Plaintiff's attorneys (who represent the client) are becoming more able to identify the case that has merit.

3. Plaintiff's attorneys are likely to name as many people as possible when filing a lawsuit. This allows them to potentially tap the pocket of the hospital and the nurse's insurance companies, as well as the physician's insurance carrier.

4. Plaintiff's lawyers are more aware that nurses are professionals and accountable for their own actions.

5. Many nurses are providing increasingly specialized and complex care that exposes the client and the nurse to greater risk (Godkin et al, 1987).

6. The nursing shortage has had an impact on the quality of nursing care.

The terms negligence and malpractice are often used interchangeably. *Negligence* is a general term referring to a deviation from the standard of care that a reasonably prudent person would use in a particular set of circumstances. *Malpractice* is a specific type of negligence that refers to deviations from a professional standard of care. Nurses, doctors, lawyers, and accountants are some of the types of professionals that may be liable for malpractice (Fiesta, 1988).

Insurance studies show that of all medical malpractice cases filed, half are dropped, one third are settled out of court, and the remainder go to trial. The third that settle out of court represent those cases that the team defending the nurse or physician believes would result in a verdict in favor of the plaintiff. The cases chosen for trial are either the ones that the defense believes it can win, or those that cannot be settled out of court because the plaintiff will not accept the dollar amount offered by the defense. The defense is successful in winning approximately 90 percent of the cases that get into court (Bokelman, 1986), although this varies from state to state. Daniels (1989) studied 1,886 malpractice cases in various geographical areas and found a 68 percent defense success rate.

Under the law each nurse is held accountable for his or her actions. A nurse cannot evade this responsibility by explaining that a physician or nursing supervisor ordered the nurse to commit the actions which injured the client. It is expected that the nurse will use judgment to question the orders that are inappropriate or likely to result in harm to the client.

Student nurses are expected to provide nursing care as would a competent registered nurse. If the nursing student fails to possess or use the degree of knowledge and skill that a registered nurse would have, the student would still be found liable for any harm to a client. While lawsuits against students are rare, the client could sue the student, instructor, facility, physician, and RN staff.

If a jury decides that a nurse is guilty of malpractice the nurse has a legally enforceable responsibility for compensating the client for the harm done. In addition, the state board of nursing may discipline the nurse (Chaney, 1987).

It is now recommended that nurses carry their own malpractice insurance policies in addition to whatever coverage may be provided by their employer. One of the reasons for having personal insurance includes needing coverage for actions outside of the employment setting, such as private duty nursing and giving advice to neighbors.

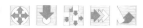

Anatomy of a Lawsuit.   When filing a lawsuit against a nurse, a client must be aware of the statute of limitations. This is a legal time limit that defines how long a suit can be filed after the client discovers an injury has occurred. For example, a client falls out of bed and breaks a hip in a state with a two-year statute of limitations. The suit must be filed within two years of the accident if the client intends to try to collect money from the nurse believed to be negligent. In another example, a client finds out four years after an operation that a clamp has been left inside. This person has up to two years after the discovery of the clamp to file a suit. The statute of limitations is often longer when the injured person is an infant or child.

After a client finds an attorney willing to consider the case the attorney may send the case to an expert witness. A nurse expert witness is someone with specialized clinical skill and knowledge who reviews the material and determines if the suspected negligent nurse violated appropriate standards of care. If the expert witness believes that the case has merit, the attorneys exchange interrogatories, which are a series of fact finding questions designed to provide information about the case.

The defense attorney who represents the nurse may also have the case reviewed by an expert witness. Depending on the expert's opinion, the defense may settle the case or proceed to the next phase. Depositions, which consist of questioning under oath, are taken from the experts and the nurses involved in the case. If the case is not dropped it proceeds to trial, which can occur two or more years after the incident. Figure 10–2 illustrates key concepts related to testifying in a deposition or trial. Figure 10–3 describes some of the strategies used by the plaintiff lawyers to unsettle a nurse.

In order to win the case the plaintiff must prove four elements:

Duty.   The plaintiff must prove that the nurse had a duty to care for the client as part of the nurse-client relationship. This relationship is established as soon as a client comes under the care of an organization by which the nurse is employed and is not difficult to prove in a lawsuit.

Breach of Duty.   A breach of duty occurs when the nurse does not deliver care according to what a similarly educated reasonably prudent nurse would have done under the same circumstances. The breach of duty may result in falls, medication errors, burns, equipment related injuries, complications, deterioration in the client's status, and so on. Standards such as the state nurse practice act or those written by professional organizations are used to evaluate the nurse's actions. Expert witnesses are utilized in most cases to establish the standard of care.

At one time a nurse's practice was evaluated against the standard of care of nurses practicing in the same geographical area. With advances in technology, communication, and transportation, the guideline has become obsolete. A nurse's performance is now evaluated on national trends and practices (Fiesta, 1986).

TESTIFYING TIPS

The following strategies provide guidelines on how to provide oral testimony during a deposition or trial. Although the judge will not be present at the deposition, the testimony in a deposition is given under oath. The transcript may be read at the trial and will be used to point out any discrepancies that may exist.

1. Plan to arrive early. This will give you a built-in time cushion if you get lost.
2. Meet with your attorney before testifying to be sure of what is covered by attorney-client privilege and what, if anything, you do not have to reveal about conversations with your lawyer.
3. On the day of the deposition or trial dress conservatively. Don't chew gum, twirl hair, or act flippant.
4. Listen to the questions being asked. Be sure you know what is being asked.
5. Maintain eye contact with the plaintiff attorney. If you don't, the lawyer may think you have something to hide.
6. Speak loudly enough to be heard so that all can hear. Don't interrupt the attorney before the question is finished. You may have incorrectly anticipated the ending of the question.
7. Display courtesy toward the plaintiff attorney. Hostile remarks can work against you.
8. Keep your answers short. Don't volunteer information.
9. Don't apologize, evade, or ramble.
10. Ask the attorney to repeat unclear questions. Sometimes the lawyer is not sure what he or she is asking.
12. Be comfortable with silence. The plaintiff attorney will use silence to encourage you to elaborate on your answer.
13. Testify only to your first-hand knowledge about an event—what you saw and did. All other information can be construed as hearsay.
14. If your lawyer says, "If you know" after the opposing attorney asks a question, that's a hint. Don't guess or speculate.
15. Listen to your attorney's objections. Think carefully before answering. If your attorney instructs you not to answer a question—DON'T.
16. Watch what you say during a break. If you are seen talking to another witness, when the testimony resumes, the plaintiff attorney may ask what you were discussing. He or she is looking for evidence that you and the other witness are agreeing on a version of the story.
17. Avoid finger pointing. Be careful to not assign blame and make the plaintiff attorney's job easier.
18. Watch your nonverbal body language. Don't fidget, look off into space, put your hand in front of your mouth, cross your arms over your chest, or act nervous when certain questions are asked. Some lawyers videotape depositions to study nonverbal body language for clues.
19. Beware of the two-part question. If you answer "yes" or "no," be sure that it is clear which part of the question you are answering.
20. Avoid humor or sarcasm. Off-the-cuff remarks may create a negative impression on the jury.
21. If the attorney repeats or rephrases your answer, be sure that it is accurate and not distorted.
22. Don't change your story to go along with the testimony of another witness. Never go along with someone else's version of the events just to keep peace. This will be construed as misrepresentation or cover-up and will destroy your credibility.
23. Avoid looking at your attorney when you are being asked questions by the plaintiff attorney. Glancing at your attorney will be interpreted that you need help in answering sensitive questions. If the question is improper your attorney will object.
24. Use your own words. Avoid inserting "lawyerese" into your responses that would indicate that you have been coached on what to say.
25. Avoid memorizing your testimony. You can refer to the medical record and incident report during the deposition.
26. After a deposition, do not discuss your testimony with other employees. The plaintiff attorney will bring this out at trial to indicate that you have all agreed on what to say.

From Iyer P, Surviving a Malpractice Suit (audiotape) Patricia Iyer Associates, P.O. Box 231, Stockton NJ 08559, 1990.

FIGURE 10–2. Surviving a deposition. (Reprinted with permission of Patricia Iyer Associates. Copyright 1990.)

1. **Flattery**—The lawyer acts very impressed with your education and experience and then lays the trap: "With all your knowledge you should have known better."

2. **Ignorance**—The lawyer deliberately mispronounces medical terms. This is designed to provoke you to educate the attorney and volunteer information. Remember that the lawyer is thoroughly versed in the subject.

3. **Leading questions**—are used to control your flow of responses and obtain a series of favorable answers. Listen to questions carefully and elaborate on your "yes" or "no" answer as needed.

4. **Use of records**—Misspellings and grammatical errors are used to embarrass you. The attorney may imply that records are inaccurate because they were not recorded on the spot. Insist that your notes are recorded as soon as possible after care, but that patient care comes first.

5. **Jumping around**—Questions are asked in no apparent order so that you won't see the traps the lawyer is trying to lay. If possible, keep track of what has been asked and try to answer each question honestly.

6. **Oh, by the way**—The last question may be a zinger. It is carefully planned to make a telling point when you are off guard, thinking your testimony is over. Don't relax until the lawyer says, "no more questions."

From Iyer P: Surviving a Malpractice Suit (audiotape) Patricia Iyer Associates, P.O. Box 231, Stockton, NJ 08559, 1990.

FIGURE 10–3. Strategies used by plaintiff attorneys. (Reprinted with permission of Patricia Iyer Associates. Copyright 1990.)

Causation.   Causation, also referred to as proximate cause, means that the plaintiff must prove that the nurse's actions actually resulted in the injury. Because there are so many factors involved this is the most difficult element to prove. In the following case the plaintiff was not able to establish proximate cause:

The nurse, in violation of the physician's orders that a postoperative abdominal surgery client should not be fed, gave the client solid food. A second operation eight days after the initial one showed the client's condition was worsening. When the client attempted to sue, there was no evidence that the feeding had made the client's condition worsen and the nurse was not held liable (Northrop and Kelly, 1987).

Damages.   The last element that the plaintiff must prove is that actual physical or emotional damages were proximately caused by the nurse's negligent actions. When the jury decides that more than one health care professional has been negligent the damages will be divided between them. A sum of money is awarded to compensate for pain, suffering, lost income, and medical bills.

Examples of Law Suits Based on the Nursing Process

Nurses are sued for malpractice because they omit one or more of the steps of the nursing process. Cases presented below illustrate how nursing actions or omissions resulted in injury to the client.

Assessment.   Angela Wickliffe was a 13 year old girl who underwent surgery on her spine. During her stay in the postanesthesia care unit she received narcotics. She was returned to the nursing unit at 11:20 AM. While Angela's nurse was at lunch, a nurse's aide checked her vital signs once—at 11:30 AM. Angela's vital signs were not checked again. She was found dead at 12:40 PM. Although she was revived she died of brain damage 12 days later. During the trial the girl's attorney pointed out that the lack of assessment for one hour was in contradiction to the hospital policy that a postop client be monitored every 15 minutes during the first hour after return to the unit. National standards also dictated that Angela should have received closer monitoring (Fiesta, 1986).

Diagnosis.   In Morreale v. Downing a critical care nurse was held to be negligent for failing to discover a hip fracture in a 13 year old boy. The boy had been in a motor vehicle accident and was hospitalized in ICU for three weeks. The nurses failed to note his impaired physical mobility when he improved to the point that he was able to walk. His mother noted a discrepancy in the length of one leg. The physician ordered an x-ray which showed a hip fracture. The nurses were held liable because they gave the boy frequent care and had ample opportunity to observe him walking and to notify the physician of unusual findings (Cushing, 1987 C).

Planning.   A 28 year old woman had a cardiac arrest in the operating room following ovarian surgery. Severe loss of oxygen to her brain resulted in permanent paralysis. At the time of the arrest, only the anesthesiologist and a scrub technician were present, despite the requirement that an RN stay with the client during this critical postop period. The surgeon had demanded that the nurse leave the room to assist in beginning another case.

The nurse should have planned a better solution to the request that she leave the client's side. The plaintiff's expert witness testified that cardiac arrest should be anticipated and planned for at any time. Short of an emergency, it was inappropriate for the surgeon to request the nurse to leave the client while in the operating room (Northrop, 1987).

Implementation.   A Kansas hospital was held liable for 55 percent of the damages of $400,000 when a three month old baby was burned by a heating pad. Before surgery the anesthesiologist asked for a heating device to prevent hypothermia during surgery. The hospital did not have a thermostatically controlled blanket and the OR nurse instead used an ordinary heating pad. The baby began to cry as soon as he was placed on the pad, which had been turned on high for one half hour before the operation, and then adjusted to the low heat position. At home the mother discovered deep burns across the baby's buttocks when she changed his diaper. The baby was readmitted with second and third degree burns and required skin grafting (Cushing, 1987 B).

Evaluation.   A New Jersey nursing home's failure to identify a weak client as a smoker requiring monitoring ultimately resulted in his death. The client

had suffered a stroke which significantly deprived him of the use of his arms and he had severe vision impairment. The nursing home's regulations required that upon admission every smoking client be described as a responsible smoker who could smoke in designated areas, or as a nonresponsible smoker who would require one to one monitoring while smoking. The regulations further provided that a client was required to be re-evaluated periodically or upon an apparent change in status.

The plaintiff's nursing home expert witness contended that irrespective of the question of whether the decedent was properly classified as a responsible smoker upon admission, the fact that he exhibited instances of apnea, falling asleep after breakfast, falling asleep with the thermometer in his mouth, and falling from his wheelchair shortly after admission, it would indicate that he should have been reclassified as a nonresponsible smoker.

The plaintiff was in the dining area with an attendant who was assisting another client. The attendant suddenly observed that the client's clothing had ignited and she observed a cigarette and lighter still in his lap. The plaintiff suffered second- and third-degree burns in the left side of his chest and his hand. He died from heart failure and shock which resulted from being placed in a cold shower (Zarin, 1987).

ETHICAL FOUNDATIONS OF NURSING PRACTICE

Ethical content is included in the nursing curriculum to assist the nurse to:

- examine commitments and values in relation to the care of clients
- engage in ethical reflection
- develop skill in moral reasoning and judgment
- develop the ability to use ethics for decision-making (Fry, 1989).

Definitions

Ethical decision-making is based on an understanding of morals and ethics. *Morals* are the beliefs which are instilled in us by our parents and society as a whole. They include our sense of what is right and wrong. For example, we learn that it is wrong to kill, steal, or tell lies. This set of beliefs forms codes of behavior based on cultural expectations.

The term *ethics* is used to describe a broader aspect of morals. Ethical thinking begins when a person goes beyond the acceptance of the rules of the social group and moves into the realm of thinking and analyzing morals (Fowler and Levine-Ariff, 1987). Nursing ethics concerns itself with a standard of behavior which reflects the profession's desire to protect or ensure the well-being of its clients (Fenner, 1980).

According to Fry (1989) the characteristics of an ethical dilemma include:

1. A conflict between human needs or the welfare of others and a need for the nurse to choose between them

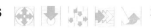

2. A choice to be made guided by moral principles

3. A choice guided by the process of weighing reasons and assigning priorities to competing values

4. A choice affected by personal feelings and values and the context of the situation.

The following are examples of ethical dilemmas that may affect nurses:

1. Abortion
2. Termination of life sustaining treatment
3. "Blowing the whistle," or exposing illegal and unethical behavior
4. Mistreatment of disabled children or retarded clients
5. Treatment decisions involving dying clients
6. Equal access to health care for all
7. Allocation of scarce health care resources which requires a decision to deny health care to a needy client (such as a kidney transplant)
8. Protecting confidentiality of client information
9. Providing treatment that conflicts with a nurse's ethical principles.

There is a difference between legal and ethical responsibilities. As described earlier in the chapter, nurses have legal responsibilities as professionals. These are defined in the nurse practice act and in other standards set by a variety of agencies. Ethical responsibilities result from the relationship which the nurse forms with the client, the employer, and other health care professionals. These ethical duties may be identical to legal responsibilities but may also oblige the nurse to perform actions beyond what the law requires. For example, the American Nurses' Association states that it is unethical for the nurse to participate in the act of killing a prisoner to fulfill a death sentence, even though the execution is legal. Table 10–1 illustrates how legal and ethical issues can be in conflict.

TABLE 10–1. EXAMPLES OF ETHICAL AND LEGAL DILEMMAS

Ethical and legal: A nurse refuses to follow a physician's order because to obey would clearly violate the nurse's ethical responsibility to the client and the nurse practice act for that state.

Ethical and illegal: A nurse informs the sexual partners of a client with AIDS of his condition without his consent after his own refusal to do so or to alter his sexual behavior, thus violating his right to privacy.

Unethical and legal: A nurse initiates CPR on a terminally ill client. The physician has not written a "do not resuscitate" order. The nurse believes that the patient would not have wanted to be resuscitated at the time of death.

Unethical and illegal: A nurse participates in the unnecessary medication of an elderly nursing home resident to make the resident less troublesome and more compliant.

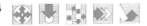

Sources of Ethics

Ethical duties are often not defined in legal statutes. The American Nurses' Association's Code for Nurses (Fig. 10–4), Standards of Nursing Practice, the Social Policy Statement, and the International Code of Nursing Ethics define the responsibilities of nurses to clients, society, and to the nursing profession. In addition, the American Nurses' Association and other specialty nursing organizations, such as the American Association of Critical Care Nurses, periodically issue statements to guide the ethical behavior of nurses. One such publication is the American Nurses' Association's statement of guidelines for withdrawing or withholding food and fluid (Ethics in Nursing, 1988).

The Code for Nurses had its beginnings as early as 1897 in the first constitution of the Nurses' Associated Alumnae, which was the forerunner of the American Nurses' Association. Over the next 88 years, the Code for Nurses was refined to its present format. In 1984 the ANA published explanations of each of the 11 points in the Code (A Code for Nurses with Interpretive Statements, 1985). The consequences of failing to follow the Code may include disciplinary action and expulsion from the ANA, as well as legal action taken against the nurse. An example of a violation of the Code was reported in 1978. Nurses were being paid by antiabortion groups for the names of women who had abortions. Members of these right to life groups then proceeded to harass the women with

---

AMERICAN NURSES' ASSOCIATION CODE FOR NURSES

1. The nurse provides services with respect for human dignity and the uniqueness of the client unrestricted by considerations of social or economic status, personal attributes, or the nature of health problems.
2. The nurse safeguards the client's right to privacy by judiciously protecting information of a confidential nature.
3. The nurse acts to safeguard the client and the public when health care and safety are affected by incompetent, unethical, or illegal practice of any person.
4. The nurse assumes responsibility and accountability for individual nursing judgments and actions.
5. The nurse maintains competence in nursing.
6. The nurse exercises informed judgment and uses individual competence and qualifications as criteria in seeking consultation, accepting responsibilities, and delegating nursing activities to others.
7. The nurse participates in activities that contribute to the ongoing development of the profession's body of knowledge.
8. The nurse participates in the profession's efforts to implement and improve standards of nursing.
9. The nurse participates in the profession's efforts to establish and maintain conditions of employment conducive to high quality nursing care.
10. The nurse participates in the profession's effort to protect the public from misinformation and misrepresentation and to maintain the integrity of nursing.
11. The nurse collaborates with members of the health professions and other citizens in promoting community and national efforts to meet the health needs of the public.

FIGURE 10–4. American Nurses' Association Code for Nurses.

abusive phone calls when they returned home from the hospital. The nurses involved in this activity violated the second point in the Code which states that the nurse safeguards the client's rights to privacy by "judiciously protecting information of a confidential nature" (Benjamin and Curtis, 1986).

Ethical Theories

The nurse is often placed in the role of client advocate in order to protect the rights of clients. While it is important for the nurse to understand the points contained in the Code for Nurses, the nurse needs more substance in order to make ethical decisions. Ethical theories describe approaches for resolving dilemmas commonly faced by nurses. "Philosophers, beginning with Socrates, Plato, and Aristotle, have for centuries attempted to answer two major questions of ethics: What is the meaning of right and of good? What ought I to do?" (Davis, 1983). Ethical theories help answer these questions.

There are two major ethical theories used to help nurses resolve health care dilemmas: deontology and utilitarianism. The *deontologic* approach states that the rightness or wrongness of actions is determined by how the interventions conform to a rule. For instance, breaking a promise to a client would be considered wrong. Deontologists use rules because they are right, irrespective of the consequences they may produce in a particular situation. This position requires the nurse to be committed to the principle of universalizability. When the nurse makes a moral judgment in one given situation, the nurse will make the same judgment in any similar situation regardless of time, place, and persons involved (Davis, 1983).

One of the flaws with this approach is that most situations have extenuating circumstances. For example, in some instances it would be better to break than to keep a promise (Fowler and Levine-Ariff, 1987). A nurse may be asked to keep a promise not to reveal that the client has brought a quart of whiskey to the hospital. After making the promise, the nurse realizes that it is better to break the promise to protect the client from the consequences of consuming alcohol while being treated in the hospital.

The *utilitarian* approach states that actions are right or wrong on the basis of the consequences of the actions. This philosophy defines "good as happiness or pleasure and right as maximizing the greatest good and least amount of harm for the greatest number of persons. This position assumes that one can weigh and measure harm and benefit and come out with the greatest possible balance of good over evil for most people" (Davis, 1983).

Utilitarians focus on the results of actions rather than on their motivations. According to this approach, the nurse would weigh the consequences of telling the truth. Other factors may take priority, such as the nurse's own survival or the continuation of the system for the benefit of future clients. In this case the nurse may not tell the truth in preference to other interests that promote greater happiness. This view is quite different from the deontologic position, which would maintain that the nurse must tell the truth without exception (Ethical Dilemmas Confronting Nurses, 1985).

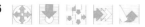

The utilitarian position is often referred to when making decisions in managing scarce health care resources.

Example.   An intensive care unit may have only one empty bed. A young father who is supporting his elderly parents and three young children is in the emergency department with chest pain. Next to him is an elderly man who lives alone and needs treatment for diabetic coma. The utilitarian position would maintain that the bed should go to the young father since it would provide the greatest good for the greatest number of people.

Critics of the utilitarian approach question "whether this position involves the total happiness for a few or the average happiness for all. A crucial question is whether or not what one does in a particular situation contributes to the greatest general good or the least amount of harm for everyone. But how can everyone's welfare really be considered? Others accuse the utilitarian of ignoring the personal nature of good, e.g., truth telling and promise keeping" (Davis, 1983).

Other philosophers have offered alternatives to deontologic and utilitarian positions. These include Franken's Theory of Obligation, Firth's Ideal Observer Theory, and Justice as Fairness by Rawls. The newer positions incorporate components of utilitarian and deontologic thinking. Nurses interested in learning more about these positions are referred to the bibliography at the end of this chapter.

Ethical Dilemmas

Nurses encounter a variety of ethical dilemmas in health care. Cassells and Redman (1989) reported on a sample of 742 nurses who described the types of ethical dilemmas they had experienced in clinical practice within a year of graduation. The most common ethical issues they had faced included the following:

1.   Issues of informed consent by clients prior to surgical procedures and hazardous tests or treatments
2.   Issues specific to initiating resuscitation when the client experienced sudden unexpected death
3.   Issues related to discontinuing life-saving treatment
4.   Moral dilemmas in caring for clients with a poor prognosis or terminal illness
5.   Evaluation of the client's level of competency to make own decisions
6.   Clients refusing treatment
7.   Issues specific to withholding information from clients
8.   Allocation of scarce resources.

Ethical Decision-Making

The steps in ethical decision-making can be compared to the nursing process.

Assessment

The nurse begins by gathering all relevant data. This includes important information on the circumstances surrounding the dilemma, the rights and duties of the individuals involved, and the factors that could influence the decision-making process such as ethical and legal dictates.

Diagnosis

Next, the ethical components of the dilemma are identified. Some of the typical conflicts involve truth telling versus withholding the truth, treating or letting die, alleviation of pain versus the preservation of life, freedom versus authority, and conflicts of rights (Curtin, 1978).

Planning

Identification of the possible solutions and selection of the best approach occurs next. The potential solutions are explored in relation to the roles of each of the individuals involved. The applicability of the ethical theories would be explored here. The phase is completed by identifying the strategies needed to implement the solution.

Implementation

Once the most acceptable solution is selected, the nurse takes action to resolve the dilemma.

Evaluation

In this final phase the nurse examines the consequences of the actions taken on behalf of the client. The results may be compared with previous experiences in similar situations.

Example of Ethical Decision-Making

During the last several years HIV infections have dramatically increased in number and given rise to a host of legal and ethical questions. Many legal concerns have arisen regarding employment practices and discrimination based on having AIDS or a positive HIV blood test. One of the ethical questions centers on the role of the nurse and physician in informing others about a client's diagnosis.

In a situation described in a recent article (Laufman, 1989), a nurse was assigned to be a case manager for a 32 year old homosexual man who had developed AIDS. (See Chapter 8 for a discussion of case management.) The client had been sexually active for only the past four years and had few partners. His family was unaware of his homosexuality and his diagnosis until a week before he died.

The client, Jose, told the nurse that he had intended to tell his family the truth about his diagnosis when his illness worsened. He expected his family to react negatively and was concerned that the nurse keep the matter confidential.

When his condition deteriorated Jose told his brother about his disease, his lifestyle, and his poor prognosis.

Jose's brother was shocked and demanded to know why the nurse had not told him about Jose's disease. The nurse explained that she could not have done so without the client's consent. Jose's brother said he and his family felt they had a right to know so that they could protect themselves from infection.

Did the client's right to confidentiality supersede the right of the family to prepare for Jose's death and to protect themselves from what they saw as the risk of AIDS?

Assessment

Information about the circumstances:

The client was living at home with his mother, brother, and two cousins. He was his mother's primary source of economic and emotional support since his father's death several years earlier. The nurse provided doses of an experimental drug to treat his eye problem. The *brother was given information about the medications Jose was receiving* but did not display curiosity or ask detailed questions about Jose's illness.

Rights and responsibilities:

Jose.   According to the Patient's Bill of Rights, *Jose had a right to considerate and respectful care.* Additionally, *he had the right to receive complete information about his condition.* The physician had told him he would probably live about two more years. Finally, *he had a right to expect that confidentiality of health information would be maintained.*

The Nurse.   The Code for Nurses specifies that *the nurse had an ethical obligation to safeguard the client's right to privacy* by protecting confidential information.

Example.   A nurse in New York was involved in a case related to protecting information about a positive AIDS blood test. A pharmacist tested positive for AIDS and was told that the results were confidential and would be kept separate from other records. The nurse from the hospital's infectious disease clinic recognized him when he was having a pre-employment physical. When the nurse told the doctor about the pharmacist's positive AIDS test, the physician decided not to recommend that the pharmacist be employed at the medical center. The pharmacist was denied the job and sued the medical center for illegal discrimination and violating the clinic's confidentiality requirement. Although the nurse was not named in the lawsuit, she could have been sued for breach of confidentiality and violation of privacy (Northrop, 1988). In Jose's case the nurse protected the confidentiality of the information concerning Jose's AIDS.

The Physician.   The position of the physician is more complex with respect to the client with AIDS. On one hand the physician is expected to maintain confidentiality of information. *"Disclosure of confidential information by a physician*

constitutes an invasion of the patient's right to privacy'' (Hirsh, 1989). However, the Tarasoff v. The Regents of California case has set a legal precedent that *the physician has a duty to warn people at risk*. In this case a psychologist was treating a client who provided the name of a former girlfriend he was intending to kill. The man carried out his threat and murdered the woman (Ms. Tarasoff). The psychologist, who protected the client's right to privacy by not sharing this information, was held liable for not warning the woman that his client intended to kill her. The court said, ''If the exercise of reasonable care to protect the threatened victim requires the therapist to warn the endangered party or those who can reasonably be expected to notify her, we see no sufficient societal interest that would protect and justify concealment. The containment of such risks lies in the public interest'' (131 California Reporter, 1976).

The American Medical Association has taken a position that *the physician should attempt to persuade the individual with AIDS to stop endangering the sexual or intravenous contacts, to notify authorities if persuasion fails, and if the authorities take no action, to notify and counsel the endangered third parties* (Closen and Issacman, 1989). However, with respect to Jose's situation, the legal precedents and advice relate to sexual and needle-sharing contacts, not to family members who are at very low risk for infection.

Factors that could influence the decision-making process:

The ethical responsibilities of the nurse and physician have been identified. Legal dictates of the state of California, where Jose lived, need to be considered. The California Health and Safety Code prohibits the willful or negligent disclosure of HIV results to any third party unless a written authorization is signed by the client. However, another statute grants immunity from civil or criminal liability to physicians who wish to warn a spouse that his or her partner has tested positive for HIV (Martello, 1989). The California laws do not require disclosure to family members other than a spouse.

Diagnosis

The ethical dilemma described in Jose's situation involves truth telling versus withholding of the truth. In this case the factors which were being balanced included the client's right to privacy versus the family's right to information.

Planning

In this phase the nurse considered the ethical theories in relation to the dilemma she experienced. The utilitarian position, which emphasizes the greatest good for the greatest number, was rejected. The nurse believed that informing the family of the diagnosis would not be in the client's best interests since they were not at high risk for infection. Rather, the nurse took the deontologic position that the decision to maintain confidentiality was right, irrespective of the consequences. Other alternatives which she rejected included refusing to care for Jose, which was inconsistent with her responsibilities as a nurse. If Jose had been irresponsible, she could have forced Jose to tell his family. Finally, she could have told the family herself but did not because this disclosure would have been illegal in California and unethical.

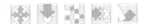

Implementation

The nurse resolved the dilemma by protecting Jose's rights and his autonomy. She provided the family with the information they needed to avoid exposure to his blood and body fluids and made sure they followed infection control procedures.

Evaluation

The greatest harm Jose could imagine was having his family relationships jeopardized by their reaction to his diagnosis and sexual orientation. When his brother learned the truth of his illness, he refused to let Jose's friends visit him in the hospital. Jose died a week later. The nurse has not had further contact with the family following Jose's death and cannot comment on the after effects of the nondisclosure on them.

Commentary

This example illustrates the complex factors which may need to be considered in resolving an ethical dilemma. Jose's case dealt with a nurse who assisted a client to keep information from family members. Another difficult aspect of the case, which the nurse did not comment on, involves the sharing of information with Jose's sexual partners. One is left with unanswered questions about what they knew about Jose's condition.

SUMMARY

Legal aspects of nursing are guided by the four principles defined above. The nurse must maintain awareness of changes in practice to ensure that the client's and the nurse's rights are protected. Ethical issues pervade many aspects of nursing practice. The effective resolution of these dilemmas rests on a foundation of knowledge concerning professional behavior and ethical theories, skill in using the nursing process, and a willingness to take risks.

REFERENCES

American Nurses' Association: Code for Nurses with Interpretive Statements. Kansas City, MO: American Nurses' Association, 1985.

American Nurses' Association: Ethical Dilemmas Confronting Nurses. Kansas City, MO: American Nurses' Association, 1985.

American Nurses' Association: Ethics in Nursing. Kansas City, MO: American Nurses' Association, 1988.

131 California Reporter 14, 27–28 (California 1976).

Baer O: Protecting your patient's privacy. Nursing Life 1985 May/June; 5:51–53.

Benjamin M, and Curtis J: Ethics in Nursing. New York: Oxford University Press, 1986.

Bokelman R: Defining the Meritorious Medical Malpractice Action in *Effective Utilization of Expert Witnesses*. Sherman Oaks, CA: Medi/Legal Institute, 1986.

Cassells J, and Redman B: Preparing students to be moral agents in clinical nursing practice. Nursing Clinics of North America 1989 Jun; 24(2):463–473.

Cazales M: Nursing and the Law. Germantown, MD: Aspen, 1978.

Champagne M, Havens B, and Swenson J: State board criteria for licensure and disciplinary procedure regarding impaired nurses. Nursing Outlook 1987; 35(2):54–57, 101.

Chaney E: Personal and vicarious liability. Journal of Pediatric Nursing 1987; 2(2):132–143.

Closen M, and Issacman S: Notifying private third parties at risk for HIV infection. TRIAL 1989 May; 50–55.

Creighton H: Legal aspects of AIDS, Part II. Nursing Management 1986 Dec; 17(12):14–16.

Creighton H: Licensure problems. Nursing Management 1986 Feb; 17(2):16, 18.

Curtin L: A proposed model for critical ethical analysis. Nursing Forum XVII 1978; 17(1):13–17.

Cushing M: Accepting or rejecting an assignment. American Journal of Nursing 1988 Nov; 88(11):1470, 1475–1476.

Cushing M: How courts look at nurse practice acts. American Journal of Nursing 1986 Feb; 86(2):131–132.

Cushing M: Keeping watch. American Journal of Nursing 1987 Aug; 87(8):1021–1022.

Cushing M: Million dollar errors. American Journal of Nursing 1987 Apr; 87(4):435–436, 440.

Cushing M: Refusing an unreasonable assignment. American Journal of Nursing 1988 Dec; 88(12):1635–1637.

Cushing M: Short staffing on trial. American Journal of Nursing 1988 Feb; 88(2):161–162.

Daniels S: Verdicts in medical malpractice cases. TRIAL 1989 May; 23–30.

Davis S: Ethical dilemmas and nursing practice. East Norwalk, CT: Appleton-Century-Crofts, 1983.

Fenner K: Ethics and the Law in Nursing. New York: Van Nostrand, 1980.

Fenner K: Nursing shortage: harbinger of increased litigation. Nursing Management 1988 Nov; 19(11):44–45.

Fiesta J: The nursing shortage: Whose liability problem? Part 1, Nursing Management January 1990, 24–25.

Fiesta J: The nursing shortage: Whose liability problem? Part 2, Nursing Management February 1990, 23–24.

Fiesta J: Look beyond your state for your standards of care. Nursing 1986 Aug; 16(8):41.

Fiesta J: The law and liability, Second edition. New York: John Wiley & Sons, 1988.

Fowler M, and Levine-Ariff J: Ethics at the Bedside. Philadelphia: JB Lippincott, 1987.

Fry S: Teaching Ethics in Nursing Curricula. Nursing Clinics of North America 1989 Jun; 24(2):485–497.

Godkin L, Wooten B, and Godkin J: The jury decides: are registered nurses legally liable for their job-related actions? Nursing Management 1987 May; 18(5):73–74, 76, 79.

Hirsh H: Hear all, see all, tell very, very little. Legal Aspects of Medical Practice, March 1989, 7–9.

How likely is a lawsuit? American Journal of Nursing, January 1990, 42.

Joint Commission Accreditation on Healthcare Organizations: Nursing Care Scoring Guidelines (Intents and Score 1s) for the 1991 Accreditation Manual for Hospitals. July/August 1990 Joint Commission Perspectives Insert, B1–B46.

Laufman J: AIDS, Ethics and the truth. American Journal of Nursing 1989 Jul; 89(7):924–930.

Markowitz L: How your state board works for you. Nursing Life 1982 May/Jun; 2:25–32.

Martello J: Can you keep a secret? AIDS: Confidentiality versus disclosure. Legal Aspects of Medical Practice, February 1989, 7–9.

Murphy J, and Connell C: Violations of the state's nurse practice act: How big is the problem? Nursing Management 1987 Sep; 18(9):44–46, 48.

Northrop C: Rights versus regulation: confidentiality in the age of AIDS. Nursing Outlook 1988 Jul–Aug; 36(4):208.

Northrop C, and Kelly M: Legal Issues in Nursing. St. Louis: CV Mosby, 1987.

Rosenfield A: A patient's bill of rights. Legal Aspects of Medical Practice, November 1988, 3–5.

Satisfaction Data: Patient perception is reality. Hospitals, July 5, 1989, 40.

Swenson J, Havens B, and Champagne M: Interpretations of state board criteria and disciplinary procedures regarding impaired nurses. Nursing Outlook 1987; 35(3):108–110, 145.

Swenson J, Havens B, and Champagne M: State board members' perceptions of impaired nurses. Nurses Outlook 1987; 35(4):154–155.

Swenson J, Havens B, and Champagne M: State boards and impaired nurses. Nursing Outlook 1989; 37(2):94–96.

Tammelleo D: The nurse practice act and deplorable nursing care. The Regan Report on Nursing Law, August 1, 1986.

The Joint Commission 1990 Accreditation Manual for Hospitals. Chicago: Joint Commission Accreditation on Healthcare Organizations, 1989.

Zarin I: $310,000 verdict, New Jersey Jury Verdict Review and Analysis, June 15–29, 1987, p. 4.

BIBLIOGRAPHY

American Nurses' Association: Social Policy Statement. Kansas City, MO: American Nurses' Association, 1982.

American Nurses' Association: Standards of Nursing Practice. Kansas City, MO: American Nurses' Association, 1973.

American Nurses' Association: Withdrawing or withholding food and fluid. American Journal of Nursing 1988 Jun; 8(6):797–798.

Bellocq J: Protecting your license. Journal of Professional Nursing 1989 Jan/Feb; 5(1):8.

Bishop A, and Scudder J: Nursing ethics in an age of controversy. Advances in Nursing Science 1987 Apr; 9(3):34–43.

Brooke P: Shopping for liability insurance. American Journal of Nursing 1989 Feb; 89(2):171–172.

Bushy A, Rauh R, and Matt B: Ethical principles: Application to an obstetric case. JOGNN 1989 May/Jun; 18(3):207–212.

Creighton H: Legal aspects of AIDS, part I. Nursing Management 1986 Nov; 17(11):14–16.

Creighton H: Legal implications of the impaired nurse, part I. Nursing Management 1988 Jan; 19(1):21–23.

Creighton H: Legal implications of the impaired nurse, part II. Nursing Management 1988 Feb; 19(2):20–21.

Curtin L, and Flaherty J: Nursing Ethics: Theories and Pragmatics. Bowie, MD: Brady, 1982.

Erickson I, and Mitchell C: Dilemmas in practice: which child gets the transplant? American Journal of Nursing 1988 Mar; 88(3):287–288.

Ethical Issues in Nursing and Nursing Education. New York: National League for Nursing, 1980.

Feutz S: Nursing and the Law, Third Edition. Eau Claire, WI: Professional Education Systems, 1989.

Frisch N: Value analysis: a method for teaching nursing ethics and promoting the moral development of students. Journal of Nursing Education 1987 Oct; 26(8):328–332.

Fry S: Toward a theory of nursing ethics. Advances in Nursing Science 1989; 11(4):9–22.

Gaul A: Ethics content in baccalaureate degree curricula. Nursing Clinics of North America 1989 Jun; 24(2):475–483.

International Council of Nurses: International Code for Nursing Ethics. In Beauchamp T, and Walters L (eds): Contemporary Issues in Bioethics. Encino, CA: Dickenson Publications, 1978.

Iyer P, and Camp N: Nursing documentation: A nursing process approach. St. Louis: Mosby. Mosby Year Book 1991.

Lind A, and Wilburn S: Power-from-within: Feminism and the ethical decision-making process in nursing. Nursing Administration Quarterly 1986 Spring; 10(3):50–57.

Munhall P: Moral development: A prerequisite. Journal of Nursing Education 1982 Jun; 21(6):11–15.

Neumann T: A nurse's guide to fail safe delegating. Nursing 1989 Sept; 19(9):63–64.

Northrop C: Legal content in the nursing curriculum: what students need and how to provide it. Nursing Outlook 1989; 34(4):200.

Nurses Associated Alumnae of the US and Canada, Constitution, 1897.

Quinley K: Twelve tips for defending yourself in a malpractice suit. American Journal of Nursing 1990 Jan; 90(1):37–40.

Ross J, and Pugh D: Limited cardiopulmonary resuscitation: The ethics of partial codes. QRB January 1988, 14(1):4–8.

Smith S, and Davis A: Ethical dilemmas: conflicts among rights, duties and obligations. American Journal of Nursing 1980 Aug; 80(8):1463–1466.

Steele S: Values Clarification in Nursing. East Norwalk, CT: Appleton-Century-Crofts, 1983.

Tammelleo D: Nurse refuses to 'float': sunk. The Regan Report on Nursing Law, December 1, 1986.

Thompson J, and Thompson H: Teaching ethics to nursing students. Nursing Outlook 1989; 37(2):84–88.

Twomey J: Analysis of the claim to distinct nursing ethics: normative and nonnormative approaches. Advances in Nursing Science 1989; 11(3):25–32.

Viens D: A history of nursing's code of ethics. Nursing Outlook 1989; 37(1):45–49.

Whiteneck M: Integrating ethics with quality assurance in long term care. QRB 1988 May; 14(5):138–143.

APPENDICES

A Head-To-Toe Assessment Criteria

General Appearance
- [ ] *Observations*—age, race, nutritional status, general health status, development
- [ ] *Color*—pink, pale, red, jaundiced, mottled, blanched, cyanotic
- [ ] *Skin*—pigmentation, vascularity, temperature, texture, turgor, lesions (type, color, size, shape, distribution), bruises, bleeding, scars, edema

Vital Signs
- [ ] Temperature
- [ ] *Pulses*—apical, radial (others when appropriate)
- [ ] Respirations
- [ ] *Blood pressure*—supine, sitting, right and left arms
- [ ] Height and weight

Head and Face
- [ ] Size, contour, symmetry, color, pain, tenderness, lesions, edema
- [ ] *Scalp*—color, texture, scales, lumps, lesions, inflammation
- [ ] *Face*—movement, expression, pigmentation, acne, tics, tremors, scars

Eyes
- [ ] *Acuity*—visual loss, glasses, contacts, prosthesis, diplopia, photophobia, color vision, pain, burning
- [ ] *Eyelids*—color, ptosis, edema, styes, exophthalmos
- [ ] *Extraocular movement*—position and alignment of eyes, strabismus, nystagmus
- [ ] *Conjunctiva*—color, discharge, vascular changes
- [ ] *Iris*—color, markings
- [ ] *Sclera*—color, vascularity, jaundice
- [ ] *Pupils*—size, shape, equality, reaction to light

Ears
- [ ] *Acuity*—hearing loss, aid, pain, tinnitus, sensitivity to sound
- [ ] *External ear*—lobe, auricle, canal
- [ ] *Inner ear*—vertigo

Nose
- [ ] Smell, nasal size, symmetry, flaring, sneezing, deformities
- [ ] *Mucosa*—color, edema, exudate, bleeding, furuncles, pain, tenderness
- [ ] Sinus tenderness, pain

Mouth and Throat
- [ ] Odor, pain, ability to speak, bite, chew, swallow, taste
- [ ] *Lips*—color, symmetry, hydration, lesions, crusting, fever blisters, cracking, swelling, numbness, drooling
- [ ] *Gums*—color, edema, bleeding, retraction, pain
- [ ] *Teeth*—number, missing, caries, caps, dentures, sensitivity to heat, cold
- [ ] *Tongue*—symmetry, color, size, hydration, markings, protrusion, ulcers, burning, swelling, coating
- [ ] *Throat*—gag reflex, soreness, cough, sputum, hemoptysis
- [ ] *Voice*—hoarseness, loss, change in pitch

Neck

☐ Symmetry, movement, range of motion, masses, scars, pain, stiffness
☐ *Trachea*—deviation, scars
☐ *Thyroid*—size, shape, symmetry, tenderness, enlargement, nodules, scars
☐ *Vessels* (carotid, jugular)—quality, strength, and symmetry of pulsations, bruits, venous distention
☐ *Lymph nodes*—size, shape, mobility, tenderness, enlargement

Chest

☐ Size, shape, symmetry, deformities, pain, tenderness
☐ *Skin*—color, rashes, scars, hair distribution, turgor, temperature, edema, crepitation
☐ *Breasts*—contour, symmetry, color, size, shape, inflammation, scars, masses (location, size, shape, mobility, tenderness), pain, dimpling, swelling
☐ *Nipples*—color, discharge, ulceration, bleeding, inversion, pain
☐ *Axillae*—nodes, enlargement, tenderness, rash, inflammation

Lungs

☐ *Breathing patterns*—rate, regularity, depth, ease, normal or adventitious, fremitus, use of accessory muscles
☐ *Sounds*—normal, adventitious, intensity, pitch, quality, duration, equality, vocal resonance

Heart

☐ *Cardiac patterns*—rate, rhythm, intensity, regularity, skipped or extra beats, point of maximum impulse
☐ Right and left cardiac borders, implanted pacemaker

Abdomen

☐ Size, color, contour, symmetry, fat, muscle tone, turgor, hair distribution, scars, umbilicus, striae, fetus, rashes, distention, abnormal pulsations
☐ *Sounds*—absent, hypoactive, hyperactive, normal, bruits
☐ Liver border, gastric air bubble, splenic dullness, air fluid, muscle spasm, rigidity, masses, guarding, tenderness, pain, rebound, bladder distention

Kidney

☐ Urinary output (amount, color, odor, sediment), frequency, urgency, hesitancy, burning, pain, dribbling, incontinence, hematuria, nocturia, oliguria

Genitalia

☐ *Female*—labia majora and minora, urethral and vaginal orifices, discharge, swelling, ulceration, nodules, masses, tenderness, pain
☐ *Male*—*penis*: discharge, ulceration, pain; *scrotum*: color, size, nodules, swelling, ulcerations, tenderness; *testes*: size, shape, swelling, masses, absence

Rectum

☐ Pigmentation, hemorrhoids, excoriation, rashes, abscess, pilonidal cyst, masses, lesions, tenderness, pain, itching, burning

Extremities

☐ Size, shape, symmetry, range of motion, temperature, color, pigmentation, scars, hematoma, bruises, rash, ulceration, numbness, paresis, swelling, prosthesis, fracture
☐ *Joints*—symmetry, active and passive mobility, deformities, stiffness, fixation, masses, swelling, fluid, bogginess, crepitation, pain, tenderness
☐ *Muscles*—symmetry, size, shape, tone, weakness, cramps, spasms, rigidity, tremor
☐ *Vessels*—symmetry and strength of pulses, venous filling, varicosities, phlebitis

Back

☐ Scars, sacral edema, spinal abnormalities, kyphosis, scoliosis, tenderness, pain

B Body Systems Assessment Criteria

General Appearance
☐ *Observations*—age, sex, race, height, weight, nutritional status, development

Vital Signs
☐ Temperature
☐ Pulse (rate)
☐ Respirations
☐ *Blood pressure*—supine, sitting, right and left arms

Neurological System
☐ Level of consciousness
☐ *Skull*—size, contour, symmetry, color, pain, tenderness, lesions, edema
☐ *Eyes*—acuity, visual loss, glasses, contacts, prosthesis, diplopia, photophobia, color vision, pain, burning, eyelid ptosis, edema, styles, exophathamos, extraocular movement, position and alignment, strabismus, nystagmus, conjunctival color, discharge, vascular changes, corneal reflex, scleral color, vascularity, jaundice, pupil size, shape, equality, reaction to light
☐ *Neck*—symmetry, movement, range of motion, masses, scars, pain, stiffness, lymph node size, shape, mobility, tenderness, enlargement
☐ *Reflexes*—Deep tendon reflexes (DTRs), Babinski, posturing

Musculoskeletal System
☐ *Activity level*—prescribed, actual, range of motion
☐ *Extremities*—size, shape, symmetry, temperature, color, pigmentation, scars, hematoma, bruises, rash, ulceration, numbness, paresis, swelling, prosthesis, fracture
☐ *Joints*—symmetry, active and passive mobility, deformities, stiffness, fixation, masses, swelling, fluid, bogginess, crepitation, pain, tenderness
☐ *Muscles*—symmetry, size, shape, tone, weakness, cramps, spasms, rigidity, tremors
☐ *Back*—scars, sacral edema, spinal abnormalities, kyphosis, scoliosis, tenderness, pain

Respiratory System
☐ *Nose*—smell, nasal size, symmetry, flaring, sneezing, deformities, mucosal color, edema, exudate, bleeding, furuncles, pain, tenderness, sinus pain
☐ *Chest*—size, shape, symmetry, deformities, pain, tenderness, expansion, crepitation, tactile fremitus
☐ *Trachea*—deviation, scars
☐ *Breathing patterns*—rate, regularity, depth, ease, use of accessory muscles, cyanosis, clubbing
☐ *Sounds*—normal, adventitious, intensity, pitch, quality, duration, equality, vocal resonance

Cardiovascular System
☐ *Cardiac patterns*—rate, rhythm, intensity, regularity, skipped or extra beats, point of maximum impulse, bruits, thrills, murmurs, rubs
☐ Precordial movements, neck veins, right and left cardiac borders, pacemaker

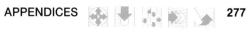

Gastrointestinal System

☐ *Mouth and throat*—odor, pain, ability to speak, bite, chew, swallow, taste, tongue size, shape, protrusion, symmetry, color, hydration, markings, ulcers, burning, swelling, coating, gum color, edema, bleeding, retraction, pain, number of teeth, absence, caries, caps, dentures, sensitivity to heat, cold, gag reflex, throat soreness, cough, sputum, hemoptysis

☐ *Abdomen*—size, color, contour, symmetry, fat, muscle tone, turgor, hair distribution, scars, umbilicus, striae, rashes, distention, abnormal pulsations, sounds: absent, hypoactive, hyperactive; tenderness, rigidity, free fluid, liver border, air bubble, splenic dullness, air rebound, muscle spasm, masses, guarding, pain

☐ *Rectum*—pigmentation, hemorrhoids, excoriation, rashes, abscess, pilonidal cyst, masses, lesions, tenderness, pain, itching, burning

Renal System

☐ *Urinary patterns*—amount, color, timing, odor, sediment, frequency, urgency, hesitancy, burning, pain, dribbling, incontinence, hematuria, nocturia, oliguria, change in stream, enuresis, flank pain, polyuria, retention, stress incontinence, bladder distention

Reproductive System

☐ *Male*—penis: discharge, ulceration, pain, size, prepuce; *scrotum*: size, color, nodules, swelling, ulceration, tenderness, pain; *testes*: size, shape, swelling, masses, absence

☐ *Female*—labia majora and minora, urethral and vaginal orifices, discharge, swelling, ulcerations, nodules, masses, tenderness, pain, pruritus, Pap smear, menstrual flow, menopause

☐ *Breasts*—contour, symmetry, color, shape, size, inflammation, scars, masses: location, size, shape, mobility, tenderness, pain; dimpling, swelling, nipples: color, discharge, ulceration, bleeding, inversion, pain; axillae: nodes, enlargement, tenderness, rash, inflammation

Integumentary System

☐ *Color*—pink, pale, red, jaundice, mottled, blanched, cyanotic

☐ *Patterns*—pigmentation, vascularity, temperature, texture, turgor, lesions (type, color, size, shape, distribution), bruises, bleeding, scars, edema, dryness, ecchymoses, masses (size, shape, location, mobility, tenderness), odors, petechiae, pruritus, bruises, bleeding, scars, edema

C Functional Health Pattern Assessment Criteria

Health Perception–Health Management
☐ Description of health (usual, current), preventive measures, previous hospitalizations and expectations of current hospitalization, description of illness (onset, cause), prior treatment (including compliance, anticipated self-care problems)

Nutritional-Metabolic
☐ Usual daily food and fluid intake, appetite, food restrictions or preferences, food supplements, recent weight change, swallowing, chewing, feeding problems

Elimination
☐ *Bowel*—usual time, frequency, color, consistency, assistive devices (laxatives, suppositories, enemas), constipation, diarrhea
☐ *Bladder*—usual frequency, problems with frequency, urgency, burning, retention, incontinence, dribbling, dysuria, polyuria, assistive devices
☐ *Skin*—condition, color, temperature, turgor, lesions, edema, pruritus

Activity-Exercise
☐ Usual daily/weekly activities, occupation, leisure-exercise patterns, limitations in ambulation, bathing, dressing, toileting, dyspnea, fatigue

Sleep-Rest
☐ *Usual sleep pattern*—bedtime, hours, sleep aids, problems falling asleep, staying asleep, feeling rested

Cognitive-Perceptual
☐ *Sensory deficits*—hearing, sight, touch, problems with vertigo, heat or cold sensitivity, ability to read, write

Self-Perception
☐ Major concerns, health goals, self-description, effects of illness on self-perception, factors contributing to illness, recovery, health maintenance

Role-Relationship
☐ *Communication*—language, clear and relevant speech, expression, understanding
☐ *Relationships*—living arrangements, support system, family life, complaints (parenting, relatives, abuse, marital problems)

Sexuality-Reproductive
☐ Changes anticipated or experienced because of condition (fertility, libido, erection, pregnancy, contraception, menstruation)

Coping–Stress Tolerance
☐ Decision-making (independent, assisted), major life changes (past, future, desired), stress management (eat, sleep, take medication, seek help), comfort/security needs

Value-Belief
☐ Sources of strength, meaning, religion (importance, type, frequency of practice), recent changes in values, beliefs, needs during hospitalization

Physical Assessment
- ☐ General appearance, weight, and height
- ☐ Eyes, appearance, drainage, pupils, vision
- ☐ Mouth, mucous membranes, teeth
- ☐ Hearing, acuity, aids
- ☐ Pulses, rate, rhythm, volume
- ☐ Respirations, rate, quality, sounds
- ☐ Blood pressure
- ☐ Temperature
- ☐ Skin color, temperature, turgor, lesions, edema, pruritus
- ☐ Functional ability, dominant hand, use of arms, legs, hands, strength, grasp, range of motion, gait, use of aids, weight-bearing
- ☐ Mental status, orientation, memory, affects, eye contact

Human Response Pattern Assessment Criteria

EXCHANGING

Cardiac—apical rate, rhythm, point of maximum impulse, blood pressure (sitting, supine, standing, right and left)

Cerebral—level of consciousness, pupils, eye opening, best verbal response, best motor response

Peripheral—pulses, skin temperature, color, capillary refill, clubbing, edema

Skin Integrity—rashes, petechiae, abrasions, lesions, bruises, surgical incisions, other

Oxygenation—respiratory rate, rhythm, depth, use of accessory muscles, dyspnea including precipitating factors, orthopnea, splinting, cough, sputum color/amount/consistency, breath sounds

Physical regulation—lymph nodes, temperature

Nutrition—eating patterns, number of meals per day, special diet, food preferences/intolerances, food allergies, caffeine intake, appetite changes, nausea/vomiting, condition of mouth/throat, height, weight, ideal body weight

Elimination—usual bowel habits, alterations from normal, constipation, diarrhea, incontinence, bowel sounds, usual urinary habits, alterations from normal, incontinence, retention, urine color/consistency/odor

COMMUNICATING

Read/write/understand English, other languages, impaired speech, other forms of communication

RELATING

Relationships—marital status, age/health of significant other, number of children/sex/ages, role in home, financial support, occupation, job satisfaction/concerns, physical/mental energy expenditures, sexual relationships, physical difficulties/effects of illness on sexuality

Socialization—quality of relationships with others, patient's description, significant other's description, staff observations, verbalization of aloneness

VALUING

Religious preference, important religious practices, spiritual concerns, cultural orientation, cultural practices

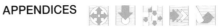

CHOOSING

Coping—client/significant other usual problem-solving methods, client/significant other method of managing stress, client affect, physical manifestations, available support systems

Participation—compliance with past/current health care regimens, willingness to comply with future health care regimen

Judgment—decision-making ability, client perspective, others' perspectives

MOVING

Activity—history of physical disability, limitations in daily activities, verbal reports of fatigue/weakness, exercise habits

Rest—hours slept per night, feeling rested upon awakening, sleeping aids, difficulty falling/remaining asleep

Recreation—leisure activities, social activities

Environmental maintenance—size and arrangement of home/stairs/bathroom, safety needs, home responsibilities

Health maintenance—health insurance, regular checkups, medications prescription/availability

Self-care—client's description of self, effects of illness/surgery on self-concept

Meaningfulness—verbalizes hopelessness, verbalizes/perceives loss of control

Sensory-perception—history of restricted environment, impaired vision, glasses, impaired hearing, hearing aid, body position/motion, taste, touch, smell, reflexes

PERCEIVING

Self-concept—client's description of self, effects of illness/surgery on self-concept

Meaningfulness—verbalizes hopelessness, verbalizes/perceives loss of control

Sensory perception—history of restricted environment, vision impaired, glasses, contact lenses, prosthesis, auditory impaired, hearing aid, body position/motion, taste, touch, smell, reflexes

KNOWING

Current health problems (client/significant other's perception)

Health history—previous illnesses/hospitalizations/surgery, diseases of heart, peripheral vascular system, lungs, liver, kidneys, cerebrovascular disorders, rheumatic fever, thyroid, others

Current medications—name, dosage, frequency, action

Risk factors—hypertension, hyperlipidemia, smoking, obesity, diabetes, sedentary lifestyle, stress, alcohol use, oral contraceptives, family history

Readiness—perception/knowledge of illness/tests/surgery, expectations of therapy, misconceptions, readiness to learn, requests for information concerning ...., educational level, learning barriers

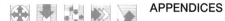

Orientation—level of alertness, orientation to person/place/time, appropriate behavior/communication

Memory—intact, recent only, remote only

FEELING

Pain/discomfort—onset, duration, location, quality, radiation, associated/aggravating/alleviating factors

Emotional integrity/status—recent stressful life events, fears, anxiety, grieving, source, physical manifestations

E

Approved Nursing Diagnoses, North America Nursing Diagnosis Association

1990

Activity intolerance
Activity intolerance, potential
Adjustment, impaired
Airway clearance, ineffective
Anxiety
Aspiration, potential for
Body image disturbance
Body temperature, potential altered
Breastfeeding, effective
Breastfeeding, ineffective
Breathing pattern, ineffective
Cardiac output, decreased
Communication, impaired verbal
Conflict, decisional
Conflict, parental role
Constipation
Constipation, colonic
Constipation, perceived
Coping, defensive
Coping, family-ineffective: compromised
Coping, family-ineffective: disabled
Coping, family: potential for growth
Coping, individual ineffective
Denial, ineffective
Diarrhea
Disuse syndrome, potential for
Diversional activity deficit
Dysreflexia
Family processes, altered
Fatigue
Fear
Fluid volume deficit (1,2)
Fluid volume deficit, potential
Fluid volume excess
Gas exchange, impaired
Grieving, anticipatory
Grieving, dysfunctional
Growth and development, altered
Health maintenance, altered
Health seeking behaviors (specify)

Home maintenance management, impaired
Hopelessness
Hyperthermia
Hypothermia
Incontinence, bowel
Incontinence, functional
Incontinence, reflex
Incontinence, stress
Incontinence, total
Incontinence, urge
Infection, potential for
Injury, potential for
Knowledge deficit (specify)
Mobility, impaired physical
Noncompliance
Nutrition, altered: less than body requirements
Nutrition, altered: more than body requirements
Nutrition, altered: potential for more than body requirements
Oral mucous membrane, altered
Pain
Pain, chronic
Parenting, altered
Parenting, altered: potential
Personal identity disturbance
Poisoning, potential for
Post-trauma response
Powerlessness
Protection, altered
Rape-trauma response
Rape-trauma syndrome: compound reaction
Rape-trauma syndrome: silent reaction
Role performance, altered
Self-care deficit: bathing/hygiene
       dressing/grooming
       feeding
       toileting
Self-esteem, chronic low
Self-esteem disturbance
Self-esteem, situational low
Sensory/perceptual alteration (specify)

(visual, auditory, kinesthetic, gustatory, tactile, olfactory)
Sexual dysfunction
Sexuality patterns, altered
Skin integrity, impaired
Skin integrity, potential impaired
Sleep pattern disturbance
Social interaction, impaired
Social isolation
Spiritual distress
Suffocation, potential for
Swallowing, impaired

Thermoregulation, ineffective
Thought processes, altered
Tissue integrity, impaired
Tissue perfusion, altered (specify type) (cardiopulmonary, cerebral, gastrointestinal, peripheral, renal)
Trauma, potential for
Unilateral neglect
Urinary elimination, altered patterns of
Urinary retention
Violence, potential for: self directed or directed at others

F

Definitions of NANDA-Approved Nursing Diagnoses, 1990

A human response pattern involving mutual giving and receiving.

Altered Nutrition: More Than Body Requirements.

The state in which the individual consumes more than adequate nutritional intake in relation to metabolic demands.

Altered Nutrition: Less Than Body Requirements.

The state in which the individual consumes inadequate nutritional intake in relation to metabolic demands.

Altered Nutrition: Potential For More Than Body Requirements.

The condition in which the individual has the potential for excessive nutritional intake in relation to metabolic demands.

Potential for Infection

The state in which an individual is at risk for being invaded by pathogenic organisms.

Potential Altered Body Temperature

The state in which the individual is at risk for failure to maintain body temperature within normal range.

Hypothermia

The state in which an individual's body temperature is reduced to below the normal range.

Hyperthermia

The state in which the individual is at risk because the body temperature is elevated above the individual's normal range.

Ineffective Thermoregulation

The state in which the individual's temperature fluctuates between hypothermia and hyperthermia.

Dysreflexia

The state in which an individual with a spinal cord injury at T7 (Thoracic 7) or above experiences a life threatening uninhibited sympathetic response of the nervous system to a noxious stimulus.

Constipation

The state in which the individual experiences decreased number of bowel movements in relation to normal elimination pattern; elimination of hard, dry stool; or absence of stool.

Perceived Constipation

The state in which an individual makes a self-diagnosis of constipation and ensures a daily bowel movement through abuse of laxatives, enemas, and suppositories.

Colonic Constipation

The state in which an individual's pattern of elimination is characterized by hard, dry stools that result from a delay in passage of food residue.

Diarrhea

The state in which the individual experiences or is at risk of experiencing a change in normal bowel movements resulting in frequent, loose, or liquid stools.

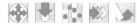
Bowel Incontinence

The state in which an individual experiences an inability to control the passage of bowel movements.

Altered Patterns of Urinary Elimination

The state in which an individual experiences or is at risk of experiencing a change in urinary function.

Stress Incontinence

The state in which an individual experiences an involuntary passage of urine less than 50 ml accompanied by increased abdominal pressure.

Reflex Incontinence

The state in which an individual experiences an involuntary passage of urine occurring at predictable intervals when a specific bladder volume is reached.

Urge Incontinence

The state in which an individual experiences involuntary passage of urine occurring soon after a strong sense of urgency to void.

Functional Incontinence

The state in which an individual experiences involuntary and unpredictable passage of urine.

Total Incontinence

The state in which an individual experiences a continuous and unpredictable passage of urine.

Urinary Retention

The state in which an individual experiences incomplete emptying of the bladder.

Altered (Specify Type) Tissue Perfusion: Renal, Cardiopulmonary, Cerebral, Gastrointestinal, Peripheral

The state in which an individual experiences or is at risk of experiencing a decrease in arterial, venous, or capillary blood flow.

Fluid Volume Excess

The state in which an individual experiences or is at risk of experiencing an excess of body fluids.

Fluid Volume Deficit, Actual or Potential

The state in which an individual experiences or is at risk of experiencing an alteration in body fluids resulting in dehydration.

Decreased Cardiac Output

A state in which an individual experiences or is at risk for experiencing cardiovascular, cerebral, or respiratory symptoms resulting from an insufficient volume of blood being pumped by the heart.

Impaired Gas Exchange

The state in which an individual experiences interference with cellular ventilation resulting from inadequate gas exchange across the alveolar–capillary membrane.

Ineffective Airway Clearance

The state in which an individual experiences interference with normal ventilation resulting from partial or complete airway obstruction.

Ineffective Breathing Pattern

The state in which an individual experiences impairment in respiratory function resulting from a change in breathing patterns.

Altered Protection

The state in which an individual experiences a decrease in the ability to guard the self from internal or external threats such as illness or injury.

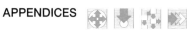

Potential for Injury

The state in which an individual is predisposed to injury because of internal or external factors.

Potential for Suffocation

The state in which an individual has accentuated risk of accidental suffocation (inadequate air available for inhalation).

Potential for Poisoning

The state in which an individual has accentuated risk for accidental exposure to or ingestion of drugs or dangerous products in doses sufficient to cause poisoning.

Potential for Trauma

The state in which an individual has accentuated risk of accidental tissue injury associated with internal or external factors.

Potential for Aspiration

The state in which an individual is at risk for entry of gastrointestinal secretions, oropharyngeal secretions, solids, or fluids into tracheobronchial passages.

Disuse Syndrome

The state in which an individual is at risk for deterioration of body systems as a result of prescribed or unavoidable musculoskeletal inactivity.

Impaired Tissue Integrity

The state in which an individual experiences damage to mucous or corneal, integumentary, or subcutaneous tissue.

Altered Oral Mucous Membranes

The state in which an individual experiences alteration of the integrity of the oral cavity.

Impaired Skin Integrity: Actual or Potential

The state in which an individual experiences or is at risk of experiencing an alteration or disruption of the skin.

COMMUNICATING

A human response pattern involving sending messages.

Impaired Verbal Communication

The state in which an individual experiences a dysfunction in ability to verbalize appropriately or interpret the meaning of words.

RELATING

A human response pattern involving established bonds.

Impaired Social Interaction

The state in which an individual participates in an insufficient quantity or quality of social exchange.

Social Isolation

The state in which an individual experiences aloneness that is perceived as imposed by others and as negative or threatening.

Altered Role Performance

The state in which an individual experiences a change, conflict, or denial of role responsibilities or inability to perform role responsibilities.

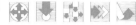

Altered Parenting
The state in which an individual experiences actual or potential alteration in ability to create an environment that promotes optimal growth and development of a child.

Sexual Dysfunction
The state in which an individual's sexual health or function is viewed as unrewarding or inadequate.

Altered Family Processes
The state experienced by a normally supportive family that is precipitated by a stressor and that results in altered family functioning.

Parental Role Conflict
The state in which a parent experiences role confusion and conflict in response to a crisis.

Altered Sexuality Patterns
The state of changed sexual health in an individual.

VALUING

A human response pattern involving the assigning of relative worth.

Spiritual Distress
The state in which an individual experiences a disturbance in religious belief or value system.

CHOOSING

A human response pattern involving the selection of alternatives.

Ineffective Individual Coping
The state in which an individual demonstrates impaired adaptive behaviors and problem-solving abilities.

Impaired Adjustment
The state in which an individual is unable to modify lifestyle/behavior in a manner consistent with a change in health status.

Defensive Coping
The state in which an individual repeatedly projects falsely positive self-evaluation based on a self-protective pattern that defends against underlying perceived threats to positive self-regard.

Ineffective Denial
The state in which an individual consciously or unconsciously attempts to disavow the knowledge or meaning of an event to reduce anxiety/fear to the detriment of health.

Ineffective Family Coping: Disabling
The state in which a family consistently responds to normal/unusual stressors with destructive behaviors.

Ineffective Family Coping: Compromised
The state in which a family temporarily responds to normal/unusual stressors with ineffective behaviors.

Family Coping: Potential for Growth
The state in which the family effectively manages adaptive tasks involved with a health challenge and exhibits desire for enhanced growth.

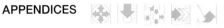

Noncompliance (Specify)
The state in which an individual is unwilling or unable to adhere to a therapeutic recommendation.

Decisional Conflict (Specify)
The state in which an individual experiences uncertainty about the course of action to be taken when choice among competing actions involves risk, loss, or challenge to personal life values.

Health-Seeking Behaviors (Specify)
The state in which an individual in stable health is actively seeking ways to alter personal health habits and/or the environment in order to move toward a higher level of health. (Stable health status is defined as age-appropriate illness prevention measures achieved, client reports good or excellent health, and signs and symptoms of disease, if present, are controlled.)

MOVING

A human response pattern involving activity.
Impaired Physical Mobility
The state in which an individual experiences limitation of physical movement because of inability or reluctance.

Activity Intolerance: Actual or Potential
The state in which an individual experiences actual or potential inability to maintain energy required for activities of daily living or to tolerate an increase in activity.

Fatigue
The state in which an individual experiences an overwhelming sense of exhaustion and decreased capacity for physical and mental work.

Sleep Pattern Disturbance
The state in which an individual experiences disruption of the quality or quantity of sleep patterns, which causes discomfort.

Diversional Activity Deficit
The state in which an individual experiences reluctance or inability to participate in activities that pass the time or provide distraction or gratification.

Impaired Home Maintenance Management
The state in which an individual experiences the inability to independently maintain a safe, growth-producing immediate environment for self or others.

Altered Health Maintenance
The state in which an individual experiences decreased ability to sustain/manage behaviors necessary to maintain or improve health status.

Feeding Self-Care Deficit
The state in which an individual experiences impaired ability to feed self independently.

Impaired Swallowing
The state in which an individual has decreased ability to voluntarily pass fluids and/or solids from the mouth to the stomach.

Ineffective Breastfeeding
The state in which a mother, infant, or child experiences dissatisfaction or difficulty with the breastfeeding process.

Effective Breastfeeding
The state in which a mother-infant dyad/family exhibits adequate proficiency and satisfaction with breastfeeding behaviors.

Bathing/Hygiene Self-Care Deficit
The state in which an individual experiences impaired ability to bathe self independently.

Dressing/Grooming Self-Care Deficit
The state in which an individual experiences impaired ability to dress self independently.

Toileting Self-Care Deficit
The state in which an individual experiences impaired ability to toilet self independently.

Altered Growth and Development
The state in which an individual deviates from the norms characteristic of age group.

PERCEIVING

A human response pattern involving the reception of information.

Body Image Disturbance
The state in which an individual experiences a negative or distorted perception of the body.

Self-Esteem Disturbance
The state in which an individual has negative self-evaluation/feelings about self or self-capabilities, which may be directly or indirectly expressed.

Chronic Low Self-Esteem
The state in which an individual has long-standing negative self-evaluation/feelings about self or self capabilities.

Situational Low Self-Esteem
The state in which an individual has negative self-evaluation/feelings about self that develop in response to a loss or change in an individual who previously had a positive self-evaluation.

Personal Identity Disturbance
The state in which an individual experiences an inability to estimate relationship of body to environment.

Sensory/Perceptual Alterations (Specify) Visual, Auditory, Kinesthetic, Gustatory, Tactile, Olfactory
The state in which an individual experiences an interruption or change in reception and/or interpretation of stimuli by receptors for sight, hearing, body position, taste, touch, or smell.

Unilateral Neglect
The state in which an individual is inattentive to a perceptually affected side.

Hopelessness
The subjective state in which an individual sees no alternatives or personal choices available and cannot mobilize energy on own behalf.

Powerlessness
The state in which an individual experiences the perception that one's own actions will not significantly affect an outcome or a perceived lack of control over a current situation or immediate happening.

KNOWING

A human response pattern involving meaning associated with information.
Knowledge Deficit (Specify)
   The state in which an individual lacks specific knowledge or skills that affect ability to maintain health.
Altered Thought Processes
   The state in which an individual experiences a disturbance in mental processes such as perception, reality orientation, memory, reasoning, and judgment.

FEELING

A human response pattern involving the subjective awareness of information.
Pain
   The state in which an individual experiences short-term pain/discomfort.
Chronic Pain
   The state in which an individual experiences pain that continues for longer than six months.
Dysfunctional Grieving
   The state in which an individual experiences an exaggerated response to an actual or potential loss of person, relationship, object, or functional abilities.
Anticipatory Grieving
   The state in which an individual experiences responses to an actual or perceived loss of a person, relationship, object, or functional abilities before the loss occurs.
Potential for Violence Self-Directed or Directed at Others
   The state in which an individual experiences a predisposition to violent, destructive acts directed toward self or others.
Post-Trauma Response
   The state in which an individual experiences a sustained painful response to an overwhelming traumatic event.
Rape-Trauma Response
   The state in which an individual experiences a trauma syndrome that results from rape and consists of an acute phase of disorganization of the victim's lifestyle and a long-term process of reorganization.
Anxiety
   The state in which an individual experiences a vague uneasy feeling, the source of which is often nonspecific or unknown.
Fear
   The state in which an individual experiences feelings of dread related to an identifiable source perceived as dangerous.

Adapted from Gordon M: Nursing Diagnosis: Process and Applications. New York: McGraw-Hill, 1982.

BUN	blood urea nitrogen
CBC	complete blood count
CC	cubic centimeter
CM	centimeter
CVP	central venous pressure
EKG	electrocardiogram
Hct	hematocrit
Hg	mercury
Hgb	hemoglobin
MM	millimeter
P	pulse
R	respirations
RBC	red blood cell
ROM	range of motion
T	temperature
WBCs	white blood cells
WNL	within normal limits

G   Exercises

Test Yourself G-1

IDENTIFICATION OF CORRECTLY AND INCORRECTLY WRITTEN CLIENT OUTCOMES

The following is a list of nursing diagnostic statements. Decide whether each statement is correctly or incorrectly written. If incorrectly stated, identify the rule(s) violated, by number, from the list below.

GUIDELINES FOR WRITING A NURSING DIAGNOSTIC STATEMENT
1. Write the diagnosis in terms of the client's response rather than nursing needs.
2. Use "related to" rather than "due to" or "caused by" to connect the two parts of the statement.
3. Write the diagnosis in legally advisable terms.
4. Write the diagnosis without value judgments.
5. Avoid reversing the two parts of the statement.
6. Avoid using single cues in the first part of the statement.
7. Be sure that the two parts of the statement do not mean the same thing.
8. Express the related factors in terms that can be changed.
9. Do not include medical diagnoses in the nursing diagnostic statement.
10. State the diagnosis clearly and concisely.

1. Spiritual distress related to challenged belief about God

2. Decisional conflict related to inability to make treatment decision

3. Activity intolerance related to persistent pain

4. Insomnia related to sleep pattern disturbance

5. Hypothermia caused by lack of appropriate clothing

6. Parental role conflict related to effects of marital separation

7. Altered patterns of urinary elimination related to benign prostatic hypertrophy

8. Poor family coping related to effects of impending death of family member

9. Fluid volume excess related to increased sodium intake

10. Altered growth and development related to the infant being taken care of by a different care giver each day

11. Body image disturbance related to loss of breast

12. Altered nutrition: less than body requirements related to lack of knowledge of diabetic diet

13. Hyperthermia related to elevated temperature

14. Potential for trauma related to failure of nurses to put up side rails

15. Social isolation related to effects of recent retirement

16. Ineffective airway clearance related to pneumonia

17. Sleep deprivation related to visual sensory perceptual alteration

18. Needs complete bed bath

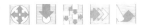
Test Answers G–1

GUIDELINES FOR WRITING A NURSING DIAGNOSTIC STATEMENT

1. Write the diagnosis in terms of the client's response rather than nursing needs.
2. Use "related to" rather than "due to" or "cause by" to connect the two parts of the statement.
3. Write the diagnosis in legally advisable terms.
4. Write the diagnosis without value judgments.
5. Avoid reversing the two parts of the statement.
6. Avoid using single cues in the first part of the statement.
7. Be sure that the two parts of the statement do not mean the same thing.
8. Express the related factors in terms that can be changed.
9. Do not include medical diagnoses in the nursing diagnostic statement.
10. State the diagnosis clearly and concisely.

	CORRECT	INCORRECT	RULE(S)
1. Spiritual distress related to challenged belief from God	√		
2. Decisional conflict related to inability to make treatment decision		√	#7
3. Activity intolerance related to persistent pain	√		
4. Insomnia related to sleep pattern disturbance		√	#5, 6, 7
5. Hypothermia caused by lack of appropriate clothing		√	#2
6. Parental role conflict related to effects of marital separation	√		
7. Altered patterns of urinary elimination related to benign prostatic hypertrophy		√	#9
8. Poor family coping related to effects of impending death of family member		√	#4
9. Fluid volume excess related to increased sodium intake	√		
10. Altered growth and development related to the infant being taken care of by a different care giver each day		√	#10
11. Body image disturbance related to loss of breast		√	#8
12. Altered nutrition: less than body requirements related to lack of knowledge of diabetic diet	√		
13. Hyperthermia related to elevated temperature		√	#7
14. Potential for trauma related to failure of nurses to put up side rails		√	#3
15. Social isolation related to effects of recent retirement	√		
16. Ineffective airway clearance related to pneumonia		√	#9
17. Sleep deprivation related to visual sensory perceptual alteration		√	#5
18. Needs complete bed bath		√	#1

Test Yourself G–2

REVISION OF INCORRECTLY WRITTEN NURSING DIAGNOSES

The nursing diagnoses that were incorrectly written in the previous exercise are listed below. Revise each nursing diagnosis to make it correct.

Nursing Diagnosis	Revision
1. Decisional conflict related to inability to make treatment decision	
2. Insomnia related to sleep pattern disturbance	
3. Hypothermia caused by lack of appropriate clothing	
4. Altered patterns of urinary elimination related to benign prostatic hypertrophy	
5. Poor family coping related to effects of impending death of family member	
6. Altered growth and development related to the infant being taken care of by a different care giver each day	
7. Body image disturbance related to loss of breast	
8. Hyperthermia related to elevated temperature	
9. Potential for trauma related to failure of nurses to put up side rails	
10. Ineffective airway clearance related to pneumonia	
11. Sleep deprivation related to visual sensory perceptual alteration	
12. Needs complete bed bath	

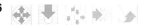

Test Answers G–2

There are a number of ways to correct the nursing diagnoses listed in this exercise. One example of a corrected revision for each nursing diagnosis is provided below.

NURSING DIAGNOSIS	REVISION
1. Decisional conflict related to inability to make treatment decision	Decisional conflict related to presence of divergent sources of information
2. Insomnia related to sleep pattern disturbance	Sleep pattern disturbance related to excessive noise
3. Hypothermia caused by lack of appropriate clothing	Hypothermia related to lack of appropriate clothing
4. Altered patterns of urinary elimination related to benign prostatic hypertrophy	Altered patterns of urinary elimination related to catheter obstruction
5. Poor family coping related to effects of impending death of family member	Ineffective family coping: disabling related to effects of impending death of family member.
6. Altered growth and development related to the infant being taken care of by a different care giver each day	Altered growth and development related to inconsistency in caregiving
7. Body image disturbance related to loss of breast	Body image disturbance related to effects of loss of breast
8. Hyperthermia related to elevated temperature	Hyperthermia related to prolonged exposure to hot environment
9. Potential for trauma related to failure of nurses to put up side rails	Potential for trauma related to decreased level of consciousness
10. Ineffective airway clearance related to pneumonia	Ineffective airway clearance related to retained secretions
11. Sleep deprivation related to visual sensory perceptual alteration	Sensory perceptual alteration (visual) related to sleep deprivation
12. Needs complete bed bath	Bathing hygiene self-care deficit related to effects of prolonged immobility

Test Yourself G–3

IDENTIFICATION OF CORRECTLY AND INCORRECTLY WRITTEN CLIENT OUTCOMES

Following is a list of nursing diagnoses and outcomes. Decide whether each *outcome* is correctly or incorrectly written. If incorrectly stated, identify, by number, the rule(s) violated from the list below.

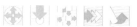

Rules

Outcomes should be:
1. Related to the human response
2. Client-centered
3. Clear and concise
4. Observable and measurable
5. Realistic
6. Time-limited
7. Determined by client and nurse together

Nursing Diagnosis	Outcome	Correct	Incorrect	Rule(s)
1. Feeding self-care deficit related to impaired physical mobility	Client will receive help to eat			
2. Ineffective breastfeeding related to decreased infant sucking	Demonstrates adequate breastfeeding as manifested by infant weight gain of 3 oz in 4 days			
3. Fear related to outcome of diagnostic studies	Less fearful			
4. Anticipatory grieving related to impending death of child	By time of child's death, family verbalizes complete acceptance			
5. Pain related to muscle spasm	Verbalizes decreased pain within 45 minutes after pain medication			
6. Potential for infection related to hazards associated with invasive equipment	Absence of redness, edema, purulent drainage, temperature elevation, and increased WBCs			
7. Potential for aspiration related to decreased level of consciousness	Prevent aspiration			
8. Ineffective denial related to perceived changes in lifestyle	Prior to discharge: realistically describes impact of disease			
9. Social isolation related to obesity, perceived unattractiveness	Losses 1 lb per week until achieves goal of 150 lbs			

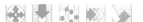

Test Answers G–3

RULES

Outcomes should be:
1. Related to the human response
2. Client-centered
3. Clear and concise
4. Observable and measurable
5. Realistic
6. Time-limited
7. Determined by client and nurse together

NURSING DIAGNOSIS	OUTCOME	CORRECT	INCORRECT	RULE(S)
1. Feeding self-care deficit related to impaired physical mobility	Client will receive help to eat		√	#3, 6
2. Ineffective breastfeeding related to decreased infant sucking	Demonstrates adequate breastfeeding as manifested by infant weight gain of 3 oz in 4 days	√		
3. Fear related to outcome of diagnostic studies	Less fearful		√	#4, 6
4. Anticipatory grieving related to impending death of child	By time of child's death, family verbalizes complete acceptance		√	#5
5. Pain related to muscle spasm	Verbalizes decreased pain within 45 minutes after pain medication	√		
6. Potential for infection related to hazards associated with invasive equipment	Absence of redness, edema, purulent drainage, temperature elevation, and increased WBCs		√	#3, 6
7. Potential for aspiration related to decreased level of consciousness	Prevent aspiration		√	#2, 6

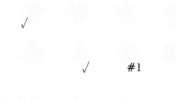

8. Ineffective denial related to perceived changes in lifestyle
   Prior to discharge: realistically describes impact of disease   √

9. Social isolation related to obesity, perceived unattractiveness
   Loses 1 lb per week until achieves goal of 150 lbs   √   #1

Test Yourself G–4

REVISION OF INCORRECTLY WRITTEN CLIENT OUTCOMES

The outcomes that were incorrectly written are listed below. A nursing diagnosis has been defined for each outcome to assist you in formulating a new outcome. Revise each outcome so that it is correctly stated.

NURSING DIAGNOSIS	OUTCOME	REVISED OUTCOME
1. Feeding self-care deficit related to impaired physical mobility	Client will receive help to eat	
2. Fear related to outcome of diagnostic studies	Less fearful	
3. Anticipatory grieving related to impending death of child	By time of child's death, family verbalizes complete acceptance	
4. Potential for infection related to hazards associated with invasive equipment	Absence of redness, edema, purulent drainage, temperature elevation, and increased WBCs	
5. Potential for aspiration related to decreased level of consciousness	Prevent aspiration	
6. Social isolation related to obesity, perceived unattractiveness	Loses 1 lb per week until achieves goal of 150 lbs	

Test Answers G–4

The following are suggested answers for the preceding exercise. Keep in mind that there is more than one way to revise an outcome.

NURSING DIAGNOSIS	OUTCOME	REVISED OUTCOME
1. Feeding self-care deficit related to impaired physical mobility	Client will receive help to eat	Prior to discharge feeds self using adaptive equipment
2. Fear related to outcome of diagnostic studies	Less fearful	Verbalizes decreased fearfulness within 24 hours
3. Anticipatory grieving related to impending death of child	By time of child's death, family verbalizes complete acceptance	Prior to child's death family verbalizes feelings regarding impending loss
4. Potential for infection related to hazards associated with invasive equipment	Absence of redness, edema, purulent drainage, temperature elevation, and increased WBCs	While CVP line in place, no evidence of infection
5. Potential for aspiration related to decreased level of consciousness	Prevent aspiration	No evidence of aspiration throughout hospitalization
6. Social isolation related to obesity, perceived unattractiveness	Loses 1 lb per week until achieves goal of 150 lbs	Interacts with peers after school at least two times per week

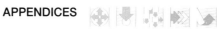

Test Yourself G–5

The following is a list of interventions. Decide whether each intervention is written correctly or incorrectly. Identify the rule violated from the list below:

RULES

Nursing Interventions Should:
1. Include precise action verbs and modifiers.
2. Specify who, what, where, how, and how much.
3. Be individualized for the client.
4. Be signed and dated.

	NURSING INTERVENTIONS	CORRECT	INCORRECT	RULE(S)
11/9 S. Wilson, Rn	1. Create a safe environment			
2/8 J. Fenton, Rn	2. Assist to cough and deep breathe q2h			
7/16 J. Adams, Rn	3. Turn client			
9/16 C. Dampier Rn	4. Irrigate wound			
9/10 S. Ricotto, Rn	5. Ambulates in room three times daily			
	6. Weigh daily prior to breakfast using bedscale			
6/10 G. Walsh, Rn	7. Encourage client to share feelings concerning loss of child			
3/7 D. West, Rn	8. ROM exercises			
2/4 L. Smith, Rn	9. Teach colostomy care			

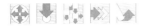

Test Answers G–5

	NURSING INTERVENTIONS	CORRECT	INCORRECT	RULE(S)
11/9 S. Wilson, Rn	1. Create a safe environment		√	1
2/8 J. Fenton, Rn	2. Assist to cough and deep breathe q2h	√		
7/16 J. Adams, Rn	3. Turn client		√	2
9/16 C. Dampu, Rn	4. Irrigate wound		√	2
9/10 S. Ricotto, Rn	5. Ambulates in room three times daily		√	This is an outcome
	6. Weigh daily prior to breakfast using bedscale		√	4
6/10 G. Walsh, Rn	7. Encourage client to share feelings concerning loss of child	√		
3/7 D. West, Rn	8. ROM exercises		√	2
2/4 L. Smith, Rn	9. Teach colostomy care		√	2, 3

Test Yourself G–6

REVISION OF INCORRECTLY WRITTEN NURSING INTERVENTIONS

	NURSING INTERVENTIONS	REVISED INTERVENTIONS
11/9 S. Wilson, Rn	1. Create a safe environment	
7/16 J. Adams, Rn	2. Turn client	
9/16 C. Dampu Rn	3. Irrigate wound	
	4. Ambulates in room three times daily	
	5. Weigh daily prior to breakfast using bedscale	
3/7 D. West, Rn	6. ROM exercises	
2/4 L. Smith, Rn	7. Teach colostomy care	

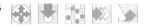

Test Answers G–6

	NURSING INTERVENTIONS	**REVISED INTERVENTIONS**
11/9 N. Wilson, Rn	1. Create a safe environment	Remove obstacles from path of ambulation
7/16 J. Adams, Rm	2. Turn client	Turn client q2h according to turning schedule
9/16 C. Dampu Rn	3. Irrigate wound	Irrigate abdominal wound with 50 cc of normal saline q shift
9/10 S. Ricotto, Rn	4. Ambulates in room three times daily	Assist to ambulate in room TID
	5. Weigh daily prior to breakfast using bedscale	Weigh daily prior to breakfast using bedscale
3/7 D. West, Rn	6. ROM exercise	Active ROM exercises to left shoulder q shift
2/4 L. Smith, Rn	7. Teach colostomy care	Teach client to apply Bongort pouch on 5/8

Test Yourself G–7

CARE PLANNING EXERCISE

Directions:

Read the following case studies. Based on the information provided identify pertinent cues, develop correctly written diagnoses, outcomes, and nursing interventions. Refer to the guidelines provided in exercises G-1, G-3, and G-5.

Case Study #1

Adam Steinman is a 75 year old gentleman confined to bed as a result of an injury to his spinal column causing some residual weakness of his lower extremities. He is referred to home care by his physician to assist in managing problems with urination. During your visit he voids 150 cc despite the fact that he has already consumed more than 600 cc of fluid. His bladder is moderately distended. You call his physician and discuss your findings. A decision is made to do a straight urethral catherization and 350 cc of urine is obtained.

Develop a care plan with one nursing diagnosis

CUES:

NURSING DIAGNOSIS: OUTCOMES: NURSING INTERVENTIONS:

Case Study Answers G–7
Case Study #1: Adam Steinman

CUES:
Bladder distention
High residual urine
Small frequent voiding

NURSING DIAGNOSIS:	OUTCOMES:	NURSING INTERVENTIONS:
Urinary retention related to diminished sensory/ motor impulses	Within one week voids at least ___ cc per void	1. Have client keep record of voiding pattern time and amounts

2. Assess and document color and consistency of urine

3. Increase oral intake to:
   1000 cc days
   $\overline{700}$ cc evenings
   $\overline{300}$ cc nights

4. Teach client/family to palpate bladder for distention q4h

5. Implement techniques that may encourage voiding: run water in bathroom

6. Consult physician to determine need for further straight catheterizations

Case Study #2

Freida Lucinda is a 76 year old woman admitted two days ago with a right-sided cerebral vascular accident. She is now alert, oriented, and able to sit up in a chair and feed herself. When clearing her tray, you notice she has eaten only the food on the right side of her plate. In addition, she did not drink her juice which she specifically requested. When questioning her, she indicates she did not see the juice on the left side of the tray. You also notice that she has combed only the right side of her hair and did not place her left arm through her robe sleeve.

Develop a care plan with one nursing diagnosis

CUES:

NURSING DIAGNOSIS: OUTCOMES: NURSING INTERVENTIONS:

Case Study Answers #2: Freida Lucinda

CUES:
Leaves food on plate on
  the affected side
Combs one side of hair
Did not place her left arm
  through her robe sleeve

NURSING DIAGNOSIS:	OUTCOMES:	NURSING INTERVENTIONS:
Unilateral neglect (left side) related to effects of impaired perception associated with hemianopsia	By time of discharge: demonstrates attention to left side	1. Bring problem to attention of client/family 2. Explain why this may be occurring 3. Approach client from the left side 4. Teach client to visually scan her environment 5. Encourage family to interact with left side: increase touching, positioning, and reference to neglected side 6. Encourage client to handle limbs on neglected side. Teach to bath, dress, and position extremities safely 7. Place all necessary equipment, food on client's right side 8. Place unnecessary items (personal) on left side and remind client to scan to left 9. Place TV on left side 10. When repositioning, remember to place client facing paralyzed extremity

Case Study #3

Mary Ann LaFleur is a 36 year old mother of three preschool children. In the sixth month of her last pregnancy, she was found to have a malignant breast tumor for which she had a left modified radical mastectomy. Eighteen months later, she found another mass in her right breast and has been admitted to your unit the morning of the surgery. The client tells you that the physician has explained the anticipated surgical options and has offered her the choice between a lumpectomy followed by radiation and chemotherapy or a second radical mastectomy. The client tells you that she really would prefer the first option but she is very concerned about her ability to handle the difficulties associated with both chemotherapy and radiation. She states "I know I have to make a decision but neither choice is appealing. If I lose my other breast I will no longer look like a woman."

Develop a care plan with at least two nursing diagnoses

CUES:

NURSING DIAGNOSIS: OUTCOMES: NURSING INTERVENTIONS:

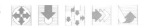

Case Study Answers #3: Mary Ann LaFleur

CUES:
Verbalized uncertainty
   about choices
Verbalized undesired
   consequences of
   treatment choices

NURSING DIAGNOSIS:	OUTCOMES:	NURSING INTERVENTIONS:
Decisional conflict (treatment option) related to unknown outcome of choices of therapy	Prior to surgery: verbalizes satisfaction with choice made	1. Encourage client to further verbalize concerns regarding both choices 2. Have client seek input from husband/family 3. Explore her fears regarding chemotherapy and radiation therapy 4. Notify physician that client is still undecided; arrange group conference

CUES:
Verbal response to
   potential change in
   appearance

NURSING DIAGNOSIS:	OUTCOMES:	NURSING INTERVENTIONS:
Potential body image disturbance related to feelings of rejection secondary to mastectomies	Verbalizes positive statements about physical appearance prior to discharge	1. Encourage client to discuss negative feelings regarding body 2. Explore feelings regarding effects of surgery and her relationship with her husband 3. Encourage her to discuss fears with her husband 4. Identify personal strengths 5. Assist client to identify other positive aspects of her physical appearance

Case Study #4

Susan Johnson is a 36 year old housewife who has been diagnosed as having rheumatoid arthritis. As the home health nurse, your initial assessment reveals an alert, oriented woman with joint swelling of the fingers and right knee. During the interview, Susan Johnson grimaces and moans slightly each time she attempts to bend her fingers. She holds her right knee and indicates that she feels best when she lies on her left side with pillows behind her back and between her legs. She states, "I feel so helpless. I'm so stiff in the morning and this pain is really getting me down. My mother has had to come to my house every day to care for my toddlers. I hate when this pain prevents me from performing my responsibilities as a mother."

Develop a care plan with at least two nursing diagnoses

CUES:

NURSING DIAGNOSIS:	**OUTCOMES:**	**NURSING INTERVENTIONS:**

Case Study Answers #4: Susan Johnson

CUES:
Grimacing/moaning
Clutching of painful knee
Feelings of helplessness
Reports of pain

NURSING DIAGNOSIS:	**OUTCOMES:**	**NURSING INTERVENTIONS:**
Acute pain related to inflammatory process	Verbalizes decreased pain within 30 minutes following initiation of comfort measures	1. Explore pain relief measures that have been helpful in the past 2. Advise client to take hot bath/shower upon arising to reduce stiffness 3. Apply cold as directed by physician 4. Explore with client times of day she can rest with joints in functional position

5. Review knowledge of medication regimen; remind not to miss dose of arthritis medications

6. Explore use of relaxation exercises to reduce stress/anxiety

7. Consult physical therapy for home physical therapy

8. Caution against exercising inflamed joints except for ROM exercises

---

CUES:
States inability to perform role expectations

NURSING DIAGNOSIS:	**OUTCOMES:**	**NURSING INTERVENTIONS:**
Altered role performance related to change in health status, effect of acute illness	Demonstrates ability to function within limitations	1. Encourage client to verbalize further regarding the effect of the change in health status on her role as wife and mother 2. Assist client to identify what part of her role she can still perform 3. Discuss plan for potential change in family member's role function during this acute episode 4. Discuss need for some temporary child care for children 5. Explore coping mechanisms that have been successful in the past and explore new options

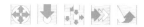

Case Study #5

Art Herbert is a 75 year old widower with no nearby relatives. He was recently discharged from the hospital after experiencing a hypertensive crisis. During the course of hospitalization he responded well to the antihypertensive medications. Three days after discharge, the home care nurse finds his blood pressure is 180/100, his weight is up by seven pounds, and he has edema of the ankles.

Art reported that he has not been taking his diuretic as prescribed, because he could not remember the instructions. He stated that he did not want to talk about those pills any more. His real concern was his bowels. He reported he had been constipated for three days, had hard dry stools, and required straining to accomplish defecation. This is especially distressing because he is accustomed to having a bowel movement daily.

Since discharge, Art has been preparing canned soups and small frozen dinners, even though his doctor prescribed a low salt diet. Prior to hospitalization, his usual diet consisted of home cooked meals prepared by his neighbor. Art said, "I don't know what is happening to me. Ever since my neighbor left for vacation I have been having all these problems. She cooked for me and reminded me to take my medicine. I can't wait until she comes home."

Develop a care plan with at least three nursing diagnoses

CUES:

NURSING DIAGNOSIS:	OUTCOMES:	NURSING INTERVENTIONS:

Case Study Answers #5: Art Herbert

CUES:
Inability to meet basic health needs: taking antihypertensive medication (diuretic), following diet

NURSING DIAGNOSIS:	OUTCOMES:	NURSING INTERVENTIONS:
Altered health maintenance related to forgetfulness, lack of support systems	By end of visit: Identifies available resources for maintaining healthy diet, taking medications as ordered	1. Provide and review medication chart noting purpose and time of medicines 2. Explore client's belief

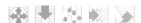

regarding medications/
physician's advice
3. Supply pill sorter and
fill on q3 day visit
4. Explore availability of
financial resources for
homemaker
5. Discuss acceptance of
assistance within the
home
6. Identify with client
other alternative support
systems
7. Write all instructions
down and place in spot
designated by client

Cues:
Hypertension
Edema of ankles
Weight gain

Nursing Diagnosis:	**Outcomes:**	**Nursing Interventions:**
Fluid volume excess related to	Within one week:	1. Call physician and notify of client's status
Excessive salt intake	Fluid balance WNL for client	2. Review with client the interaction of excessive salt on body system
Noncompliance with medication regimen	Absence of peripheral edema	3. Explore in further detail types of foods he has been eating. Do a refrigerator and pantry review
	Return to baseline weight	4. Caution against food with hidden sodium
		5. Instruct client to weigh self on his scale each morning. Start a flow sheet
		6. Review and write down when he should call his doctor: increasing shortness of breath, weight gain, more edema
		7. Explore with physician possibility of antiembolism stockings

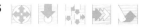

8. Instruct client to
elevate feet when sitting
9. Emphasize importance
of adhering to medication
regimen

CUES:
Hard dry stools
Straining
Decreased frequency of
  bowel movements

NURSING DIAGNOSIS:
Colonic constipation
  related to changes in
  dietary intake, change
  in daily routine

OUTCOMES:
Within two weeks
  resumes daily bowel
  movement

NURSING INTERVENTIONS:
1. Evaluate present diet
for fiber and fluid content
2. Explore knowledge of
role of fluids, fiber, and
exercise in management of
constipation
3. Investigate possibility
of antihypertensive
medication contributing to
constipation
4. Suggest adding fiber
and natural bran to diet
5. Make out fluid intake
plan to remind client to
drink fluids within his
restrictions (1500 cc)
6. Explore temporary use
of natural laxatives;
instruct on consequences
of long-term laxative
usage
7. Explore alternatives to
providing well balanced
meals:
    Neighbors
    Meals On Wheels
    Temporary homemaker
8. Explore plan for
increasing activity level

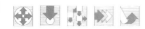

Case Study #6

Helen O'Brien is a 76 year old white woman admitted to your unit. Your assessment reveals the following data: vital signs T = 101 F, B/P = 96/70 mm Hg, P = 110 beats/minute, R = 18 breaths/minute (no abnormal breath sounds), height = 5 ft 5 in, weight = 96 lb. Helen's skin is dry, pale, and warm to touch with decreased skin turgor and dry oral mucous membranes. She looks emaciated, has dark circles under her eyes, and reports that she has lost 15 lbs in the last two months since her husband died. She has no obvious open areas on her skin; however, you observe a 3 cm erythemic (reddened) area on her coccyx.

She has full range of motion but is unable to walk without assistance since she is weak and dizzy. Helen indicates that she has fallen twice at home; however, there is no evidence of injury. She is alert and oriented but is obviously tense throughout the interview. She moves her hands continuously and changes position frequently. She cries intermittently and is particularly tearful when her husband is mentioned. She states, "I'm not surprised this happened—I knew I'd get sick if I didn't eat more." She reveals that she has had no appetite and has been unable to sleep more than three hours a night since her husband's death. Helen shares that she is extremely lonely and feels worried and helpless most of the time. All she has is her cat.

Lab data reveal
—CBC: decreased Hgb and RBC, increased hematocrit
—Urinalysis: concentrated dark amber urine with increased specific gravity, urine culture negative
—Chest x-ray and EKG: normal

Develop a care plan with at least five diagnoses

CUES:

NURSING DIAGNOSIS: OUTCOMES: NURSING INTERVENTIONS:

Case Study Answers #6: Helen O'Brien

CUES:

Body weight 20% or more less than ideal for height and frame

Decrease Hgb and RBC

Decreased skin turgor

Reported inadequate food intake

NURSING DIAGNOSIS:	OUTCOMES:	NURSING INTERVENTIONS:
Altered nutrition: less than body requirements related to decreased appetite secondary to depression	Consumes 2000 calories daily	1. Determine food likes and dislikes 2. Offer small frequent feedings every four hours at 8 AM, 12 PM, 4 PM, and 8 PM 3. Encourage the client to drink milkshakes at 10 AM and 6 PM 4. Closely observe the client's food and fluid intake 5. Give the client positive feedback for adhering to prescribed diet 6. Explore possibility of family/friends visiting at mealtime

CUES:

Difficulty remaining asleep
Dark circles under eyes

NURSING DIAGNOSIS:	OUTCOMES:	NURSING INTERVENTIONS:
Sleep pattern disturbance related to fear/anxiety, depression	Sleeps at least four hours each night without interruption	1. Assess and document sleeping pattern 2. Encourage client to verbalize underlying causes of sleeplessness 3. Provide a quiet peaceful time for resting 4. Provide a nighttime routine to encourage sleep 5. Reduce caffeine intake during the evening hours 6. Discourage sleeping during the day

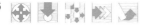

7. Schedule activities at night to allow for at least four hours of uninterrupted sleep

---

CUES:
Report of two falls
Unable to walk without
    assistance

NURSING DIAGNOSIS:	**OUTCOMES:**	**NURSING INTERVENTIONS:**
Potential for trauma related to dizziness and weakness	Throughout hospitalization, no evidence of trauma Calls for assistance before ambulating	1. Keep room free of obstacles 2. Side rails up at all times 3. Keep items within reach on bedside stand (telephone, call bell) 4. Instruct client to call for help before getting OOB 5. Encourage use of railings when in bathroom and hall

---

CUES:
Dryness
Evidence of 3 cm
    erythemic area on
    coccyx

NURSING DIAGNOSIS:	**OUTCOMES:**	**NURSING INTERVENTIONS:**
Impaired skin integrity related to altered nutritional state and immobility	By time of discharge: No further evidence of skin breakdown 3 cm area of erythema decreased in size	1. Instruct client to turn and do small pressure shifts 2. Apply egg crate mattress to bed 3. Inspect skin for redness, tenderness, maceration and edema 4. Apply skin barrier dressing to 3 cm erythemic area 5. Massage body prominences gently with lotion q4h 6. Keep skin clean and dry, and bed free from wrinkles

7. Monitor nutritional and fluid intake, monitor serum protein, albumin level, and CBC

CUES:
Decreased BP
Decreased skin turgor
Dry skin, oral mucous
  membranes

NURSING DIAGNOSIS:	**OUTCOMES:**	**NURSING INTERVENTIONS:**

Fluid volume deficit related to loss of appetite, decreased fluid intake	Balanced I/O
	Vital signs within desired limits
		1. Monitor I/O q8h
		2. Assess skin turgor, mucous membranes, dryness, and skin temperature q8h
		3. Monitor VS q4h
		4. Administer IV fluids as ordered 2000 cc q24h
		5. Encourage po fluid intake to 2000 cc:
		    7–3 1000 cc,
		    3–11 700 cc,
		    11–7 300 cc
		6. Keep fluid of choice at bedside (specify)
		7. Monitor electrolyte, BUN, creatinine and Hgb + Hct

CUES:
Weight loss
Changes in sleep patterns
Feelings of sorrow
Crying when husband is
  mentioned

NURSING DIAGNOSIS:	**OUTCOMES:**	**NURSING INTERVENTIONS:**
Dysfunctional grieving related to lack of resolution of grieving response, decreased support systems	By time of discharge: Verbalizes feelings about husband's death	1. Encourage the client to verbalize her feelings 2. Let her know you will listen and accept what she is expressing 3. Allow her to cry if desired; stay with and support her or provide privacy for brief periods 4. Assist the client to identify available support systems in the community 5. Support the client when she is making choices

Nursing Care Plans

See the beginning of Appendix G for a listing of abbreviations. The following are additional abbreviations used in Appendix H

ABGs	arterial blood gases
ADLs	activities of daily living
H&H	hemoglobin and hematcrit
HOB	head of bed
ICP	intracranial pressure
IPPB	intermittent positive pressure breathing
LOC	level of consciousness
O_2	oxygen
s/s	signs and symptoms
TENS	transcutaneous electrical nerve stimulation
UTI	urinary tract infection

DISUSE SYNDROME H–1 *See Appendix F for definition

NURSING DIAGNOSIS:
Potential for disuse
  syndrome related
    to
—immobility
—severe pain
—altered LOC

OUTCOMES:
Throughout period of
  immobilization:
—Joint ROM at same
  level as prior to illness
—Muscle size/strength
  WNL for client
—No evidence of joint
  contractures

NURSING INTERVENTIONS:
a. Assess and record base
line function of muscles
and joints
b. Consult physical/
occupational therapy (date
_____)
c. Passive/active ROM to
all joints q _____ h.
Adhere to schedule:_____

_____

—Coordinate with
  physical therapy
—Instruct significant
  other to do scheduled
  exercises
d. Maintain body in
alignment using rolls,
pillows, etc. Specify _____

_____

e. Use supportive devices
(specify) to keep hands/
arms/feet in functional
position. Use according to
schedule. Specify _____

_____

—Remove splints and
  assess skin for s/s
  pressure q _____ h

OUTCOMES:

NURSING INTERVENTIONS:

f. Dangle at bedside as tolerated

g. Encourage participation/independence in self-care within limitations of client

h. Consider use of specialized bed Rotorest, Mediscus, etc, to assist in managing musculoskeletal problems

Throughout period of immobilization:

No evidence of s/s of:

—venous thrombosis/ pulmonary embolism

—orthostatic hypotension

—peripheral edema

a. Evaluate and report s/s of thrombus formations: sustained pain or tenderness, unusual warmth and redness

☐ Calf/thigh measurements at same place q _____

☐ Assess lower extremities for Homans' sign q _____

b. Maintain antiembolic hose ☐ knee high, ☐ thigh high. Remove for _____ min q shift to perform assessment and reapply

c. Maintain intermittent venous compression device if available

d. Assist client to perform active/passive dorsiflexion and plantar flexion exercises _____ times q _____

e. Change position q _____ hr

—Avoid positions that might compromise blood flow

—When placing client upright, raise slowly and assess for dizziness, drop in BP

f. Refrain from placing pillows or constricting object under knees. Do not gatch bed

DISUSE SYNDROME H–1

OUTCOMES:

NURSING INTERVENTIONS:

g. Monitor for sudden chest pain, cough with hemoptysis, dyspnea, cyanosis

h. Maintain hydration to 2–3 L/24 hr unless contraindicated
7–3 _____ 3–11 _____
11–7 _____

ı. Assess peripheral pulses q _____

j. Assess for peripheral edema on feet, hands, and sacrum q _____

k. When placing client upright raise slowly and assess for dizziness and drop in BP

l. Administer and monitor the effects of prophylactic anticoagulation as prescribed: aspirin, low-dose heparin, or Coumadin.

Throughout period of
  immobilization:
—Lung sounds clear
—Rate, rhythm, depth of
  respirations WNL for
  client
—Pulmonary function
  studies WNL for client
—Expectorates secretions

a. Assess breath sounds q _____. Note: areas of hypoventilation and adventitious breath sounds

b. Evaluate and record rate, rhythm, and depth of respirations, and use of accessory muscles q _____

c. Position client to promote optimal breathing. Specify _____
  —Evaluate HOB within
  limitation of client
  —Sit OOB/chair.
  Specify _____
  _____

d. Assess ability to cough and expectorate secretions

e. Suction using aseptic technique as indicated

f. Assist to cough and deep breath q _____ h

g. Assist and evaluate effects of IPPB and incentive spirometry q __ h

DISUSE SYNDROME H–1

OUTCOMES:

Throughout period of
   immobilization:
—No evidence of skin
   breakdown

NURSING INTERVENTIONS:

a. Reposition q _____ h.
Initiate a repositioning
schedule
b. Teach client/family to
perform pressure shifts
and reliefs
c. Inspect pressure points
q _____ h
d. Assess for redness,
tenderness, echymosis,
maceration, edema, and
skin breakdown
e. Keep heels off bed.
Specify _____
_____
f. Initiate use of pressure
relieving devices (egg
crate, air mattress, air
fluidized bed, gel pads).
Specify _____
_____
g. Administer gentle
massage at position
changes to pressure points
h. Keep skin clean and
dry, and bed free from
wrinkles
i. Take measure to control
bowel and bladder
incontinence if present.
Specify _____
j. Monitor protein and
fluid intake
k. Monitor serum protein,
albumin level and CBC

Throughout period of
   immobilization:
—Normal bowel
   movement at least q ___
   days
—No evidence of gastric
   distress

a. Obtain information
about prior elimination
patterns or rituals
b. Assess for indications
of constipation
c. Provide high fiber/
roughage diet as tolerated
d. Encourage fluid intake
by providing fluids of
choice. Specify _____
e. Administer and
evaluate effectiveness of
stool softener/laxatives

DISUSE SYNDROME H–1

OUTCOMES:	NURSING INTERVENTIONS:
	f. Observe for signs of gastric distress: heartburn, nausea and check stools/gastric secretions for occult blood q _____
SG between 1.010–1.030 —Urine output WNL —No evidence of infection, calculi	a. Monitor intake and output q24h b. Evaluate color, clarity, and consistency of urine c. Assess for s/s renal calculi, flank pain, hematuria d. Monitor serum calcium level and presence of calcium crystals in urine e. Incorporate cranberry juice in diet f. Utilize bathroom or commode for voiding, defecating as tolerated g. Provide privacy during voiding/defecation
Throughout period of immobilization: —Oriented to time, place, and person	a. Assess level of orientation b. Provide appropriate sensory stimulation: —Encourage family/friends to visit patient and become involved in care —Provide access to radio, TV, reading material —Discuss current events —Encourage socialization with other clients and group activities as appropriate —Encourage family/friends to speak with client even if client is unable to respond
—Utilizes learned coping mechanisms within _____	a. Answer client/family's questions b. Explore coping mechanisms used in past and ability to use in present situation

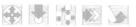

DISUSE SYNDROME H–1

OUTCOMES:

NURSING INTERVENTIONS:

c. Assist client (when appropriate) to identify and test new coping mechanisms

d. Keep patient informed of condition and progress

e. Allow client to make decisions in daily care

f. Assist client to set realistic goals

Throughout period of immobilization:

—Reports pain promptly

—Verbalizes decreased pain within 30 min following initiation of comfort measures

a. Help identify pain relief measures that have been helpful in the past

b. Explore with client feelings/attitudes regarding fear of addiction

c. Instruct client/family
—To report pain promptly
—To describe using 0–10 scale
—Regarding prescribed regimen for pain relief
—To evaluate and report effectiveness of interventions

d. Assess for pain q _____ using verbal and nonverbal cues, including location, quality, intensity, duration, precipitating/aggravating/relieving factors, and associated symptoms

e. Explain source of pain if known

f. Collaborate with physician to establish a pain control regimen
☐ Medications:
☐ Apply ice to surgical site
☐ TENS
☐ Patient-controlled analgesia

g. Provide therapeutic comfort measures
☐ Massage
☐ Relaxation

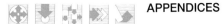
DISUSE SYNDROME H–1

NURSING DIAGNOSIS:	OUTCOMES:	NURSING INTERVENTIONS:
		☐ Diversional activities
		———
		h. Reassure and support client/family during episodes of pain
		i. Provide quiet environment and organize care to promote periods of uninterrupted rest
		j. Medicate prior to activities to promote participation
		k. Assess and document findings and effectiveness of interventions

POTENTIAL FOR INFECTION H–2

Potential for infection related to —effects of chronic illness —inadequate immune system —hazards associated with invasive equipment —effects of chemotherapy —other	Throughout period of immobilization: —No evidence of local/systemic infection	a. Assess risk for potential infection b. Assess for s/s of infection (Specify) ——— and document all findings ☐ Monitor oral/rectal temp and pulse q ——— h ☐ Auscultate breath sounds q ——— ☐ Monitor body fluids for changes in color, consistency, and odor ☐ Observe wounds, incisions, catheter, and monitoring sites for redness, swelling, and drainage ☐ Assess for lethargy, malaise, and chills c. Obtain cultures as indicated d. Maintain aseptic technique when assisting with or performing invasive procedures, dressing changes, and monitoring the integrity of invasive lines/equipment

POTENTIAL FOR INFECTION H–2

NURSING DIAGNOSIS:	OUTCOMES:	NURSING INTERVENTIONS:
		e. Change dressing at ____ site q ____
		f. Use reverse isolation when indicated
		g. Take measures to minimize client's exposure to other infected clients, nurses, or visitors
		h. Maintain integrity of closed urinary drainage system, perform catheter care per institutional policy
		i. Instruct/assist client with procedure to minimize risk of infection
		☐ Coughing and deep breathing exercises q ____
		☐ Incentive spirometry q ____
		☐ Position change q ____
		☐ Ambulation q ____
		☐ Performance of personal and oral hygiene. Specify ____
		☐ Choosing well-balanced diet
		Administer medications and monitor effects of:
		☐ Antipyretics
		☐ Prophylactic antibiotics

KNOWLEDGE DEFICIT (IN HOSPITALIZED CLIENT) H–3

Knowledge deficit (disease process, diet, activity, medication, support systems, follow-up care, procedure, pre-/postop care)	Prior to procedure: —Describes procedure —Describes usual pre/ postop care	a. Assess client/family learning needs, level of knowledge, intellectual ability, barriers to teaching/learning process
		b. Provide for physical comfort of learner prior to teaching session
		c. Distribute teaching materials appropriate to learning needs and client's level of understanding
	Prior to discharge: —Defines disease process	d. Instruct client/family regarding:

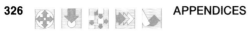
KNOWLEDGE DEFICIT H–3

OUTCOMES:
(Specify) _____

NURSING INTERVENTIONS:
☐ _____ structure and function
☐ pathology of _____
☐ procedure (reinforce physician's explanation in terms client/family can understand)
☐ preop care (anesthesia, premed, prcp, NPO)
☐ postop care (postanesthesia care unit, monitoring, specialized equipment, pain regimen)
☐ other identified learning needs (specify) _____

—Selects _____ foods from menu

e. Consultation with dietician _____ (date)
f. Assist client/family to select appropriate foods from menu

—Names own medications and describes action, dosage, and major side effects

g. Provide medication information for each postdischarge medication. (Specify) _____
h. Review medication schedule

—Identifies appropriate postdischarge activity

i. Review with client/family:
☐ recommended activity levels
☐ symptoms requiring activity reduction/cessation
☐ alternative activities
☐ activities to avoid

—Identifies postdischarge resources

j. Provide information regarding postdischarge resources:
☐ wellness program
☐ support group
k. Review symptoms requiring notification of physician:
☐
☐
☐
☐
☐

KNOWLEDGE DEFICIT H–3

NURSING DIAGNOSIS:	OUTCOMES:	NURSING INTERVENTIONS:
	—Explains importance of and states plans for followup care	l. Instruct client to make follow-up appointment with physician _____ (date) m. Reinforce teaching as necessary. Obtain verbal or written feedback n. Document progress in nursing notes/teaching record

POSTOPERATIVE COLOSTOMY H–4

Potential for injury related to complications of surgical procedure: obstruction	—Nasogastric (NG) tube drainage within normal limits q8h —Passage of flatus/ discharge from the stoma by _____ postop day —By time of discharge, return of bowel function through the stoma	a. Check NG tube patency. Irrigate with 30 cc normal saline solution q _____ h and prn b. Monitor NG tube contents. Chart color/ amount of drainage q ____ h c. Assess bowel activity q _____ h ☐ Passage of flatus/ drainage ☐ Bowel sounds q ____ ☐ Stool (amount, consistency, color, odor, frequency) d. Monitor for changes in stool consistency as nutritional intake progresses
Potential altered tissue integrity related to —decreased perfusion to stoma —contamination of wound site by ostomy drainage/surgical drain —risk of wound dehiscence	—Throughout hospitalization, pink to red colored stoma —Demonstrates wound healing by time of discharge	a. Monitor stoma q _____ b. Notify physician immediately if stoma color is dusky or blackened c. Contain stomal drainage with appliance. Keep dressing over surgical site when changing ostomy appliance or emptying drainage d. Observe wound site q _____ for signs of redness, swelling, induration, tenderness, and dehiscence

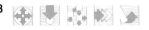
POSTOPERATIVE COLOSTOMY H-4

NURSING DIAGNOSIS:	OUTCOMES:	NURSING INTERVENTIONS:
Potential altered skin integrity (peristomal) related to irritating stomal drainage	Throughout postop period: —Peristomal skin free from excoriation —Stomal drainage contained by ostomy appliance	a. Initiate peristomal care and apply ostomy appliance and skin barrier as soon as possible postop. (Specify) _____ b. Change pouch q ____ day and prn, before leakage occurs ☐ Cleanse peristomal area with warm water and mild soap. Pat skin dry ☐ Measure stoma for correct opening size at each appliance change; size should be $\frac{1}{8}$ inch larger than stoma ☐ Protect area immediately surrounding stoma with ostomy paste before applying skin barrier and appliance c. Empty pouch when bag is $\frac{1}{3}$ full to avoid pulling on appliance seal and leakage d. Document condition of peristomal skin e. Consult with ostomy therapist (Date) _____
Pain related to effects of surgery	Reports pain promptly when experiencing it Verbalizes decreased pain within 30 min following initiation of comfort measures Participates in postop care within ____	a. Instruct client/family: ☐ to report pain promptly and to describe using 0–10 scale ☐ regarding prescribed regimen for pain relief ☐ regarding sensations that are likely to result from procedures b. Assess for pain frequently q ____ c. Collaborate with physician to establish a pain control regimen. Administer analgesics or narcotics per order

POSTOPERATIVE COLOSTOMY H–4

NURSING DIAGNOSIS:	OUTCOMES:	NURSING INTERVENTIONS:
		d. Provide therapeutic comfort measures: ☐ Position change (Specify position of comfort or position to avoid) _____ ☐ Back rub ☐ Diversional activities e. Provide quiet environment and organize care to promote periods of uninterrupted rest f. Reassure and support client/family during episodes of pain g. Assess and document findings and evaluate effectiveness of interventions
Body image disturbance related to effect of change in body function: —stoma —loss of fecal continence	Within _____: —Verbalizes feelings about altered bowel function; stoma —Express positive statements about self and ability to deal with change	a. Assess client's perception of body changes and perceived impact of the change in their lifestyle b. Note verbal remarks to stoma and altered bowel elimination c. Acknowledge feelings of anger/depression/denial as normal emotional response at this time d. Assist client/family member to view, touch, and care for stoma when ready e. Encourage client/family to express feelings regarding stoma ☐ Spend at least _____ min in room q shift to allow for verbalization ☐ Ask open-ended questions f. Provide all care in a positive manner. Avoid all mannerisms connotating distaste g. Assist client to maintain own personal

POSTOPERATIVE COLOSTOMY H–4

NURSING DIAGNOSIS:	OUTCOMES:	NURSING INTERVENTIONS:
		hygiene, bedclothes, apply make-up
		h. Offer to arrange for visitor with ostomy to provide realistic support
Potential altered sexuality patterns related to effects of presence of ostomy	By time of discharge client and partner will verbalize concerns and explore alternatives	a. Assess perceptions of how ostomy will affect sexual activity
		b. Offer realistic information to prevent misconceptions
		c. Encourage communication with significant other and explain need to share feelings
		d. Explain that near-normal sexual activity can be resumed when physical condition allows; instruct to avoid pressure on ostomy site
		e. Encourage client/partner to seek professional guidance as needed, or if impotency is a problem
Knowledge deficit: —care of ostomy	By time of discharge: —Client or family member will be able to demonstrate care of the ostomy appliance —Client/family will be able to describe dietary management for proper regulation of ostomy	a. Assess for readiness to learn ostomy care
		b. Initiate teaching plan and provide teaching packet (Date) _____
		c. Give step-by-step explanation to client
		d. Include family members(s) in teaching
		e. Provide list of ostomy equipment and suggested places of purchase
		f. Social Service referral for follow-up by home care (Date) _____
		g. Review prescribed diet. Dietary consult if necessary
		h. If no specific diet order, review foods to avoid for gas, odor formation, and blockage

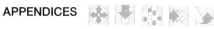

TOTAL HIP REPLACEMENT (POSTOP) H–5

NURSING DIAGNOSIS:

Potential for injury (dislocation) related to unstable hip joint

OUTCOMES:

At time of discharge demonstrates healing with extremity in proper alignment

NURSING INTERVENTIONS:

a. Keep _____ hip abducted at all times using

_____

☐ Splints
☐ Abduction pillows
☐ Two pillows
☐ Traction

b. Encourage periodic elevation of HOB no greater than _____ degrees per physician order.

c. Instruct client to use overbed trapeze for weight shifts, linen changes, and use of fracture pan (keep HOB elevated at least 20 degrees when on fracture pan)

d. Perform gluteal and quadriceps exercises and dorsiplantar flexion exercise of ankles. Specify

_____

e. Turn client to unoperative side only, unless otherwise ordered with operative leg maintained in abduction and extension

f. OOB/chair. Specify date and method _____. Keep within flexion restrictions.

☐ No weight bearing __ leg
☐ Elevate sitting surface with pillows
☐ Use elevated toilet seat or elevated commode

g. Coordinate with physical therapy instructions on transfer technique and ambulation

TOTAL HIP REPLACEMENT (POSTOP) H–5

NURSING DIAGNOSIS:	**OUTCOMES:**	**NURSING INTERVENTIONS:**

NURSING DIAGNOSIS:

Potential for infection related to
—effects of anesthesia/ surgery
—hazards associated with invasive equipment

OUTCOMES:

Throughout period of immobilization:

No evidence of local/ systemic infection

NURSING INTERVENTIONS:

a. Assess risk factors for potential infection

b. Assess for s/s of infection (Specify) ———— and document all findings

☐ Monitor temperature oral/rectal and pulse q ——— h

☐ Auscultate breath sounds q ————

☐ Monitor body fluids for changes in color, consistency, and odor

☐ Observe wounds, incisions, and catheter, for redness, swelling, and drainage

☐ Assess for lethargy, malaise, and chills

c. Obtain cultures as indicated

d. Maintain aseptic technique when assisting with or performing invasive procedures, and dressing changes.

e. Change dressing at —— site q ————

f. Use reverse isolation when indicated

g. Take measures to minimize client's exposure to other infected clients, nurses, or visitors

h. Maintain integrity of closed urinary drainage system. Perform catheter care per institutional policy

i. Instruct/assist client with procedure to minimize risk of infection

☐ Coughing and deep breathing exercises q ——

☐ Incentive spirometry

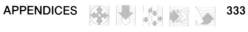

TOTAL HIP REPLACEMENT (POSTOP) H–5

NURSING DIAGNOSIS:	OUTCOMES:	NURSING INTERVENTIONS:
		q —— ☐ Position change q —— ☐ Ambulation q —— ☐ Performance of personal and oral hygiene. Specify —— ☐ Choosing well-balanced diet j. Administer medications and monitor effects of: ☐ Antipyretics ☐ Prophylactic antibiotics
Impaired physical mobility related to —effect of surgery —prescribed restrictions	During postop period: No loss of muscle tone/ strength in unaffected extremities	a. Initiate active ROM exercises to unaffected extremities q —— b. Encourage participation in self-care activities c. Coordinate with physical therapy instructions on transfer technique and ambulation
Potential impaired skin integrity related to decreased mobility	No evidence of skin breakdown at time of discharge	a. Initiate turning schedule turn q —— h (specify) —— b. Massage bony prominence q —— h c. Inspect skin for redness, swelling, and breakdown d. Keep skin clean and dry at all times e. Relieve pressure on both heels with bilateral heel protectors f. Initiate pressure relieving devices (eggcrate air mattress, air fluidized bed, gel, pad). Specify —— g. Keep heel of bed (specify) ——. Instruct to use overbed trapeze to shift weight q ——. h. Monitor protein and fluid intake

TOTAL HIP REPLACEMENT (POSTOP) H–5

NURSING DIAGNOSIS:	OUTCOMES:	NURSING INTERVENTIONS:
Potential for altered tissue perfusion: peripheral related to —immobility —compromised circulation —excessive bleeding	Throughout hospitalization: —Peripheral pulses within normal limits —No evidence of venous thrombosis, peripheral edema, bleeding	a. Assess operative extremity for excessive edema b. Maintain antiembolic stockings, Ace bandages —Remove q ____ and evaluate for constriction, bunching, and signs of pressure c. Neurovascular check of both extremities q ____ h × ____ h, then ____ h d. Assess lower extremities for Homans' sign q ____ e. Assist client to perform active/passive dorsiflexion and plantarflexion exercises ____ times q ____, starting ____ f. Evaluate and report s/s of thrombus formation: (Sustained pain or tenderness, unusual warmth, and redness) g. Calf, thigh measurements at same place q ____ h. Administer and monitor effects of prophylactic anticoagulants as prescribed: aspirin, low dose heparin, Coumadin i. Avoid positions that might compromise blood flow. Do not gatch bed j. Refrain from placing pillows or constricting objects under knees k. Monitor VS and Hgb and Hct l. Maintain suction-drainage system at wound site m. Chart amount and consistency of drainage q shift. Note: excessive bleeding/wound drainage

TOTAL HIP REPLACEMENT (POSTOP) H–5

NURSING DIAGNOSIS:

Pain related to
—effects of surgery
—inflammatory process

OUTCOMES:

Reports pain promptly
Verbalizes decreased pain
    within 30 min following
    initiation of comfort
    measures

NURSING INTERVENTIONS:

a. Help identify pain relief measures that have been helpful in the past

b. Explore with client feelings/attitudes regarding fear of addiction

c. Instruct client/family
  ☐ To report pain promptly
  ☐ To describe using 0–10 scale
  ☐ Regarding prescribed regimens for pain relief
  ☐ To evaluate and report effectiveness of interventions

d. Assess for pain q _____ using verbal and nonverbal cues, including location, quality, intensity, duration, precipitating/ aggravating/relieving factors, and associated symptoms.

e. Explain source of pain if known

f. Collaborate with physician to establish a pain control regimen
  ☐ Medications
  ☐ Apply ice to surgical site
  ☐ TENS
  ☐ Patient controlled analgesia

g. Provide therapeutic comfort measures
  ☐ Massage
  ☐ Relaxation
  ☐ Diversional activities _____
  ☐ Alteration in environment _____

h. Reassure and support client/family during episodes of pain

i. Provide quiet environment and organize care to promote periods of uninterrupted rest

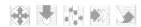
TOTAL HIP REPLACEMENT (POSTOP) H–5

NURSING DIAGNOSIS:	OUTCOMES:	NURSING INTERVENTIONS:
		j. Medicate prior to activities to promote participation
		k. Assess and document findings and effectiveness of interventions
Potential altered health maintenance related to lack of knowledge re: postdischarge care	Prior to discharge: Demonstrates proper positioning and transfer techniques	a. Have client demonstrate transfer techniques
	Verbalizes discharge instructions regarding activity, care of incision and medications	b. Reinforce information given by physician, physical therapist
		c. Stress that the client should not —Flex hip more than 90 degrees —Sit on low chair, stool, or toilet seat —Bend to tie shoes —Cross legs when sitting, standing, or lying —Get up from a chair without moving to the edge first —Lie on "good side" without a pillow between legs —Pick up any objects from the floor or reach into lower cupboard or drawers
		d. Care of incisional area: Specify _____
		e. Explain medication doses, schedule, and side effects: Specify _____

ACUTE CEREBRAL VASCULAR ACCIDENT H–6

NURSING DIAGNOSIS:	OUTCOMES:	NURSING INTERVENTIONS:

Altered tissue perfusion: cerebral related to
—impaired circulation
—changes in intracranial pressure
—decreased cerebral oxygenation
	Stable neuro signs throughout hospitalization	a. Assess and monitor neuro signs including LOC/mental status, pupillary response, motor, and sensory function q ___ h × _____, then q _____
		b. Monitor vital signs q _____
		c. Administer medications to maintain normotension
		d. Take measures to maintain patent airway
		e. Administer oxygen via _____ at _____ L/min
		f. Promote venous outflow:
		  ☐ Elevate HOB _____
		  ☐ Keep head and neck in alignment
		g. Maintain fluid intake at _____ cc q 24 h. Avoid overhydration (may increase ICP)
		h. Administer and monitor effects of medications:
		  ☐ Heparin, Coumadin, aspirin
		  ☐ Steroids
		  ☐ Antiseizure
		  ☐ Diuretic
		i. Organize care to allow for rest periods

Impaired physical mobility related to L/R hemiplegia, hemiparesis, decreased LOC	—Maintains ROM to joints at same level as prior to illness
	—Client and family demonstrate ability to perform ROM exercises on affected side and to position correctly within _____ days
	—Demonstrates transfer techniques with assistance by time of discharge
		a. Assess and record baseline function of muscles/joints
		b. Coordinate plan with physical and occupational therapy
		c. Maintain correct body alignment and support hand and feet in functional position using assistive devices (Specify)
		  ☐ Splints
		  ☐ Pillows

ACUTE CEREBRAL VASCULAR ACCIDENT H–6

NURSING DIAGNOSIS:	OUTCOMES:	NURSING INTERVENTIONS:
		☐ Sandbags
		☐ Footboard
		☐ Trochanter rolls
		☐ Foot drop protectors
		d. Active/passive ROM exercises to joints q _____ h. (Specify) _____
		e. Utilize trapeze bar over bed to assist with position changes
		f. Instruct client and family in:
		☐ ROM exercises
		☐ Bed to chair transfer
		☐ Position in bed (avoid high Fowler's position—leads to hip flexion)
Impaired verbal communication related to dysarthria, dysphagia, aphasia	During hospitalization: —Utilizes alternative methods to communicate —Exhibits minimal frustration when communicating	a. Assess client's mental status and ability to express self and understand others
		b. Try to anticipate client's needs
		c. Keep call signal within reach of unaffected side
		d. Maintain eye contact when communicating
		e. Diminish external distractions when communicating
		f. Use short, simple yes-and-no questions and gestures when communicating
		g. Speak slowly and allow adequate time for response
		h. Use all interactions to stimulate speech
		i. Use communication aid (Specify) _____
		j. Obtain speech therapy consult (Date) _____

ACUTE CEREBRAL VASCULAR ACCIDENT H–6

NURSING DIAGNOSIS:	OUTCOMES:	NURSING INTERVENTIONS:
Potential for aspiration related to —retained secretions —effect of impaired gag reflex —decreased LOC	Throughout hospitalization able to maintain oral intake without evidence of aspiration	a. Assess status of gag reflex, ability to swallow prior to each eating attempt b. Avoid clear liquids. Introduce foods slowly, starting with semisolids (oatmeal, Jell-o, sherbet) c. Assist with oral intake as needed, instruct family on proper feeding technique d. Refrain from giving client large amounts of fluids po which may increase risk of vomiting and aspiration e. Position client with HOB elevated 30 degrees at least during each feeding and for at least one hour after meal f. Monitor respiratory status, rate depth and rhythm q _____ g. Assess for and report adventitious breath sounds, restlessness, pallor, and agitation h. Keep suction equipment on standby in case of aspiration or if client is unable to clear secretions i. If aspiration occurs, stop oral intake, maintain oxygen as prescribed. Prepare for chest x-ray and EKGs
Potential impaired skin integrity related to —prolonged immobility —incontinence —decreased nutritional intake	Throughout hospitalization no evidence of skin breakdown	a. Reposition q _____ h. Initiate a repositioning schedule b. Teach client/family to perform pressure shifts c. Inspect pressure points q _____ h with special attention to splints and affected limbs

ACUTE CEREBRAL VASCULAR ACCIDENT H–6

NURSING DIAGNOSIS:	OUTCOMES:	NURSING INTERVENTIONS:
		d. Assess for redness, tenderness, ecchymosis, maceration, edema, and skin breakdown
		e. Keep heels off bed (Specify) _____
		f. Initiate use of pressure relieving devices (eggcrate air mattress, air fluidized bed, gel pads). (Specify)
		g. Administer gentle massage at position changes to pressure points
		h. Keep skin clean and dry and bed free from wrinkles
		i. Take measures to control bowel and bladder incontinence if present
		j. Monitor nutritional and fluid intake
		k. Monitor serum protein, albumin, and CBC
Potential altered patterns of urinary elimination related to —effects of sensorimotor impairment —impaired communication	By time of discharge experiences decreased episodes of incontinence/retention	a. Monitor urinary output. Assess for incontinence or retention
		b. Ascertain if client is aware of need to void
		c. Assess if client is able to communicate need to void
		d. Assure client that urinary problems are common and could be temporary
		e. Offer bed pan/urinal after meals and at regular intervals (Specify) _____
		f. Palpate bladder to assess for distention
		g. Implement measures to stimulate voiding: ☐ Maintain privacy ☐ Running water ☐ Bedside commode if possible ☐ Comfortable position ☐ Credé maneuver

ACUTE CEREBRAL VASCULAR ACCIDENT H–6

NURSING DIAGNOSIS:	OUTCOMES:	NURSING INTERVENTIONS:
		h. Use disposable incontinence pads, external/internal urinary system as necessary i. Provide catheter care if retention catheter is in place j. Maintain fluids at least _____ cc/24 hr. Limit fluid intake after 8 PM k. Assess color, consistency of urine to determine concentration and presence of UTI l. Obtain urine specimens as ordered
Constipation related to —diminished nutrition —immobility —impaired communication —lack of response to defecation impulse	Bowel movement without incontinence q _____ day	a. Determine previous bowel habits and measures to maintain them b. Assess if client is aware or able to communicate need to defecate c. Assess and record frequency and character of stool and incontinence d. Monitor for fecal impaction q _____ days e. When client can tolerate, consult dietician to add high fiber and roughage to diet f. Encourage fluids _____ cc/24 hr g. Administer and monitor effects of: ☐ Stool softeners ☐ Suppositories ☐ Enemas h. Encourage/assist with ambulation and increase activities as tolerated i. Implement measures to stimulate evacuation: —Maintain privacy —Comfortable position —Commode at bedside —Warm fluids

ACUTE CEREBRAL VASCULAR ACCIDENT H–6

NURSING DIAGNOSIS:	OUTCOMES:	NURSING INTERVENTIONS:

Potential for trauma related to
—decreased mobility
—visual/perceptual impairment
—decreased sensation
—change in mental status/ LOC
	By time of discharge no evidence of trauma	a. Assess client's visual and sensory function and document deficits
		b. Keep frequently used objects within reach on unaffected side
		c. Approach from unaffected side. Encourage family to do same
		d. Teach client and family to:
		  —Safeguard areas of diminished sensation (e.g., heat/cold, pain, pressure)
		  —Monitor temperature of food, bathwater to prevent accidental injury
		e. Assist client/teach family how to safely assist with ADL's and mobility as needed
		f. Avoid use of restraints whenever possible; agitation causes an increase in ICP

Altered thought process: confusion related to effects of cerebral ischemia	—When reoriented, correctly identifies person, place, and time —Responds appropriately to others	a. Orient conscious client to person, place, time b. Explain all activities, procedures, and events c. Have family bring in familiar objects from home d. Place clock/calendar within client's visual field e. Implement a constant routine, encourage family/ staff to abide by it

PNEUMONIA H–7

Ineffective airway clearance related to —increased production of viscous secretions —dehydration	Breath sounds WNL within _____	a. Monitor breath sounds _____ b. Administer humidified O$_2$ at _____ L/min via _____ c. Encourage/assist client

PNEUMONIA H–7

NURSING DIAGNOSIS:	OUTCOMES:	NURSING INTERVENTIONS:

—fatigue; decreased energy level		to cough and deep breathe using splinting as necessary q _____
		 d. Assist with and monitor effects of chest physiotherapy and breathing treatments
		 e. Maintain adequate hydration at _____ cc IV and po q4h
		      _____ cc Days
		      _____ cc Evenings
		      _____ cc Nights
		 f. If client unable to cough, suction prn
		 g. Utilize artificial airway as needed
		 h. Administer and monitor the effects of expectorants, antibiotics

Ineffective breathing pattern related to persistent pain, fatigue	Rate, rhythm, and depth of respiration WNL within _____ ABGs within desired limits throughout hospitalization No evidence of respiratory distress	a. Assess respiratory rate, rhythm, and use of accessory muscles b. Monitor for s/s of hypoxia, respiratory distress c. Auscultate breath sounds q _____ d. Monitor ABG results and report significant deviations e. Administer O_2 at _____ L/min via _____ f. Position client for optimal breathing g. Initiate pain management regimen. Specify _____ h. Organize activities to minimize fatigue
Potential for fluid volume deficit related to decreased circulating volume secondary to decreased fluid intake, diaphoresis, hyperthermia	Within _____ BP WNL for client Balanced I & O Urine output >30 cc/hr within _____ Urine specific gravity 1.010–1.030 within ___	a. Assess VS, skin turgor q _____ h b. Monitor I and O q ___ and report output <30 cc for two consecutive hours to physician c. Measure specific gravity

PNEUMONIA H–7

NURSING DIAGNOSIS:	OUTCOMES:	NURSING INTERVENTIONS:
		q _____ d. Monitor for s/s dehydration e. Administer po and IV fluids/medication per physician order and document response f. Monitor lab values and report significant changes in H & H, electrolytes
Hyperthermia related to —dehydration —decreased fluid intake —effects of infection —altered metabolism	Body temperature <101 degrees F within _____	a. Monitor oral/rectal temperature q _____ h b. Obtain blood/sputum cultures and sensitivity as ordered c. Remove excess blankets. Administer tepid bath, ice bag to groin, axilla d. Use hypothermia blanket as ordered for temperature greater than _____ following unit protocol e. Administer antipyretics q _____ h for temperatures greater than _____ degrees f. Administer antimicrobials per physician order, monitor and document effects
Altered nutrition: less than body requirements related to decreased caloric intake, increased metabolic needs	Weight loss of no more than _____ lb throughout hospitalization	a. Weigh daily at _____ using _____ scale b. Monitor nutritional intake, initiate caloric count c. Monitor serum protein albumin d. Minimize activity level to decrease metabolic needs e. Increase activity as tolerated f. Assess food likes and dislikes g. Provide frequent small high protein/high carbohydrate diet

PNEUMONIA H–7

NURSING DIAGNOSIS:	OUTCOMES:	NURSING INTERVENTIONS:
		h. Encourage food from home if permitted i. Provide enteral and parenteral nutrition as ordered j. Administer vitamin supplements as ordered

Pain related to pleuritic inflammation, persistent cough	Verbal or nonverbal indication of pain relief within 30 min following initiation of comfort measures	a. If applicable instruct client/family to report pain promptly, to describe using 0–10 scale and regarding prescribed regimen for pain relief
		b. Assess for pain frequently q _____ including location, intensity, duration, precipitating/aggravating factors, and associated symptoms
		c. Collaborate with physician to establish a pain control regimen. Avoid over medication in order to avoid depressing respirations
		d. Administer appropriate medications to treat the cough
		   ☐ Do not suppress a productive cough
		   ☐ Administer cough suppressants and humidity for a dry hacking cough
		e. Provide therapeutic comfort measure:
		   ☐ Position change (specify position of comfort) _____
		
		   ☐ Diversional activities
		   ☐ Relaxation exercises
		f. Assess and document findings and effectiveness of interventions

Implementation Using Functional Health Patterns Model

The client's physical and emotional needs are identified in the assessment phase of the nursing process. A nursing diagnosis and outcomes are formulated, and individualized nursing interventions are written. During the implementation phase, the nurse initiates these interventions. The following subsections discuss the type of interventions used based on the 11 functional health patterns identified by Gordon (1982). Table A–1 divides the patterns into physical or emotional categories. A definition and description are provided for each pattern. Commonly associated nursing diagnoses are listed based on the work of Gordon (1982) and Carpenito (1983). Additionally, contributing factors are identified for each pattern. The focus for interventions in each area is presented, along with sample methods of implementation.

TABLE A–1. CATEGORIES OF FUNCTIONAL HEALTH PATTERNS

BIOPHYSICAL	EMOTIONAL
Health perception–health management	Self-perception–self-concept
Nutritional-metabolic	Role-relationship
Elimination	Sexuality-reproductive
Activity-exercise	Coping–stress tolerance
Sleep-rest	Value-belief
Cognitive-perceptual	

Biophysical Patterns

Those patterns identified as biophysical include health perception–health management, nutritional-metabolic, elimination, activity-exercise, sleep-rest, and cognitive-perceptual. The following will define and describe each pattern, identify associated nursing diagnoses, and describe nursing interventions.

Health Perception—Health Management

Definition. This pattern describes individual, family, or community perceptions of health and defines the usual practices utilized to promote or maintain health. This identification assists the nurse to develop nursing interventions that are (1) consistent with positive health practices, (2) designed to clarify the client's incorrect perceptions, and (3) directed toward identification of alternative health strategies.

ASSOCIATED NURSING DIAGNOSES	RELATED FACTORS
1. Altered health maintenance	Lack of knowledge, existing unhealthy lifestyle, inaccessibility to necessary resources, anxiety, nontherapeutic relationships or environment, physical or perceptual deficits, age, changes in self-image
2. Noncompliance	
3. Potential for infection	
4. Altered protection	
5. Potential for injury	
6. Potential for trauma	
7. Potential for poisoning	
8. Potential for suffocation	
9. Health-seeking behaviors (specify)	

Interventions. The implementation of nursing interventions may be directed toward (1) identification of unhealthy patterns through assessment or screening, (2) provision of health education, including formal and informal teaching approaches involving the client, family, or community at large, (3) identification of available resources, including personnel, finances, and equipment, and (4) initiation of environmental changes, if required.

Example. Al Rogers, a 42 year old man, is seen in his physician's office with a diagnosis of urinary tract infection. In assessing this client's perception of health, the nurse identifies that he considers himself to be basically healthy and feels that this problem can be managed effectively by careful attention to prescribed orders, minor lifestyle changes, and regular follow-up.

In this case, the nurse's approach will include reinforcement of the client's positive perceptions and careful explanation of therapeutic approaches.

Example. Pat O'Brien, age 42, is admitted to a same day surgery unit for a biopsy of her left breast. The nurse's assessment indicates that the client's mother died eight years ago from metastatic breast cancer. The nurse also determines that Pat does not perform breast self-examination or have regular gynecological check-ups.

The nurse's interventions in this case will focus on identifying the risk factors associated with malignant breast disease, particularly age and familial history. Additionally, the nurse must communicate the need for regular preventive approaches.

Nutritional-Metabolic

Definition. This pattern describes the client's usual pattern of consumption of food or fluids. The client's status is based on the identification of metabolic needs and a subsequent comparison of the client's food and fluid intake as well as nutritional supplements, height, weight, skin, and mucous membranes. This allows the nurse (1) to identify incorrect perceptions regarding food and fluid consumption, (2) to anticipate potential problems, and (3) to determine definitive approaches to prevent or correct them.

ASSOCIATED NURSING DIAGNOSES	RELATED FACTORS
1. Potential fluid volume deficit 2. Fluid volume deficit 3. Fluid volume excess 4. Altered nutrition: less than body requirements 5. Altered nutrition: more than body requirements 6. Altered nutrition: potential for more than body requirements 7. Altered oral mucous membrane 8. Impaired skin integrity 9. Ineffective breastfeeding 10. Effective breastfeeding 11. Potential for aspiration 12. Impaired swallowing 13. Impaired tissue integrity 14. Potential altered body temperature 15. Ineffective thermoregulation 16. Hyperthermia 17. Hypothermia	Elevated temperature, burns, irritating or excessive drainage, infection, nausea or vomiting, nasogastric suction, anorexia, blood loss, weakness, effects of therapy, diarrhea, excessive sodium intake, immobility, swallowing difficulties, wired jaw, lack of knowledge, loneliness, boredom, sedentary lifestyle, inadequate oral hygiene

Interventions. Nursing interventions will be directed toward (1) identification of specific unhealthy patterns, (2) determination of the factors precipitating their potential or actual occurrence, (3) initiation of specific approaches to prevent or correct individual nutritional problems, (4) provision of specific education, when required, and (5) identification of available resources.

Example. Carla Ramirez is seen for the first time in a prenatal clinic. She is 17 years old and is pregnant with her second child. Her first baby was delivered two months prematurely and died three days after birth. Carla indicates that she is unmarried and on welfare and lives with her parents and nine siblings.

The nurse identifies that this client has specific nutritional needs because of her pregnancy. Assessment also indicates a number of factors that will interfere with the client's ability to satisfy these needs. Therefore, the nurse will implement interventions designed to increase the potential for Carla to obtain the food, milk, and vitamin supplements required during pregnancy.

Example. Glenn Stevens, age 86, is admitted with a fractured humerus, which requires skeletal traction. The nurse identifies that Mr. Stevens is thin and slightly dehydrated and has limited mobility as a result of the continuous traction.

In this case, the nurse recognizes that the client's decreased nutritional and fluid status in combination with immobility exposes him to the potential for altered skin integrity. The nurse's approach would include nutritional supplementation, increased fluid intake, and skin protection measures.

Elimination

Definition. This pattern describes the client's ability to eliminate body wastes, including those of bowel and bladder. Critical indicators focus on regularity and control. The nurse evaluates usual patterns of bowel and bladder elimination, including the existence of alternative routes (e.g., ostomy). This allows the nurse (1) to identify incorrect perceptions related to bowel or bladder function, (2) to anticipate actual or potential deficits, (3) to propose alternative approaches to facilitate elimination or correct known deficits, and (4) to assess the effects of existing deviations.

ASSOCIATED NURSING DIAGNOSES	RELATED FACTORS
1. Constipation 2. Perceived constipation 3. Colonic constipation 4. Diarrhea 5. Bowel incontinence 6. Altered patterns of urinary elimination 7. Functional incontinence 8. Reflex incontinence 9. Stress incontinence 10. Urge incontinence 11. Total incontinence 12. Urinary retention	Immobility, effects of therapy, pregnancy, pain, lack of privacy, decreased fluid intake, stress, lack of knowledge, use of laxatives, irritating foods, tube feedings, dehydration, infection, diminished bladder capacity, barriers to ambulation

Interventions. The implementation of nursing approaches may be directed toward (1) defining normal elimination patterns and comparing them with current patterns, (2) identifying specific contributing factors, (3) developing preventive or corrective approaches to ensure positive elimination, and (4) providing education as required.

Example. James Balfour is a 49 year old man admitted for cervical strain. His treatment modality includes bedrest, moist heat, ultrasound therapy, and the use of analgesics (acetaminophen [Tylenol] with codeine). Mr. Balfour identifies that he is constipated.

The nurse recognizes that the treatment regimen required to manage Mr. Balfour's back problem predisposes him to bowel elimination problems. This is the result of a combination of immobility and the effects of codeine. The nurse implements interventions designed to reduce or eliminate this problem, which include providing adequate roughage in his diet, increasing fluid intake, and suggesting the need for stool softeners.

Example. Joan Terrence is seen in the community health clinic for follow-up after a temporary colostomy for diverticulitis. The client indicates that her ostomy functions regularly every other day, and the nurse finds that the condition of her stoma and skin is excellent.

Although this client's method of elimination is altered, the nurse is able to assess that the client perceives her ostomy to be functioning normally. Additionally, the nurse determines that the client's normal pattern of elimination has resumed. Therefore, the interventions in this case will focus on reinforcing the client's perceptions and providing additional resources as required.

Activity-Exercise

Definition. This pattern includes a broad range of concerns that focus on specific activities requiring the expenditure of energy. These consist of the common activities of daily living, such as eating, hygiene, grooming, and toileting, as well as leisure and recreation. Critical indicators also include mobility and respiratory and cardiac functions, since alterations in these areas may predispose the client to activity and exercise problems.

ASSOCIATED NURSING DIAGNOSES	RELATED FACTORS
1. Potential activity intolerance	Prolonged immobility, pain, fatigue,
2. Activity intolerance	effects of therapy, retained secretions,
3. Ineffective airway clearance	weakness, decreased oxygenation,
4. Ineffective breathing patterns	depression, sedentary lifestyle, effects of
5. Impaired gas exchange	surgery, lack of motivation, smoking,
6. Decreased cardiac output	high-risk environment, fear, absent or
7. Impaired physical mobility	nonfunctioning body parts, presence of
8. Potential for disuse syndrome	invasive lines, hypothermia, infection,
9. Fatigue	inadequate nutritional intake, decreased
10. Bathing/hygiene self-care deficit	physical activity, lack of knowledge,
11. Dressing/grooming self-care deficit	limited range of motion
12. Feeding self-care deficit	
13. Toileting self-care deficit	
14. Diversional activity deficit	
15. Impaired home maintenance management	
16. Altered (specify) tissue perfusion (renal, cerebral, cardiopulmonary, gastrointestinal, peripheral)	
17. Dysreflexia	
18. Altered growth and development	

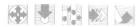

Interventions.   The implementation of nursing approaches may be directed toward (1) identifying usual activity–exercise patterns, (2) evaluating client responses to activity based on findings, (3) implementing preventive, supportive, or therapeutic approaches to minimize effects on lifestyle, and (4) providing client and family education as required.

Example.   Carlton Henning is a 58 year old man with metastic cancer of the lung who is being followed at home by the visiting nurse. As a result of his disease process, Mr. Henning's activity is restricted to bedrest at this time. In addition, he is home alone a large amount of time, since his wife must work to support the family. The nurse often observes the client looking out of the window and staring for prolonged periods of time.

Mr. Henning obviously has a number of problems of concern. His mobility and respiratory functions are impaired, and his activity tolerance is limited. In this case, the nurse may also focus on the provision of diversional activities designed to alter his limited routine. These could include reading, playing cards, watching television, or listening to classical music.

Example.   Cathy Sizemore is a 37 year old woman admitted to the hospital with advanced multiple sclerosis. She is divorced and lives with her elderly mother, who has chronic congestive heart failure. With the progression of her disease, Cathy is now confined to a wheelchair and verbalizes concern about her ability to manage the upkeep of her apartment.

Here, the nurse recognizes that an active diagnosis of impaired home maintenance management exists. At this point, the nurse will explore available resources to assist Cathy and her mother in their present living situation. Subsequently, it may be necessary to discuss long-term arrangements in alternative settings, should they be required.

Sleep-Rest

Definition.   This pattern focuses on the client's ability to obtain sleep, rest, or relaxation. The nurse attempts to define the client's normal sleep patterns and their subsequent effects on the activities of daily living. Critical factors include identification of sleep requirements, additional restful activities, and the client's ability to implement relaxation techniques when appropriate.

ASSOCIATED NURSING DIAGNOSIS	RELATED FACTORS
Sleep pattern disturbance	Pain, anxiety, impaired elimination, hospitalization, effects of therapy, pregnancy, depression, stress, unfamiliar environment

Interventions.   The implementation of nursing interventions may be directed toward (1) identifying the client's normal sleep-rest pattern, (2) determining the client's perception of the effects of the usual pattern, (3) initiating measures to increase the duration or quality of sleep and rest, (4) promoting relaxation through physical or mental techniques, and (5) providing health teaching for the client and family as necessary.

Example.   Ken Slater is a truck driver who is hospitalized for surgery to repair a hiatal hernia. He is frequently observed walking in the hall or watching television during the night. However, he sleeps at long intervals during the day.

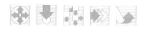

The nurse's initial assessment of this client's behavior suggests a sleep pattern disturbance. However, further discussion with the client reveals that he usually drives for long periods at night when traffic is lighter and sleeps during the day. Therefore, the nurse would attempt to maintain his normal pattern and provide frequent rest periods during the day.

Example.   Andrew Hardy is a 52 year old man admitted to the hospital with recurrent angina. He has been pain-free for two days. However, he is unable to sleep for longer than a two-hour interval. The client indicates that he usually sleeps about six hours nightly. Mr. Hardy states that he is concerned about losing his job, since this is his third hospitalization this year.

In this case, the nurse recognizes both short- and long-term sleep-rest implications. The initiation of relaxation techniques may be utilized immediately to increase the duration of the client's sleep pattern. Additionally, the nurse should incorporate health teaching strategies, including stress management to alleviate usual job demands.

Cognitive-Perceptual

Definition.   This pattern describes the client's sensory abilities (hearing, seeing, taste, smell, and touch) as well as higher level cognitive functions (language, memory, decision-making, problem-solving). The nurse attempts to identify usual patterns, specific deficits, and compensatory mechanisms utilized by the client.

ASSOCIATED NURSING DIAGNOSES	RELATED FACTORS
1. Pain 2. Chronic pain 3. Sensory perceptual alterations (specify—visual, auditory, kinesthetic, gustatory, tactile olfactory) 4. Unilateral neglect 5. Knowledge deficit (specify) 6. Altered thought processes 7. Decisional conflict	Effects of surgery, anxiety, social or cultural barriers, ineffective coping patterns, age, unfamiliar environment, effects of therapy, substance abuse, immobility, pregnancy, sensory overload or deprivation, isolation, fear, depression, conflict

Interventions.   The implementation of nursing approaches may be directed toward (1) determining the source of the client's deficits in sensation or perception, (2) identifying positive mechanisms currently utilized as well as other potential approaches, (3) providing specific education regarding temporary measures and long-term potential for managing problems, and (4) obtaining additional resources when required.

Example.   Nina Tallone had a stroke five days ago. The nurse notes that she has difficulty in expressing her thoughts and experiences short-term memory losses. As a result, Mrs. Tallone is hesitant to respond to questioning or to participate in conversations with unfamiliar people. She is also frustrated by her inability to recall recent events.

The nurse's approach to the management of this client's problems may focus on educating her about the disease process and effects of stroke. Additional strategies for managing memory loss and utilization of approaches suggested by a speech therapist may be of value.

Example. Tom Gorski is a policeman who is being seen in the physician's office for persistent hypertension. The nurse's interactions with this client reveal a total lack of knowledge regarding the disease process, the need for frequent monitoring, the effects of high salt intake, and the relationship between stress and the occurrence of hypertension.

Here, the nurse's action is clearly defined—the development and implementation of a comprehensive teaching plan. Consideration must be given to incorporating some of the client's usual patterns to ensure compliance with the prescribed strategies.

Emotional Patterns

Those patterns identified as a reflection of the emotional component of the client's needs are *self-perception–self-concept, role-relationship, sexuality-reproductive, coping–stress tolerance,* and *value-belief.*

Self-Perception–Self-Concept

Definition. This pattern defines the client's perception of self in terms of four predominant variables–body image, self-esteem, role performance, and personal identity (Carpenito, 1983). The nurse attempts to identify the effects of change, loss, or threat on the client's self-perception.

ASSOCIATED NURSING DIAGNOSES	RELATED FACTORS
1. Anxiety 2. Fear 3. Powerlessness 4. Hopelessness 5. Body image disturbance 6. Personal identity disturbance 7. Self-esteem disturbance 8. Chronic low self-esteem 9. Situational low self-esteem	Feelings of hopelessness, change, actual or perceived threat, loss of body part or function, hospitalization, terminal disease, disability, effects of therapy, pain, lack of knowledge, inadequate coping, loss of job, divorce, pregnancy, stress

Interventions. The implementation of nursing interventions may be directed toward (1) assisting the client to define perception of self and its relationship to health, (2) identifying specific variables contributing to the client's problems, (3) assisting the client to develop problem-solving skills to deal with the effects of change, loss, or threat, and (4) providing education or referral to additional resources when required.

Example. JoEllen Parker is a 12 year old girl who visits the school nurse's office frequently with vague somatic complaints. The nurse's approach has been to investigate each complaint and to reassure JoEllen. During these conversations, the nurse learns that this client feels awkward because she is about five inches taller than all of her friends, including the boys in class. She also has begun to menstruate and is afraid that others will find out and make fun of her.

The nurse recognizes that this client's self-image has been affected by rapid body changes associated with puberty. Nursing approaches will focus on continuing their trusting relationship and assisting JoEllen to deal with rapid physical changes compounded by peer pressure.

Example. Frank Nichols is an elderly client who is transferred from the coronary care unit following a myocardial infarction (heart attack) complicated by heart failure. The nurse notes that he is apathetic and depressed and refuses to make decisions regarding his care. Eventually, the client reveals that he feels frustrated by the lack of information provided by his physician. He also indicates that "It doesn't matter what I think—they'll do what they want anyway."

This client is exhibiting behaviors that are typical of one who feels powerless in a health care setting. The nurse's role here is that of client advocate. Interventions will focus on improving communication, educating the client about his rights in the health care system, and determining strategies to increase his degree of control over this situation.

Role-Relationship

Definition. This pattern describes the client's individual, family, and social roles. The client's perceptions of roles and relationships are important because they form a component of identity. Individuals require a variety of roles and levels of relationships to be self-actualized. The client's degree of satisfaction with roles and relationships and the level of independence attained are also important considerations.

ASSOCIATED NURSING DIAGNOSES	RELATED FACTORS
1. Anticipatory grieving 2. Dysfunctional grieving 3. Altered role performance 4. Social isolation 5. Impaired social interaction 6. Altered family processes 7. Potential altered parenting 8. Altered parenting 9. Parental role conflict 10. Impaired verbal communication 11. Potential for violence: self-directed or directed at others	Language barrier, aphasia, decreased level of consciousness, intubation, pain, lack of privacy, illness or loss of family member, financial crisis, lack of support systems, loss of body part or function, hospitalization, divorce, lack of knowledge, impaired bonding, stress, suicidal tendencies, anger, fear, drug or alcohol abuse

Interventions. The implementation of nursing approaches may be directed toward (1) assisting the client to identify individual, family, or social roles that are of concern, (2) examining the associated relationships to identify supporting or distressing features, (3) providing education or additional resources when necessary, and (4) assisting the client to develop strategies for managing those areas that are unsatisfying or undesirable.

Example. Lucy Caron is a 54 year old woman with a progressive neuromuscular disease. Over a period of five months, she has had progressive paralysis, which resulted in respiratory problems requiring a tracheostomy. At this point, Mrs. Caron is unable to speak and has such limited movement in her left arm that she is unable to write. It is therefore extremely difficult for her to communicate with her family or the nursing staff.

In this case, the nurse recognizes the client's severe communication deficits. Therefore, the nurse requests the assistance of the occupational therapist. A computer is provided that allows the client to select a message that is printed on a screen for the family or staff. This enhances the client's personal and therapeutic relationships.

Example. Tony Angeli is a navy submarine officer who is frequently at sea for prolonged periods of time. Therefore, his interactions with his youngest son, age eight months, have been minimal. He verbalizes his frustration and feelings of parental failure in a conversation with the clinic nurse.

Here, the nurse's interventions focus on counseling to assist the father to achieve a more positive feeling about his parental role.

Sexuality-Reproductive

Definition. This pattern reflects the client's sexual identity and involves the client's ability to express sexuality and achieve satisfying individual or interpersonal relationships. This pattern also includes the status of the client's reproductive capabilities.

Associated Nursing Diagnoses	Related Factors
1. Sexual dysfunction	Lack of knowledge, effects of therapy,
2. Altered sexuality patterns	hospitalization, loss of body part,
3. Rape-trauma syndrome	unwilling partner, stress, lack of privacy,
4. Rape-trauma syndrome: compound reacton	abuse, violent episode
5. Rape-trauma syndrome: silent reaction	

Interventions. The implementation of nursing interventions may be directed toward (1) assisting the client to clarify individual perceptions related to sexuality and sexual identity, (2) identifying barriers to adequate sexual expression or feeling to reproduction, (3) providing education regarding sexual or reproductive concerns, and (4) allowing the client to develop viable alternatives with nursing support.

Example. Chris Spoko is a 17 year old runaway seen in the community health clinic with symptoms of depression, withdrawal, and multiple sleep disturbances. He tells the nurse that he was raped by a male homosexual four months ago. He describes feelings of guilt and disgust and indicates that this was probably his punishment for running away.

The nurse's interventions in this case are directed toward providing psychological support to this traumatized client. The therapeutic relationship should be maintained, and the nurse should reassure the client, help him to resolve his guilt feelings, and assist him to develop a realistic plan for the future. Additional counseling or therapy may be recommended if necessary.

Example. Pam Bernhardt is a 52 year old client seen in the doctor's office six weeks following a hysterectomy. She verbalizes her concern about resuming sexual relations with her husband, indicating that "it just won't be the same."

In this example, the nurse utilizes a supportive approach, explains the normalcy of the client's response, and encourages open dialogue between the client and her spouse. Her fears may be unfounded, and in fact, their relationship may improve as a result of this type of dialogue.

Coping-Stress Tolerance

Definition. This pattern involves the identification of the types and degree of stress associated with the client's lifestyle. The coping mechanisms utilized by the indi-

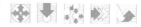

vidual and the family are identified as well as the client's ability to manage various levels of stress. The client's perception of these variables is particularly important in this pattern, because interventions must be directed to what the client perceives to be problematic.

ASSOCIATED NURSING DIAGNOSES	RELATED FACTORS
1. Ineffective individual coping	Loss of job, divorce, relocation, sensory
2. Ineffective family coping: compromised	overload or deprivation, persistent stress, loss of body part, feelings of helplessness,
3. Ineffective family coping: disabling	hospitalization, terminal illness, domestic
4. Family coping: potential for growth	violence
5. Defensive coping	
6. Ineffective denial	
7. Impaired adjustment	
8. Post-trauma response	

Interventions. The implementation of nursing interventions may be directed toward (1) assisting the client to identify personal patterns of response to individual or family stress, (2) identifying the sources of stress for the client as an individual, (3) developing positive coping strategies to avoid distress, (4) providing education regarding identified variables and the use of relaxation, and (5) obtaining additional resources when required.

Example. Ken Cord is an elderly client hospitalized in an intensive care unit as a result of respiratory failure secondary to chronic obstructive lung disease. He has been in the unit for three weeks and suddenly begins screaming that he can't take it anymore. He states that all the noises are "driving me crazy, I never get any rest, and I'm tired of all this fussing and these newfangled machines."

This is a classic response to the sensory overload associated with critical care areas. In this situation, the nurse utilizes interpersonal skills to assist the client to identify alternate coping strategies. The use of relaxation techniques may be particularly beneficial if accompanied by a reduction in environmental stimulation.

Example. Marilyn Holcombe, a 32 year old woman, is examined in the emergency department following a beating by her husband. Marilyn states that her husband becomes abusive when he drinks. "I'd like to leave him, but I'm afraid he'll find me," she says.

The nurse recognizes the need to assist Marilyn in coping with her husband's behavior. This may involve encouraging the client to discuss her feelings about this current situation, her desire for a change, and the availability of support systems.

Value-Belief

Definition. This pattern defines the client and family belief systems. These include what the client believes to be correct and valuable based on personal knowledge, individual and community norms, or faith. The client's perception of the value of preventive care, treatment modalities, or even life itself may influence individual ability to manage the problems associated with conflicting beliefs or value systems.

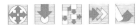

ASSOCIATED NURSING DIAGNOSIS	RELATED FACTORS
1. Spiritual distress	Hospitalization, conflicting value systems, inability to practice spiritual rituals, effects of therapy, isolation

Interventions. Nursing interventions will be directed toward (1) identifying the specific value or belief pattern involved, (2) determining particular sources of conflict, when appropriate, (3) obtaining available resources to facilitate the practice of religious beliefs or the resolution of conflicts, and (4) providing information regarding health management to assist the client in making informed choices regarding continued health practices.

Example. John and Carrie Davis are Jehovah's Witnesses. Their 16 year old daughter, Nancy, was involved in a sleding accident that resulted in a compound fracture of the ankle with bleeding into the joint. Mr. and Mrs. Davis oppose the use of blood transfusions on a religious basis and refuse to allow the administration of a transfusion during surgery.

The nurse recognizes the conflict between the parents' religious beliefs and the desire to save their child's life. In this case, the nurse ensures that the family is well-informed regarding alternative treatment modalities and possible adverse reactions. Additionally, the nurse supports the parents while they resolve this conflict.

REFERENCES

Carpenito, LJ: Nursing Diagnosis—Application to Clinical Practice. Philadelphia, J.B. Lippincott, 1983.
Gordon, M: Nursing Diagnosis: Process and Application. New York: McGraw-Hill, 1982.

INDEX

Note: Page numbers followed by letter f refer to figures; those followed by t refer to tables.